Positional Release Techniques

For Churchill Livingstone:

Editorial Director, Health Professions: Mary Law
Project Development Manager: Katrina Mather
Head of Project Management: Ewan Halley
Design Direction: George Ajayi / Judith Wright

Positional Release Techniques

 with accompanying CD-ROM

Leon Chaitow ND DO
Registered Osteopathic Practitioner and Senior Lecturer, School of Integrated Health,
University of Westminster, London, UK

with contributions from

Ed Wilson BA (Hons) MCSP SRP (Chapter 11 The Mulligan concept: NAGs, SNAGs, MWMs, etc.)
Senior Physiotherapist, Highthorn Physiotherapy Clinic, York, UK

Dylan Morrissey MSc MMACP MCSP (Chapter 12 Unloading and proprioceptive taping)
Physiotherapist, London, UK

Foreword by

John McPartland DO MS
Adjunct Assistant Professor, Department of Biomechanics,
Michigan State University College of Osteopathic Medicine,
East Lansing, Michigan, USA

Postgraduate Programme Director, Osteopathic Medicine,
UNITEC, Auckland, New Zealand

Illustrated by

Graeme Chambers BA (Hons)
Medical Artist

SECOND EDITION

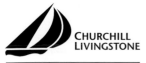 CHURCHILL LIVINGSTONE

EDINBURGH LONDON NEW YORK PHILADELPHIA ST LOUIS SYDNEY TORONTO 2002

CHURCHILL LIVINGSTONE
An imprint of Harcourt Publishers Limited

© Pearson Professional Limited 1997
© Harcourt Publishers Limited 1999, 2002

🞓 is a registered trademark of Harcourt Publishers Limited

First edition 1997
Second edition 2002

ISBN 0 443 07081 4

British Library Cataloguing in Publication Data
A catalogue record for this book is available from the British Library

Library of Congress Cataloging in Publication Data
A catalog record for this book is available from the Library of
Congress

Note
Medical knowledge is constantly changing. As new information
becomes available, changes in treatment, procedures, equipment and
the use of drugs become necessary. The author, contributors and the
publishers have taken care to ensure that the information given in this
text is accurate and up to date. However, readers are strongly advised
to confirm that the information, especially with regard to drug usage,
complies with the latest legislation and standards of practice.

Neither the publishers nor the author will be liable for any loss or
damage of any nature occasioned to or suffered by any person acting
or refraining from acting as a result of reliance on the material
contained in this publication.

The
publisher's
policy is to use
**paper manufactured
from sustainable forests**

Printed in China

Contents

The CD-ROM accompanying this text includes video sequences of all the techniques indicated in the text by the ⊙ icon. To look at the video for a given technique, click on the relevant icon in the contents list on the CD-ROM. The CD-ROM is designed to be used in conjuction with the text and not as a stand-alone product.

Abbreviations

AIIS:	anterior inferior iliac spine	OA:	occipito atlantal
AK:	applied kinesiology	OMT:	osteopathic manipulative therapy
ASIS:	anterior superior iliac spine	PIR:	postisometric relaxation
CCP:	common compensatory pattern	PNF:	proprioceptive neuromuscular facilitation
CFS:	chronic fatigue syndrome		
CNS:	central nervous system	PR:	positional release
DTP:	dominant tender point	PRT:	positional release technique
FMS:	fibromyalgia syndrome	PSIS:	posterior superior iliac spine
FPR:	facilitated positional release	SBIS:	silicone breast implant syndrome
INIT:	integrated neuromuscular inhibition technique	SCS:	strain/counterstrain
		SE:	scanning evaluation
ME:	myalgic encephalomyelitis	SF:	sacral foramen
MET:	muscle energy technique/therapy (US)	SNAGs:	sustained NAGs
MPS:	myofascial pain syndrome	TART:	texture, assymetry, range of motion, tenderness
MWM:	mobilisation with movement		
NAGs:	natural apophyseal glides	TMJ:	temporomandibular joint

Foreword

With this second edition of *Positional Release Techniques,* Leon Chaitow develops the topic in four or more directions: he expands on the history of positional release techniques, extends the nomenclature, unfolds new theoretical constructs, and adds techniques from an augmented variety of sources – sources varied by discipline and by geography. *Positional Release Techniques* has gone global. Chaitow even expands the duration of treatment, beyond Jones's classic '90-second rule', to include treatments ranging from four seconds (in Schiowitz's facilitated positional release – FPR) to those lasting hours or days (Morrissey's taping methods).

For me, positional release was a revelation when I first met Larry Jones in 1984. He was one of those grand old innovators of the osteopathic profession, on a par with his teachers Bill Sutherland, Harold Hoover, and Fred Mitchell. Jones developed strain/counterstrain (SCS) in the 1950s. SCS was the culmination of 20 years of independent clinical tinkering in Jones's rural clinical practice. The technique he developed is simple yet powerful. SCS is now used by a panoply of practitioners. Many of Jones's students adapted his ideas and coined new methods. Jones encouraged these modifications. He did not want to become the guru of a static SCS cult, but preferred to be the originator of an evolving system. With Jones's passing in 1996, Leon Chaitow has assumed the mantle of *modus evolutionari.*

Chaitow's genius is synthesis: he puts together ideas from different thinkers, including DOs, DCs, PTs, NDs, MDs, and practitioners from several trademarked schools of bodywork. He has extracted pearls from some very esoteric journals. With his fresh eye, he also pulls pearls from mainstream sources, often from articles that I have read but misunderstood. Re-reading this literature has imbued me with new enthusiasm.

In Chapter 2, the author reviews the many theories underpinning positional release techniques. He includes Jones's original proprioceptive hypothesis, Korr's facilitation model, Ward's myofascial 'tight-loose' concepts, the importance of nociception (as emphasized by Dick, Van Buskirk, and Willard), Zink's compensatory pattern and its new corollary, Myers' 'anatomy trains,' and finally, Chaitow's own circulatory concepts. One SCS hypothesis omitted by the author but worthy of mention is the axiom of *non-sequential motion.* It is described by McPartland and Zigler, and relates to their diagnostic approach of 'Any painful point as a starting point for SCS' (on page 8). *Non-sequential* or *non-communicative* motion is a biomechanical theory that explains the classic 'healthy person bends over and a cripple stands up.' When someone bends over and then twists, they must reverse the sequence to return to their original position. If someone returns to their position in an altered sequence, they may end up in a different, often painful, place. Early in the evolution of SCS, Jones emphasized the importance of placing patients in a position of strain, then unwinding patients in a biomechanically proper sequence of movements. This concept is worth resurrecting.

Diagnostic approaches vary, as alluded to above. Chaitow again performs a yeoman's service, synthesizing a wide variety of approaches for presentation to a wider audience. Although some wags have called SCS diagnosis 'indirect and circuitous,'a double-blind controlled trial (described and illustrated on pages 16-17) found that SCS diagnosis was *more accurate* than standard osteopathic and chiropractic assessments of patients with neck pain.

Positional release techniques, despite the term 'positional,' actually take practitioners away from structure, and into the realm of function: how tissues feel, how they behave, and how they react to different stresses and loads. A practitioner undergoing this evolution of thought recapitulates a process experienced by many other practitioners, such as Andrew Taylor Still, Charlotte Weaver, George Goodheart, Janet Travell, Marsh Morrison, and Chaitow's familiar mentors, Boris Chaitow and Stanley Lief. They all moved away from the direct manipulation of misaligned structure to the indirect treatment of 'dysfunctional function.' These indirect techniques subtly allow the body to correct and heal itself. As such they are superior to direct kinds of bodywork that forcibly impose themselves upon dysfunctions. As Chaitow says in his Preface, 'Excessive adaptive demands [direct techniques] simply load the system more heavily, and symptoms are likely to worsen.'

That is not to say positional release techniques do not have side-effects! I recall treating a patient with a bulging disc, coupled with psoas spasm. SCS completely eliminated his psoas distress. Joyfully pain-free, he leaped off the table, and promptly herniated his disc! Thus, indirect techniques can cause 'indirect iatrogenesis.' But misapplied SCS can *directly* generate mishaps: the treatment of cervical extension strains (Figs 3.15, 3.16, 7.4) must be approached with caution, because exaggerated cervical extension, coupled with rotation, can compromise the vertebral arteries. To wit, some of Jones's SCS techniques for treating the cranium are not designed for the light-hearted or light-headed.

Positional Release Techniques is filled with concrete examples, fine line drawings, and careful guidelines, which make the techniques easy to learn and apply. The text illustrates a plethora of tutorial exercises. Chaitow begins with exercises developed by Jones, designed for practitioners who want exact results. Some of the illustrated treatments have passed down directly from Jones (e.g. Fig. 3.26, complete with Jones's superfluous finger spread). Other illustrated treatments depart from Jones's suggested positions, and these adaptations are much easier to perform for practitioners not 6'4" (193 cm) tall like Jones. Other worthwhile exercises include Woolbright's famous 'box' tutorial, Dickey's 'tissue preference patterns,' and several self-treatment techniques.

For practitioners not adept at memorizing points and positions, Chaitow outlines several empiric approaches. Empiric approaches are useful for 'maverick' patients who do not respond to rote positioning. Here is where functional rises to the fore. Chaitow translates the functional empiricisms of Hoover, Bowles, and Johnston into easily comprehended techniques. The author subsequently illustrates refinements in functional and SCS techniques developed by Goodheart, Greenman, Schiowitz, Morrison, Stiles, Di Giovanna, Chaitow and others. Chaitow also presents some direct methods that nevertheless agree with some positional release principles. Highlighted concepts include Wilson and Mulligan's 'mobilization with movement' (NAGS and SNAGs), the Spencer shoulder sequence, and the 'unloading' taping concepts as described by Dylan Morrissey.

Positional Release Techniques is an excellent text for *all levels* of beginners. The treatment methods described in this book are powerful. The diagnostic techniques are accurate. Many patients prefer positional release treatments. There are far fewer side-effects. The methods are easy to learn. Positional release techniques, as my mentor John Goodridge says, 'are the future.' Leon Chaitow is to be congratulated, once again, for combining his tireless scholarship and seamless composition into an outstanding book of pearls.

UNITEC   John M. McPartland
Auckland, New Zealand   DO MS

Preface

The ideas that permeate positional release technique (PRT) methodology can be equated with non-invasive, non-interventionist, passive and gentle approaches that 'allow' change to emerge, rather than forcing it do so. Despite the apparently general nature of PRT methods, clinical experience within the osteopathic profession shows that they can be intensely practical and specific.

Two main themes emerge from PRT in its original form. The strain/counterstrain approach derives from the original work of osteopathic physician Lawrence Jones. It uses a pain monitor to find optimal positioning (i.e. when pain is no longer felt at the monitoring point). Functional technique also emerged out of osteopathic medicine; this PRT approach is based on positioning whilst sensing/palpating the tissues involved, so that they achieve their greatest degree of comfort or ease, without using pain as a guide.

In order to gain a sense of the underlying concepts involved in PRT application it is necessary to accept that the self-regulating mechanisms of the body are always the final determinants as to what happens following any form of intervention. For example, a high velocity thrust adjustment (HVT), or application of a muscle energy technique (MET) or myofascial release (MFR), or almost any other procedure, acts as a catalyst for change. If the treatment is appropriate the body produces an adaptive response that will allow enhanced function and therapeutic benefit. The adaptive response is the key to whether or not

benefit follows treatment. Excessive adaptive demands simply load the system more heavily, and symptoms are likely to worsen, while if there is inadequate therapeutic stimulus little value emerges from the exercise. The methods mentioned above (HVT, MET and MFR) are all 'direct', that is to say, a barrier (or several barriers) will have been identified, and the therapeutic objective will be to push the barrier(s) back, in order to mobilise a restricted joint, or to lengthen a shortened myofascial structure (for example).

Consider another way of addressing the restriction problem – an indirect one: reflect on whether, if the barrier is 'disengaged', the inherent tendency towards normality, demonstrated in the natural propensity for dysfunction to normalise (broken bones mend, tissues heal), is capable of restoring normality to the types of dysfunction to which HVT, MET and MFR (as examples) are being applied.

Is it possible for self-regulating, homeostatic mechanisms to be encouraged to act when the load on dysfunctional tissues is temporarily eased? Can a restricted joint release without force? Can an excessively tight, muscular condition release spontaneously? And can pain sometimes be relieved instantaneously, merely by holding the painful tissues in an 'eased' position?

Clinical PRT evidence shows that all these questions can be answered affirmatively, at times. If restriction – whether of joint or soft tissue – involves hypertonicity and relative circulatory deficit (ischaemia, etc.), then is it possible that an opportunity for spontaneous change may occur by holding these same restricted tissues in a way that reduces the tone and allows (albeit temporarily) enhanced circulation through the tissues, and a chance for neural resetting (involving proprioceptors and nociceptors), to take place?

PRT methodology suggests that this is the case and a number of variations have evolved that incorporate the concept of 'offering an opportunity for change', as distinct from 'forcing a change', as is the case with HVT and MET for example.

There are particular settings and contexts in which PRT is probably the treatment method of first choice – as in extreme pain, recent trauma (for example whiplash, or immediately following a sporting or everyday strain), post surgery, extreme fragility (for example advanced osteoporosis). In addition, PRT is sufficiently versatile, with numerous variations, to be useful as a part of a sequence involving other interventions, for example before or following HVT application, or as part of a sequence involving MET and neuromuscular technique in trigger point deactivation, or as a means of easing hypertonicity during a massage therapy treatment.

The ideas that underpin PRT are also to be found in craniosacral methodology, in which disengagement of restrictions, moving away from restriction barriers, is a common approach. Of particular interest in this second edition is the inclusion of chapters that discuss two physiotherapy-derived methods that have strong links to the underlying concepts of PRT. First there is the approach that 'proprioceptively unloads' dysfunctional joints and tissues and then tapes the structures into their 'ease' state for hours or days, in contrast to the minutes of 'ease' used in osteopathic PRT methodology. Dylan Morrissey has described this effective alternative in Chapter 12.

In Chapter 11 Ed Wilson presents a description of those aspects of the work of Brian Mulligan, the New Zealand physiotherapist whose mobilisation with movement (MWM) concepts have been so widely adopted in physiotherapy settings. There are specific variations within MWM that have close similarities with PRT ideas and Wilson has performed the invaluable task of moving beyond descriptions of methods to evaluation of underlying mechanisms.

The cross-fertilisation and interdisciplinary possibilities that are exemplified by the coming together of osteopathic and physiotherapeutic methods and ideas highlight the potential for the future, as barriers and rivalries give way to co-operation, collaboration and ultimately integration, for the benefit of all.

Corfu 2001   LC

Acknowledgements

My sincere thanks go to the many osteopathic and physiotherapeutic practitioners whose work has resulted in positional release methods coming to the forefront of integrative body-work approaches. In particular my thanks go to Ed Wilson and Dylan Morrissey for contributing their specialised knowledge to this book.

1

Spontaneous positional release variations

POSITIONAL RELEASE (PR)

This chapter contains a review of a variety of ways in which the practical application of positional release methodology can be used therapeutically. The idea behind the techniques is very simple indeed, although the application can itself require great skill and delicacy of touch. If tissues are inappropriately tense, indurated, hypertonic, shortened or contracted, the therapeutic intent is usually to release these undesirable states in order to encourage a retreat of restriction barriers. The methods which can achieve this are commonly of a direct nature. The soft tissue in question may be stretched, massaged, mobilised and manipulated using any of dozens of perfectly appropriate techniques. However, if the tissues are painful, in spasm, inflamed, or have recently been traumatised, or if the available manual method induces discomfort, then an alternative approach is called for. Ideally one is required which causes little discomfort while allowing a spontaneous resolution of the tense, dysfunctional state of the tissues. The cluster of methods which can be grouped as positional release techniques, and which this text attempts to describe, offer precisely these opportunities.

A number of different methods exist involving the positioning of an area of the body, or the whole body, in such a way as to evoke a therapeutically significant physiological response which helps to resolve musculoskeletal dysfunction. The means whereby these beneficial changes occur seems to involve a combination of the neurological and circulatory changes which

1

take place when a distressed area is placed in its most comfortable, its most 'easy', most pain-free position. The theoretical basis for the efficacy of positional release will be outlined in Chapter 3.

The developer of functional technique, one of the major methods of spontaneous positional release (discussed in this chapter and in Ch. 8), was Harold V. Hoover. He used the term 'dynamic neutral' (Hoover 1969) to describe what was being achieved as the tissues relating to a structurally disturbed joint or area were positioned in a state of 'ease'. Charles Bowles (1969) has discussed dynamic neutral further. He states:

Dynamic neutral is a state in which tissues find themselves when the motion of the structure they serve is free, unrestricted and within the range of normal physiological limits … Dynamic neutral is not a static condition … it is a continuing state of normal, during living motion, during living activity … it is the state and condition to be restored to a dysfunctional area.

As explanations and descriptions are offered for the spontaneous physiological responses which take place when tissues are placed in a balanced state, in this and later chapters, the terms 'ease' and 'bind' will frequently be used to simplistically describe the extremes of restriction and freedom of movement. The term 'dynamic neutral' may be considered as being interchangeable with 'ease'.

The impetus towards the use of this most basic and non-invasive of treatment methods in a coherent, rather than a hit-and-miss manner, lies in the work of Lawrence Jones, who developed an approach to somatic dysfunction (Jones 1981) which he termed 'strain and counterstrain' (SCS) (described in detail in Ch. 2). Walther (1988) describes the moment of discovery in these words:

Jones's initial observation of the efficacy of counterstrain was with a patient who was unresponsive to treatment. The patient had been unable to sleep because of pain. Jones attempted to find a comfortable position for the patient to aid him in sleeping. After 20 minutes of trial and error, a position was finally achieved in which the patient's pain was relieved. Leaving the patient in this position for a short time, Jones was astonished when the patient came out of the position and was able to stand comfortably erect. The relief of pain was lasting and the patient made an uneventful recovery.

The position of 'ease' which Jones found for this patient was an exaggeration of the position in which spasm was holding him, which provided Jones with an insight into the mechanisms involved.

Over the years since Jones first made his valuable observation that a position which exaggerated a patient's distortion could provide the opportunity for a release of spasm and hypertonicity, many variations on this basic theme have emerged, some building logically on that first insight, with others moving in new directions. The summary of variations of positional release methods found in this chapter, and in Box 1.1, are as comprehensive as possible at the time of writing; however, new versions are regularly appearing, and the author acknowledges that it may have been impossible to exhaustively detail all variations.

Common basis

The commonality of all of these approaches is that they move the patient or the affected tissues away from any resistance barriers and towards positions of comfort.

The shorthand terms used for these two extremes are 'bind' and 'ease' – which anyone who has handled the human body will recognise as extremely apt descriptors.

The need for the many variations to be understood should be obvious. Different clinical settings require the availability of a variety of therapeutic approaches. An example described in more detail in Chapter 7 (pp. 125–126) is a case in which severely ill pre- and postoperative, bedbound patients were treated for their current pain and discomfort, without leaving their beds. In such a setting, no rigid application of procedures can be adhered to, and flexibility can best be achieved via easy access to different ways of reaching the same ends (Schwartz 1986).

Jones's approach requires verbal feedback from the patient as to tenderness in a 'tender' point which is being used as a monitor, and which the operator is palpating while attempting to find a position of ease.

One can imagine a situation in which the use of Jones 'tender points as a monitor' method (Ch. 3) would be inappropriate or actually impossible, for example in the case of someone who had lost the ability to communicate verbally, or who did not speak the same language, or who was too young or too ill to cooperate in the manner required. In such a case a need would be apparent for a method which allowed the operator to achieve the same ends without verbal communication.

This is possible, as will be demonstrated, using either 'functional' methods or 'facilitated positional release' approaches, which involve the operator finding a position of maximum ease by means of palpation alone, assessing for a state of 'ease' in the tissues. This approach is described below in brief (p. 8) and in later chapters in more detail.

As we examine a number of the variations on the same theme of positional release, release by placing the patient, or area, into 'ease', the diverse clinical and therapeutic potentials for the use of this approach will become clearer.

It is important to note that if positional release methods are being applied to chronically fibrosed tissue the result would produce a reduction in hypertonicity, but would not result in any reduction in fibrosis. Pain relief or improved mobility may therefore be only temporary or partial in such cases. This does not nullify the usefulness of PRT, but emphasises the need when treating chronic problems to use PRT methods as part of an integrated approach. This will be seen to be of particular value in deactivation of myofascial trigger points, using a combination of manual methods in a sequence known as integrated neuromuscular inhibition technique – INIT (see Chapter 6).

'Unlatching' restrictions

Upledger and Vredevoogd (1983) give a practical explanation of indirect methods of treatment, especially as related to cranial therapy. The idea of moving a restricted area in the direction of ease is, they say, 'a sort of "unlatching" principle.

Often in order to open a latch we must first exaggerate its closure'. The application of positional release methods in cranial structures is explored further in Chapter 10.

In normal tissues there exists in the midrange of motion an area of 'ease' or balance, where the tissues are at their least tense. When there is a restriction in the normal range of motion of an area, whether of osseous or soft-tissue origin, the now limited range will almost always still have a place, a moment, a point, which is neutral, of maximum comfort, or ease, usually lying somewhere between the new restriction barrier in one direction, and the physiological barrier in the other. Finding this balance point, also known as 'dynamic neutral', is a key element in PRT. Staying in this 'ease' state for an appropriate length of time (see below) offers restrictions a chance to 'unlatch', release, normalise. In this way it can be seen that the positioning element of the process is the preparation for the treatment to commence, and that the 'treatment' itself is self-generated by the tissues, in response to this careful positioning. This helps to explain Jones' original name for what became strain/counterstrain, which he first termed 'spontaneous release by positioning' (Greenman 1996).

All of the variations on the theme of positional release, described briefly below and in the summary at the end of this chapter (Box 1.1), are discussed in greater detail in later chapters.

PR VARIATIONS

1. Exaggeration of distortion

One of the first observations made by Jones was that a position of 'comfort' or ease, commonly (usually) was an exaggeration of whatever adaptive distortion patterns were present. Stated simply, the tissues which were already shortened were made comfortable by being supported in an even shorter state, so allowing neurological and circulatory mechanisms to operate and to assist in resolution of the dysfunctional state.

If we consider the example of someone bent forward in psoas spasm/lumbago. The person would probably be in considerable discomfort or pain, and would be posturally distorted – bent into flexion together with rotation and side-bending. Any attempt to straighten towards a more physiologically normal posture would be met by increased, possibly severe, pain.

Engaging the barrier of resistance would therefore not be an ideal first treatment option in an acute setting such as this. However, moving the area away from the restriction barrier would usually be relatively painless. In strain/counterstrain methodology the position required to find 'ease' for someone in this state normally involves painlessly increasing the degree of distortion displayed, placing the person (in the case of the example given) into some variation based on forward bending and rotation, until pain is found to reduce or resolve. After 90 seconds or more, in this position of ease, a slow return to neutral would be carried out and theoretically – and commonly in practice – the patient would be somewhat, or completely, relieved of pain and spasm. If, therefore, it is possible to recognise an acute or chronic distortion of tissues from their normal position, an exaggeration of this, following guidelines which will be outlined in Chapter 3, is likely to prove helpful in resolving the situation.

Researcher and massage therapist Sandy Fritz (personal communication 2000) has adapted this concept of exaggerating distortion. She evaluates the overall postural pattern of patients and encourages them to increase the levels of their overall postural model of rotation, flexion or whatever, and she then holds them firmly in that exaggeratedly distorted position. After a short while, during which time positional release effects will have been operating (see Chapter 3 and 4) she asks the patient actively, against her resistance, to attempt to return to their neutral (starting) position. This effectively employs reciprocal inhibition of shortened structures (a muscle energy technique procedure), subsequently allowing a more normal position to be adopted.

2. Replication of position of strain

Jones was also able to correlate reported positions of strain with the ultimate 'position of ease' used in successful treatment.

Take, for example, someone bending to lift a load when an emergency stabilisation is required and strain, and perhaps spasm, results (perhaps the person slips, or the load shifts – see notes on the mechanisms involved in strain/counterstrain (SCS) in Chapter 3). The patient would then be locked into the same position of lumbago-like distortion as was noted in example 1, above.

If, as SCS suggests, the position of ease often equals the position of strain – then the patient needs to go back (or rather be taken back) into flexion, in slow motion, until tenderness vanishes from a tender point which was being monitored, and/or until a sense of ease was perceived in the previously hypertonic shortened tissues.

Flexion would be the first direction tested and small 'fine-tuning' positioning towards a final position of ease would usually achieve a situation in which there is a maximum reduction in pain. This position is held for 90 seconds or more (see notes on timing in this and in Chapter 4) before slowly returning the patient to neutral at which time, as in example 1 above, a partial or total resolution of hypertonicity, spasm and pain should be noted.

It should be obvious that the position of strain, as just described, is often going to be an exact duplication of the position of exaggeration of distortion – as in example 1.

These two elements of SCS are of considerable clinical value – when the patient can report on the exact position in which strain occurred. While obvious spasm such as torticollis or acute anteflexion spasm ('lumbago') is not the norm, distorted adaptation patterns are extremely common, and once recognised can be used to guide the practitioner towards appropriate positioning of tissues, when these are being treated using PRT.

3. Using Jones' tender points as monitors

There are two main variants in which the practitioner utilises changes reported by the patient, as to the degree of palpated pain ('tender points'), as a means of identifying the ideal final position of the part, or whole body.

3A Jones' strain/counterstrain (SCS)

Over many years of clinical experience Jones (1981) compiled lists of specific tender-point areas relating to every imaginable strain of most of the joints and muscles of the body. There are just over 200 such charted tender points which have been 'proven' (by clinical experience) to relate to particular strain patterns (flexion, extension, etc.) or structures (muscles, ligaments, joints). The tender points are usually found in tissues which were in a shortened state at the time of strain (whether acute or chronic), rather than those which were (or are being) at stretch. New tender points are periodically reported in the osteopathic literature – for example a cluster of sacral points relating to sacroiliac strains (Ramirez et al 1989) and low back pain.

Jones and his co-workers have also provided strict guidelines for achieving ease in any tender points which are being palpated (the position of ease usually involving a 'folding' or crowding of the tissues in which the tender point lies). These and other guidelines will be detailed in Chapters 3 and 4.

The treatment method usually recommended involves maintaining pressure on the monitor tender point, or periodically probing it, as a position is achieved in which:

- There is no additional pain in whatever area is symptomatic, and
- The monitor-point pain has reduced by at least 70%, and
- No new or additional pain is created.

This position of comfort (ease) is held for an appropriate length of time (90 seconds, according to Jones; however, there are marked variations of opinion as to the ideal length of time required in the position of ease, as will become apparent in discussion of the many variables available in positional release methodology – specifically see notes in Chapter 4 on 'Timing and PRT'. Weiselfish (1993) as well as D'Ambrogio and Roth (1997) suggest that different mechanisms and timings are involved in the use of positional release methodology when treating neuromuscular, as opposed to neurological, problems.

In the example of the person with acute low back pain who is locked in flexion, the tender point would be expected to be located on the anterior surface of the abdomen, in the muscle structures which were short at the time of strain (when the patient was in flexion), and the position which removes tenderness from this point will, as in previous examples, require flexion, probably accompanied by some fine-tuning involving rotation and/or side-bending.

If there is a problem with Jones' somewhat formulaic approach it is that, while he is frequently correct as to the position of ease recommended for particular points, he is nevertheless sometimes wrong – or, to put it differently, the biomechanics of the particular strain (acute or chronic adaptation) with which the operator is confronted may not coincide with Jones' guidelines. An operator who relies solely on these 'menus', or formulae, could find difficulty in handling a situation in which Jones' prescription failed to produce the desired results. Reliance on Jones' menu of points and positions can therefore lead to the operator becoming dependent on them, and it is suggested that a reliance on palpation skills, and other variations on Jones' original observations, offers a more rounded approach to dealing with strain and pain.

Fortunately, Goodheart (1984) and others have offered less rigid frameworks within which to work using positional release mechanisms.

3B Positional release therapy (D'Ambrogio & Roth 1997)

Positional release therapy (PRTherapy) is a derivative evolution from Jones' SCS, based on the work of a number of manual therapists including Kerry D'Ambrogio PT and George Roth DC. PRTherapy uses many of the basic Jones concepts and findings, but has evolved various modifications. One is for a systematic scanning evaluation in which all or most of the tender points are assessed prior to treatment. A great deal of emphasis is placed on this element of diligent evaluation prior to treatment,

PRT treatment differs from that described by Jones … with conventional counterstrain and other forms of positional release, a patient with shoulder pain is treated using the same general rules and principles. Therapy is mainly localized to that upper quadrant, and six to eight points might be treated for a total of 90 seconds each. With global PRT sessions, only one to three points are usually treated. The goal is to spend more time on evaluation and less time on treatment. If the most dominant point of the body is located and treated, a majority of the other tender points (which may be adaptations to the dominant lesion) will often be eliminated.

The scanning for tender points, grading these to find the most dominant ones for treatment, and the period of holding time once a position of ease has been achieved, are the key differences between PRT (where the 'T' stands for 'therapy' and not 'technique', as in the title of this book) and Jones' SCS methodology. PRTherapy suggests that 90 seconds of holding is an adequate holding period for positional release of straightforward musculoskeletal dysfunctions; however, it is suggested that a longer 5 to 10 (and sometimes up to 20) minutes is necessary for fascial release to occur. Holding-time issues will be discussed further in Chapter 4. In most other particulars PRTherapy is identical to Jones' SCS.

4. Goodheart's approach

(Goodheart 1984, Walther 1988)

Both Jones' SCS methodology and that of PRTherapy require a somewhat 'cookbook' approach, in which specific sites are predicted for the location of tender points in relation to particular muscles and joints. The fact is that while these point locations are commonly very accurate, they are not universally so. Anatomical individuality has dictated that many structures vary in their location in different people. The strains to which the body is subject are also extremely variable. As a result there are many instances clinically in which reliance on the maps of tender points developed by Jones may be unhelpful (who was it who said 'the map is not the territory'?).

Fortunately a practical solution has been devised by George Goodheart (the developer of applied kinesiology) who has described an almost universally applicable formula, which relies more on the individual features displayed by the patient, and less on rigid recipes as used in Jones', and less so in PRTherapy, approaches.

Goodheart suggests that a suitable tender point be searched for (using palpation techniques described in Chapter 4) in the tissues opposite those 'active' when pain or restriction is noted. If pain or restriction is reported, or is apparent on any given movement, the antagonist muscles to those operating at the time pain is noted will be those that house the tender point(s).

Thus, for example, pain (wherever it is felt) which occurs when the neck is being turned to the left will require that a tender point be located in the muscles which would turn the head to the right.

In the earlier examples of a person locked in forward bending with acute pain and spasm, using Goodheart's approach, pain and restriction would usually be experienced as the person straightened up (i.e. as they move towards extension) from their position of enforced flexion. This action (straightening up) would usually cause pain in the back but, irrespective of where the pain is noted, a tender point would be sought (and subsequently treated by being taken to a state of ease) in the muscles opposing those working when pain was experienced – i.e. the appropriate tender point would be located in the flexor muscles (probably psoas) in this example.

It is important to emphasise that tender points, which are going to be used as 'monitors' during the positioning phase of this approach, are not sought in the muscles opposite those where pain is noted, but in the muscles opposite those which are actively moving the patient, or area, when pain or restriction is noted.

The general region in which such tender points are eventually located would often be very similar to the prescribed Jones points. There are, however, distinct advantages in using Goodheart's approach:

- The point will relate specifically to the individual's problem, having been located in response to identified pain or restriction, and not by means of a formula.
- Because a variety of movements may produce pain or restriction in any given dysfunctional

situation, a variety of tender points may be identified and treated using this approach.

- Patients can be taught to use this concept for self-treatment and first aid. The author has found this particularly useful in chronic pain conditions where patients have been taught within a few minutes to be able to achieve relief from pain for significant periods, using the formula devised by Goodheart.

Goodheart has added a number of modifications to the application of counterstrain methodology which will be elaborated on in later chapters. These relate primarily to the use of a neuromuscular stretch technique, applied to the tissues around the apparently dysfunctional muscle spindle during the holding of the position of ease. This refinement is said to reduce the amount of time the position of ease needs to be maintained, from 90 seconds (Jones) to 30 seconds. See the Spencer sequence (pp.79–83), which demonstrates the principles of the Goodheart approach.

5. Functional technique

(Bowles 1981, Hoover 1969)

In many ways functional technique is the most revolutionary of the positional release techniques. The practitioner engages in a subtle and detailed evaluation of the quality of motion in dysfunctional tissues, rather than attempting to engage and reduce restrictions directly. Unlike Jones' counterstrain methods osteopathic functional technique does not use alterations in reported pain as its guide to the position of ease and relies instead on achieving optimal reduction in palpated tone in stressed (hypertonic/spasm) tissues, as the body (or part) is positioned, or fine-tuned, using all available directions of movement in a given region. Greenman (1996) summarises:

The working hypothesis for functional technique is the premise that dysfunction results in altered neural activity. The abnormal dysfunction stimulates aberrant afferent impulses from mechanoreceptors and nociceptors … Functional techniques can be described as afferent reduction procedures.

There are two main variants in functional technique known as (A) 'balance and hold', and (B) 'dynamic functional'.

5A Balance and hold functional technique

When employing 'balance and hold' a position of combined ease is achieved in tissues using what is known as a 'stacking' sequence, explained and described in detail in a later chapter (Ch. 8, pp. 140–144). One hand palpates the affected tissues (molded to them, without invasive pressure). This is described as the 'listening' hand since it assesses changes in tone as the operator's other hand guides the patient (or part) through a sequence of positions which are aimed at enhancing ease and reducing bind.

A sequence of evaluations is carried out, each involving different directions of movement (flexion/extension, rotation right and left, side-bending right and left, etc.) with each new sequence starting at the point of maximum ease discovered during the previous evaluation, or combined points of ease of a number of previous evaluations. In this way, one position of ease is 'stacked' onto another until all directions of movement have been assessed for ease.

In the case of an individual with a low back problem, such as the one discussed above, the tense tissues in the low back would be the ones being palpated and treated. Following a sequence of flexion/extension, side-bending and rotating in each direction, followed by translation (a 'shunt' or glide movement) right and left, translation anterior and posterior, and compression/distraction – so involving all available directions of movement of the area – a position of maximum ease would be arrived at. At this stage respiration influences are evaluated, as the patient breathes fully in and out and the response of the tissues is monitored. The patient is asked to maintain the breath at the position which produces the greatest 'ease' in the palpated tissues, for as long as is comfortable and then to breathe normally. The combined position of ease is held for 90 seconds or more, in order to facilitate a release of hypertonicity and reduction in pain. Following this a re-evaluation of dysfunction is carried out and the entire procedure may be repeated one or more times.

It is important to note that the precise sequence in which the various directions of motion are evaluated is irrelevant, as long as all possibilities are included.

Theoretically (and usually, in practice) the position of palpated maximum ease (reduced tone) in the distressed tissues should correspond with the position which would have been found were pain being used as a guide, as in either Jones' or Goodheart's approach, or using the more basic 'exaggeration of distortion' or 'replication of position of strain'. While extremely effective, the 'balance and hold' approach is somewhat static in that it fails to take account of the likelihood that while in the 'held' position changes will usually occur in the tissues (referred to as 'unwinding') to which the practitioner could respond with accommodating positioning. The advantage of 'balance and hold' is that it is more easily applied than the 'dynamic functional procedure' (below).

5B Dynamic functional technique

When using dynamic functional procedures, a more fluid approach is initiated as the practitioner applies a 'listening' hand to dysfunctional tissues and the other ('motor') hand guides the tissues in minute increments towards maximum ease.

In effect, precisely the same end-point should be achieved as in the balance and hold method, with the only variant being the constant monitoring and balancing of feedback from dysfunctional tissues, as the ease–bind status is assessed, as movement towards ease and away from bind continues (Johnstone 1997).

Exercises in this form of palpation (which, when complete, produces the 'combined' position of ease) will be found in Chapter 8 (pp. 145–146).

6. Any painful point as a starting place for SCS (McPartland & Zigler 1993)

It is reasonable to assume that all areas which palpate as unnaturally painful are responding to, or are associated with, some degree of imbalance, dysfunction or reflexive activity, which may well involve acute or chronic strain.

Jones commenced his approach from the viewpoint of identifying the likely position of tender points relating to particular strain positions, usually in tissues shortened during acute or chronic strains. It makes just as much sense to work from the opposite direction, so that any painful point elicited during soft-tissue evaluation, massage or palpation, including a search for trigger points, may be usefully treated by positional release, whether the strain which produced the pain (or which is maintaining it) can be identified or not, irrespective of whether the problem is acute or chronic.

Experience and simple logic tell us that the response to positional release of a chronically fibrosed area will be less dramatic than from tissues held in simple spasm or hypertonicity. Nevertheless, even in chronic settings, a degree of release and ease can be produced in dysfunctional tissues, allowing for improved function and easier access to the deeper fibrosis.

This approach, of being able to treat any painful tissue using positional release, is valid whether the pain is being monitored via feedback from the patient (using reducing levels of pain in the palpated point as a guide) or whether the concept of assessing a reduction in tone in the tissues is being used (as in functional technique as described above).

Again, a lengthy period of up to 90 seconds is recommended as the time for holding the position of maximum ease – although some (such as Marsh Morrison – see variation 8 below) suggest just 20 seconds, and advocates of facilitated positional release (below) have reduced the 'holding time' to under 5 seconds.

7. Facilitated positional release (FPR)

(Schiowitz 1990)

This variation on the theme of functional and SCS methods involves the positioning of the distressed area into the direction of its greatest freedom of movement, starting from a position of 'neutral' in terms of the overall body position.

As an example, the seated patient's sagittal posture might be modified to take the body, or the part (neck for example), into a more 'neutral' position – a balance between flexion and extension – to 'unload the facets' (Schiowitz 1997). After this, an application of a facilitating force (usually a crowding or a torsion of the tissues) is introduced. No pain monitor is used but rather a palpating/listening hand is applied (as in functional technique) which senses for changes in ease and bind in distressed tissues as the body/part is carefully positioned and repositioned. The final 'crowding' or torsioning of the tissues, to encourage a 'slackening' of local tension, is the facilitating aspect of the process, according to its theorists.

This 'crowding' might involve compression applied through the long axis of a limb perhaps, or directly downwards through the spine via cranially applied pressure, or some such variation.

The length of time the position of ease is held is usually suggested at less than 5 seconds. It is claimed that altered tissue texture, either surface or deep, can be successfully treated in this way. Schiowitz (1997) states, 'The order of the two steps, first placing tissue into its position of ease and then applying the facilitating force, may be reversed'.

The mechanisms involved are thought to relate to modifications in neural activity which reduces hypertonicity (Carew 1985). No explanation is offered for the discrepancy between the proposed holding time (under 5 seconds), as compared with Jones' work, or functional technique methodology (90 seconds as a rule). FPR will be evaluated and discussed in greater detail in Chapter 9.

8. Induration technique

Marsh Morrison (1969) suggested very light palpation, using extremely light touch, as a means of feeling a 'drag' sensation (see notes on palpation in Chapter 4, p. 76) alongside the spine (as lateral as the tips of the transverse processes). The 'drag' sensation relates to increased hydrosis, which is a physiological response to increased sympathetic activity, and is an almost invariable factor in skin overlying a trigger and other forms of reflexively induced dysfunction, or prolonged hypertonicity. Once drag is noted, carefully applied pressure into the tissues normally evinces a report of pain.

The operator stands on the contralateral side of the prone patient to that in which pain has been discovered in these paraspinal tissues.

Once located, tender or painful points (lying no more lateral than the tip of the transverse process) are palpated for the level of their sensitivity to pressure (Fig. 1.1). Pressure on the tender point is held by firm thumb or finger contact while, with the soft thenar eminence of the other hand, the tip of the spinous process most adjacent to the tender point is very gently eased towards the pain (ounces of pressure only), so crowding and slackening the tissues being palpated, until pain reduces by at least 70%. Direct pressure of this sort (lightly applied) towards the pain should slacken the paraspinal musculature transversely, and lessen the degree of sensitivity.

If it does not do so, then the angle of push on the spinous process towards the tender point should be varied slightly so that, somewhere within an arc embracing a half circle, an angle will be found to abolish the pain totally, as well as lessening the palpated feeling of tissue tension. This position is held for 20 seconds (according to Morrison) after which the next point is treated. A full spinal treatment is possible using this extremely gentle approach which incorporates the same principles as SCS and functional technique. Enhanced spinal function and pain reduction are the objectives.

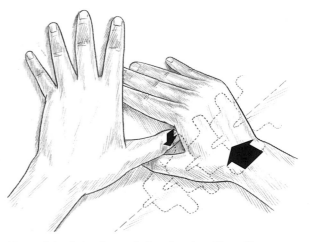

Figure 1.1 Induration technique hand positions. Pressure used on the spinous processes is measured in ounces (grams) at most.

9. Integrated neuromuscular inhibition technique (INIT)

INIT (Chaitow 1994) involves using a 'position of ease' for tissues housing a trigger point as part of a sequence of its deactivation. The sequence commences with the location of a tender/pain/trigger point, followed by application of ischaemic compression (this is optional and is avoided if pain is too intense or the patient too fragile or sensitive), followed by the introduction of positional release. After an appropriate length of time, during which the tissues are held in 'ease', the patient is asked to introduce an isometric contraction into the affected tissues for 7 to 10 seconds, after which these are stretched (or they may be stretched at the same time as the contraction, if fibrotic tissue calls for such attention). Subsequently, a further position of ease period may be instigated, or other variations which facilitate activation of the antagonists to the muscles involved, may be introduced.

This efficient trigger-point treatment will be described in greater detail in Chapter 6.

10. Proprioceptive taping

A quite different approach, practical aspects of which will be touched on in Chapter 11, and more fully explained in Chapter 12, is 'unloading' taping, a physiotherapy variant on PRT (Fig. 1.2). This is a method which seems to incorporate many of the principles associated with PRT. In recent years, for example, specific conditions, commonly involving knee and/or shoulder dysfunction, have been treated by physiotherapists by means of application of supportive taping to 'unload' the affected joints (spinal unloading is also used at times). Morrissey (2000) explains:

Proprioception is a critical component of coordinated shoulder movement with significant deficits having been identified in pathological and fatigued shoulders (Carpenter 1998). It is an integral part of rehabilitation programs to attempt to minimize or reverse these proprioceptive deficits. Taping is a useful adjunct to a patient-specific integrated treatment approach aiming to restore full pain-free movement to the shoulder girdle. Taping is particularly useful in addressing movement faults at the scapulo-thoracic, gleno-humeral and acromio-clavicular joints. The exact mechanisms by which

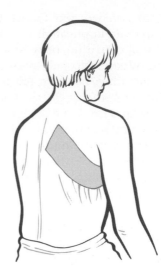

Figure 1.2   Proprioceptive taping for serratus anterior facilitation and inferior angle abduction.

shoulder taping is effective is not yet clear but the suggestion is that the effects are both proprioceptive and mechanical.

It is interesting to note that some of the methods used in taping deliberately place distressed joints and tissues into ease positions for hours, or even days, with marked benefit. Additional information regarding this approach will be found in Chapters 4, 10 and 11.

11. Mobilisation with movement (MWM)

In Chapter 11 physiotherapist Ed Wilson outlines the features of mobilisation with movement (MWM) and its variants, as developed by New Zealand physiotherapist, Brian Mulligan (1992), which has elements which equate closely with positional release principles. Features of the MWM methods as used in treatment of cervical and upper thoracic facet joint dysfunctions are as follows:

- The methods carry the acronym SNAGs, for 'sustained natural apophyseal glides'.
- SNAGs are used to treat restriction or pain, experienced on flexion, extension, side-flexion or rotation of the cervical spine, usually from C3 and lower.

- It is essential to be aware of the facet angles of the segments being treated.
- Patient is weight-bearing, usually seated.
- Movements are actively performed by the patient, in the direction of restriction, while the practitioner passively holds an area (in the cervical and thoracic spine it is the segment immediately cephalad to the restriction) in anterior translation.
- This passive light pressure represents the positional release element of the method.
- In the cervical spine the facet plane is towards the eyes.
- Residual stiffness/soreness is to be anticipated on the following day.
- The patient may usefully apply 'overpressure' to reinforce movement towards the restriction barrier.
- The same procedure is performed several times.
- Instant functional improvement is likely.
- At no time should pain be experienced.

The mechanisms whereby MWM methods achieve their effects are as yet uncertain. Wilson hypothesises that all joint abnormalities create afferent output which sensitises (facilitates) the CNS, particularly wide dynamic range (WDR) cells of the dorsal horn (Korr 1976). This creates efferent discharge to, and alters tone in, muscles controlling the joint, creating a vicious circle.

In the absence of intra- or extra-articular pathology, if the CNS can be offered normal afferent input for a period, muscle contractile power may alter, realigning joint biomechanics and helping to break into the cycle of dysfunction. By halting the excitatory barrage a previously painful movement may become pain-free. Additionally, normal mechanoreceptor input from active muscles (as in SNAGs) should enhance normal function.

12. Other approaches

There are a variety of methods involving positional release which do not quite fit into any of the categories listed above. These range from an effective rib-release technique devised by the founder of cranial osteopathy, WG Sutherland, and described by PE Kimberley (1980) to various cranial techniques described by John Upledger (Upledger & Vredevoogd 1983) and others, as well as fascial restriction techniques described by Jerry Dickey (1989) and variations modified by George Goodheart (Walther 1988). Some of these methods will be described in Chapter 10, with others being outlined in Chapter 7, which focuses on hospital use of SCS and its variations.

COMMONALITIES AND DIFFERENCES

What all PRT methods have in common is that they have as an objective a reduction in the tone of the distressed tissues associated with the dysfunction being treated. The means whereby this is achieved vary, some using reduced pain levels as a guide to the comfort/ease position, and others using variations on palpated change. The differences between the various methods relate largely to details as to how long the ease position should be held, ranging from under 5 seconds (facilitated positional release) to 20 minutes (positional release therapy) and even days (physiotherapy taping). The issues will be explored in Chapters 3 and 4.

In the next chapter some of the main theories which help to explain the success of PRT will be evaluated.

Box 1.1 Summary of PR variations

All methods require PRT positioning to be performed slowly without introducing any additional pain to the patient. In all variations, a slow return to neutral is advised following the holding of the position of ease. Most of the positional release methods involve motion into ease, away from bind, utilising a slackening, crowding or 'folding' of dysfunctional tissues, in order to facilitate muscle spindle resetting and improved function.

Despite the gentleness of the methods there is commonly a reaction involving stiffness and possibly discomfort on the day following treatment, as tissues adjust to their new situation and adaptation processes accommodate these changes.

SCS
- Seeks tender points which are utilised for monitoring in tissues shortened at the time of acute or chronic strain.
- Tender points are used as guides to the 'ease' position, as pain reduces during positioning.
- Normally uses flexion to ease strains on the front of the body and extension to ease pain on the back of the body (see specific guidelines in Chapter 3).
- The position of ease once established (at least 70% reduction in pain from tender point) is held for 90 seconds as a rule.
- Commonly replicates the position of strain in order to find the position of ease.
- Commonly exaggerates existing deviations/distortions in order to achieve ease in tender palpated tissues.
- Tender points are usually situated in muscles antagonistic to those involved in motion which is painful or restricted.
- Goodheart adds various facilitating methods in order to reduce the time required for tissue release (see Chapter 4 for more details).
- Positional release therapy suggests holding for up to 20 minutes to achieve enhanced tissue changes, but agree with Jones' '90 second rule' for simple musculoskeletal dysfunction treatment.

Functional techniques
- With one hand monitoring (listening) and the other acting to introduce movement, the joint is taken to its position of maximal ease in all available directions of motion – a point of dynamic neutral – in which one position of ease has been 'stacked' on another.
- The process of stacking involves subsequent assessments for ease in different directions of movement, commencing at the point of ease revealed by the previous assessment.
- Following the holding of the position of dynamic neutral until a sense of warmth or pulsation or greater ease is noted (90 second minimum suggested), the whole sequence is repeated at least once more, with variations in the positions of ease being evident as a consequence of changes resulting from the previous 'treatment'.

Facilitated positional release
- In treating soft-tissue dysfunction, FPR uses a sequence involving neutralising the anteroposterior curve, followed by creation of a position of ease, followed by crowding and/or torsion to produce a sense of greater ease in palpated tissues (Note: this sequence can be varied).
- In treating joint restriction the same approach is used, but the joint involved is also guided towards its directions of most-free motion.
- The time the position of ease is held in FPR is 3 to 4 seconds only before retesting.
- If no improvement is noted the condition is considered to require more direct approaches of treatment.

Fascial release
- Soft tissues are held in the direction of greatest ease until 'release' occurs.
- The process is repeated until there exists symmetry of motion in all directions.

Cranial manipulation (applicable anywhere on the body)
- The restricted structure/tissues will be taken towards their direction of greatest ease, at which time this position is held until there is a sense of an attempt by the structure/tissues to return towards the direction from which they have been moved. This is resisted.
- Subsequently, the barrier usually retreats and the tissues are taken into greater ease. The process is repeated.

Proprioceptive taping
- Use of supportive taping to unload dysfunctional, stressed tissues and joints, for long enough to allow re-education processes to take place, as a result of proprioceptive modifications.

Mobilisation with movement (MWM) including SNAGs
- Gentle short-term positioning of joints, including spinal, in order to allow active pain-free movement to be performed by the patient, in order to restore normal function.

REFERENCES

Bowles C 1969 'Dynamic Neutral' – a bridge. Academy of Applied Osteopathy Yearbook: 1–2
Bowles C 1981 Functional technique – a modern perspective. J American Osteopathic Association 80(3): 326–331

Carew T 1985 The control of reflex action. In: Kandel E (ed) Principles of Neural Science, 2nd edn. Elsevier, New York
Carpenter J 1998 The effects of muscle fatigue on shoulder joint position sense. American Journal of Sports Medicine 26: 262–265

Chaitow L 1994 Integrated neuromuscular inhibition technique. British Journal of Osteopathy 13: 17–20

D'Ambrogio K, Roth G 1997 Positional Release Therapy. Mosby, St. Louis

Dickey J 1989 Postoperative osteopathic manipulative management of median sternotomy patients. J American Osteopathic Association 89(10): 1309–1322

Goodheart G 1984 Applied Kinesiology Workshop Procedure Manual, 21st edn. Privately published, Detroit

Greenman P 1996 Principles of Manual Medicine, 2nd edn. Williams & Wilkins, Baltimore

Hoover H V 1969 Collected papers. Academy of Applied Osteopathy Year Book

Johnstone W L 1997 Functional technique. In: Ward R (ed) Foundations for Osteopathic Medicine. Williams & Wilkins, Baltimore

Jones L 1981 Strain and Counterstrain. Academy of Applied Osteopathy, Colorado Springs

Kimberley P (Ed) 1980 Outline of Osteopathic Manipulative Procedures. Kirksville College of Osteopathic Medicine, Kirksville, Missouri

Korr I 1976 Spinal Cord as organizer of disease process. Academy of Applied Osteopathy Yearbook

McPartland J H, Zigler M 1993 Strain-counterstrain course syllabus, 2nd edn. St Lawrence Institute of Higher Learning, East Landing, MI

Morrison M 1969 Lecture notes presentation/seminar. Research Society for Naturopathy, London

Morrissey D 2000 Proprioceptive shoulder taping. Bodywork and Movement Therapies 4(3): 189–194

Mulligan B 1992 Manual Therapy. Plane View Services, Wellington, New Zealand

Ramirez M et al 1989 Low back pain – diagnosis by six newly discovered sacral tender points and treatment with counterstrain technique. J American Osteopathic Association 89(7): 905–913

Schiowitz S 1990 Facilitated positional release. J American Osteopathic Association 90(2): 145–156

Schiowitz S 1997 Facilitated positional release. In: Ward R (ed) Foundations for Osteopathic Medicine. Williams & Wilkins, Baltimore

Schwartz H 1986 The use of counterstrain in an acutely ill in-hospital population. J American Osteopathic Association 86(7): 433–42

Upledger J, Vredevoogd J 1983 Craniosacral Therapy. Eastland Press, Seattle

Walther D 1988 Applied Kinesiology Synopsis. Systems DC, Pueblo

Weiselfish S 1993 Manual Therapy for Orthopedic and Neurologic Patients. Regional Physical Therapy, Hartford, Connecticut

2

The evolution of dysfunction

DYSFUNCTION VARIABLES

Biomechanical changes sometimes occur dramatically, suddenly, traumatically. Strains, sprains, twists and blows are incidents which, depending on the degree of force involved and the tissues affected, have largely predictable consequences (inflammation, etc.). By far the majority of somatic dysfunctional conditions, however, occur gradually. They evolve over time as the tissues locally, and the body generally, adapt to and absorb the stresses being imposed. A combination commonly occurs in which stress is suddenly applied to already adaptively compromised tissues, for example when an action such as bending or lifting, which would 'normally' be well coped with, results in injury due to the chronically modified state of the tissues involved.

Therapeutic interventions need to take account of these variables, since it is patently undesirable to perform the same manual methods which might be suitable for chronic indurated tissues to acutely irritated ones.

Positional release methods are applicable to both acute and chronic dysfunctional states. However, as will become clear, some PRT variations are more useful in acute, painful conditions, or for frail, sensitive individuals, than in chronic situations.

PALPATORY LITERACY

Skilful palpation allows for discrimination between the various states and stages of dysfunction, with some degree of accuracy. Lord and Bogduk (1996) state:

There have been many claims regarding the accuracy of manual diagnosis but few data. Only one study (Jull & Bogduk 1988) compared manual diagnosis to the criterion standard of local anaesthetic blocks. The authors found the sensitivity and specificity of the manual examination technique to be 100%. The manual therapist correctly identified all patients with proven joint pain, the symptomatic and asymptomatic segments. The ability of other manual examiners to replicate these results has not been tested.

This study of the skills of (albeit) one (physio) therapist's ability to localise dysfunction suggests that isolating a segment or joint which is dysfunctional is well within the potential of manual therapists, if palpation skills are adequately refined. The application of positional release methodology requires a high degree of palpatory literacy, since the ability to 'read' tissue responses to positioning is critical, especially in application of functional methodology.

Osteopathic assessment of somatic dysfunction

Gibbons and Tehan (2001) explain the basis of osteopathic palpation when assessing for somatic dysfunction (particularly spinal dysfunction) as follows (using the acronym ARTT).

A relates to asymmetry DiGiovanna (1991) links the criteria of asymmetry to a positional focus stating that the 'position of the vertebra or other bone is asymmetrical'. Greenman (1996) broadens the concept of asymmetry by including functional in addition to structural asymmetry.

R relates to range of motion Alteration in range of motion can apply to a single joint, several joints or a region of the musculoskeletal system. The abnormality may be either restricted or increased mobility and includes assessment of quality of movement and 'end-feel'.

T relates to tissue texture changes The identification of tissue texture change is important in the diagnosis of somatic dysfunction. Palpable changes may be noted in superficial, intermediate and deep tissues. It is important for clinicians to recognise normal from abnormal.

T relates to tissue tenderness Undue tissue tenderness may be evident. Pain provocation and reproduction of familiar symptoms are often used to localise somatic dysfunction.

Comparing SCS palpation with standard methods

McPartland and Goodridge (1997) tested the value of osteopathic palpation procedures (modifying the acronym ARTT to TART) specifically to evaluate the accuracy of positional release palpation, using Jones' strain/counterstrain methodology.

This study addresses five questions:

- What is the inter-examiner reliability of diagnostic tests used in strain/counterstrain technique?
- How does this compare with the reliability of the traditional osteopathic examination ('TART' exam)?
- How reliable are different aspects of the TART exam?
- Do positive findings of Jones' points correlate with positive findings of spinal dysfunction?
- Are osteopathic students more reliable with SCS diagnosis or TART tests?

In this study examiners palpated for tender points which corresponded to those listed by Jones (1981) for the first three cervical segments (Fig. 2.1). These points were located by means of their anatomical position as described in Jones' original strain/counterstrain textbook, and were characterised as being areas of 'tight' nodular myofascial tissue.

The TART exam comprised assessment for:

- Tender paraspinal muscles
- Asymmetry of joints
- Restriction in ROM
- Tissue texture abnormalities.

Of these, zygapophyseal joint tenderness and tissue texture changes were the most accurate. In Jones' methodology the location of the tender point is meant to define the nature of the dysfunction. However, McPartland and Goodridge found that, 'Few Jones points correlated well with the cervical articulations that they presumably represent'. They did find that overall use of Jones' tender points (i.e. soft-tissue tenderness) was a more accurate method of localising dysfunction in symptomatic patients than use of

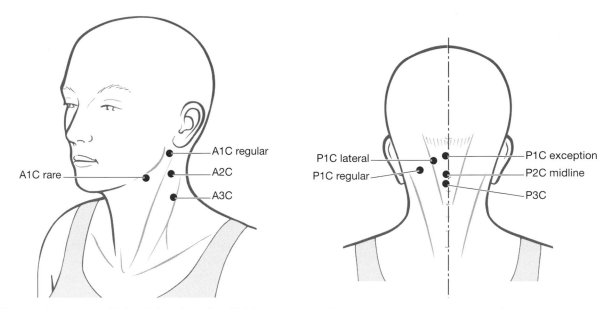

Figure 2.1 Location of left-sided tender points. Right-sided tender points are located at mirror-image positions. A = anterior; P = posterior.

joint tenderness evaluation in the TART exam, and that 'students performed much better at SCS diagnosis than TART diagnosis'.

In manual medicine it is vital that practitioners and therapists have the opportunity to evaluate and palpate normal individuals, with pliable musculature, mobile joint structures and sound respiratory function, so that dysfunctional examples can be more easily identified. Apart from standard functional examination it is important that practitioners and therapists acquire the abilities to assess by observation and touch, relearning skills familiar to older generations of 'low-tech' health care providers.

Information gained from a thorough history, clinical examination and segmental analysis will direct the practitioner towards any possible somatic dysfunction and/or pathology. This depth of diagnostic deliberation is essential if one is to assess which treatment approach might be the most effective.

IS THERE AN OPTIMAL POSTURE AND FUNCTION?

If structural modifications (restricted joints, shortened or weakened muscles, etc.) result

from, as well as reinforce, functional imbalances in posture, respiration and in other functions, it is of some importance to establish whether an optimal, ideal state is a clinical reality.

Kuchera and Kuchera (in Ward 1997) describe what they see as an 'optimal posture'.

Optimal posture is a balanced configuration of the body with respect to gravity. It depends on normal arches of the feet, vertical alignment of the ankles, and horizontal orientation (in the coronal plane) of the sacral base. The presence of an optimum posture suggests that there is perfect distribution of the body mass around the centre of gravity. The compressive force on the spinal disks is balanced by ligamentous tension; there is minimal energy expenditure from postural muscles. Structural and functional stressors on the body, however, may prevent achievement of optimum posture. In this case homeostatic mechanisms provide for 'compensation' in an effort to provide maximum postural function within the existing structure of the individual. Compensation is the counterbalancing of any defect of structure or function.

This concise description of postural reality highlights the fact that there is hardly ever an example of an optimal postural state, and by implication of respiratory function. However, there can be a well-compensated mechanism (postural or respiratory) which, despite asymmetry and adaptations, functions close to optimally. This is clearly the ideal, that systems and mechanisms should 'work' effectively. Unless due notice is taken of emotional states, gravitational influences, proprioception and other neural inputs, inborn characteristics (such as short leg), as well as habitual patterns of use (upper chest breathing, for example) and wear and tear, whatever postural and functional anomalies are observed will remain signs of 'something' abnormal happening, of ongoing compensation or adaptation, but the chance of understanding just what the 'something' is, will be remote. It is useful to be able to evaluate and assess patterns of function, which indicate just how close, or far, the individual is from an optimal postural state.

A wider perspective

Whatever efforts are directed towards removal of the causes of any functional imbalance (dysfunction), whether this involves medication, surgery, or manual rehabilitation strategies, there is likely to be a benefit if identifiable biomechanical, structural constraints can be modified towards normal.

While specific restrictions (such as shortened muscles, restricted joints, etc.) may be identified and treated, a wider perspective may also be employed in order to determine the presence of global restriction patterns. There are few local biomechanical problems which are not influenced by distant features. A fallen arch may impact via a chain of interacting influences on a stiff neck. Murphy (2000) discusses the work of Moss (1962), who demonstrated that TMJ and cranial distortion, including nasal obstruction, was commonly associated with, 'forward head carriage, abnormal cervical lordosis, rounded shoulders, a flattened chest wall and a slouching posture'. The question might well be asked as to where such a chain begins – with the facial and jaw imbalance, or in the overall postural distortion pattern, which impacted on the face and jaw?

Making sense of dysfunction on a global, whole-body scale requires that particular features be evaluated and in some coherent way formed into a rationale for whatever is being observed and presented, in terms of symptoms. In other words a 'story' needs to be constructed out of the evidence available. In relation to positional release a useful construct relates to the relative freedom of movement, or lack of it, as noted by palpation and assessment.

TIGHT–LOOSE CONCEPT

The so called 'tight–loose' concept is one way of visualising the three-dimensionality of the body, or part of it, as it is palpated and assessed (Ward 1997) This might involve seeking evidence for large or small areas in which interactive asymmetry exists, involving structures which are inappropriately 'tight' and/or 'loose', relative to each other.

For example:

- a 'tight' sacroiliac/hip is commonly noted on one side, while the contralateral side is 'loose'
- a 'tight' SCM and 'loose' scalenes are frequently noted ipsilaterally
- one shoulder may test as 'tight' and the other 'loose'.

Areas of dysfunction commonly involve vertical, horizontal and 'encircling' (also described as crossover, or spiral, or 'wrap-around') patterns of involvement.

Ward describes a 'typical' wrap-around pattern associated with a tight left low back area (which ends up involving the entire trunk and cervical area) as 'tight' areas evolve to compensate for loose, inhibited, areas (or vice versa). 'Tightness' in the posterior left hip, SI joint, lumbar erector spinae and lower rib cage, associated with:

- looseness on the right low back
- tightness of the lateral and anterior rib cage on the right
- tight left thoracic inlet, posteriorly, as well as
- tight left craniocervical attachments (involving jaw mechanics).

Clinical choices

Treatment choices involve a wide range of possibilities when addressing tightness. In bodywork in general the most common approach is to attempt, using one means or another, to push back the boundary, to engage the restriction barrier in order to force it to retreat, whether by means of stretching, or articulation, or direct manual pressure, or massage, or by reflex influences on restricted tissues. Barrier issues are discussed further later in this chapter.

Positional release methodology calls for disengagement from the restriction barrier, moving towards the point of balance between the tight and the loose structures. As tight areas are freed or loosened, even if only to a degree, at any given treatment session, so would inhibiting influences on 'loose', weak areas diminish, allowing a restoration of more normal tone and therefore relative balance. In positional release terminology, terms and words are used which describe relative balance, including 'dynamic neutral', 'position of ease', 'comfort zone', 'position of comfort' and 'tissue preference'.

D'Ambrogio and Roth (1997) suggest that the range within which such a balanced state can be achieved in dysfunctional tissues is very small, within 2 to 3 degrees. 'It may be speculated that positioning beyond its ideal range places the antagonistic muscles or opposing fascial structures under increased stretch, which in turn causes proprioceptive/neural spillover, resulting in reactivation of the facilitated segment. (See later this chapter for discussion of facilitation.)

Pain and the 'tight–loose' concept

Paradoxically, pain is often noted in the 'loose' rather than the 'tight' areas of the body, which may involve hypermobility and ligamentous laxity at the 'loose' joint or site. More commonly pain is associated with tight and bound, tethered structures, resulting from local overuse/misuse/abuse factors, scar tissue or to reflexively induced influences, or to centrally mediated neural control.

Myofascial trigger points may exist in either 'tight' or 'loose' structures, but the likelihood is that they will appear more frequently, and be more stressed, in those which are tethered, restricted, tight and where tissues are therefore relatively ischaemic.

It is axiomatic that unless these myofascial trigger points are deactivated they will help to sustain the dysfunctional postural patterns which emerge. Also axiomatic is the fact that myofascial trigger points will continue to evolve if the aetiological factors, which created and maintained them, are not corrected (Simons et al 1998).

Such deactivation may involve removing the biomechanical and other stress patterns, which create and maintain trigger points, or by direct manual intervention. A sequence of integrated methods for trigger-point deactivation is described in Chapter 6 which involves positional release (see also description of INIT in Chapter 1).

Barriers, and other terminology

In osteopathic positional release methodology (strain/counterstrain, functional technique, etc.) the terms 'bind' and 'ease' are often used to describe what is noted as unduly 'tight' or 'loose' (Jones 1981).

In manual medicine, when joint and soft-tissue 'end-feel' is being evaluated, a similar concept is involved in the area being evaluated and it is common practice to make sense of such findings by comparing sides (Kaltenborn 1985).

The characterization of features described as having a soft or hard end-feel, or as being 'tight or loose', or as demonstrating feelings of ease or bind, may be one deciding factor as to which therapeutic approaches are introduced, and in what sequence.

These findings (loose–tight, etc.) have an intimate relationship with the concept of barriers, which need to be identified in preparation for direct (i.e. where action is directed towards the restriction barrier, towards bind, tightness) and indirect techniques (where action involves movement away from barriers of restriction, towards ease, looseness).

Ward (1997) states, 'tightness suggests tethering, while looseness suggests joint and/or soft tissue laxity, with or without neural inhibition'.

However, it is worth recalling that the tight side may be the normal side, and also that clinically it is possible that tight restriction barriers may best be left unchallenged, in case they are offering some protective benefit.

As an example, van Wingerden (1997) reports that both intrinsic and extrinsic support for the sacroiliac joint derives in part from the hamstring (biceps femoris) status. Intrinsically the influence is via the close anatomical and physiological relationship between biceps femoris and the sacrotuberous ligament (they frequently attach via a strong tendinous link).

Force from the biceps femoris muscle can lead to increased tension of the sacrotuberous ligament in various ways. Since increased tension of the sacrotuberous ligament diminishes the range of sacroiliac joint motion, the biceps femoris can play a role in stabilisation of the SIJ (Vleeming 1989).

Van Wingerden (1997) also notes that in low-back patients, forward flexion is often painful as the load on the spine increases. This happens whether flexion occurs in the spine or via the hip joints (tilting of the pelvis). If the hamstrings are tight and short they effectively prevent pelvic tilting. 'In this respect, an increase in hamstring tension might well be part of a defensive arthrokinematic reflex mechanism of the body to diminish spinal load.'

If such a state of affairs is long-standing the hamstrings (biceps femoris) will shorten, possibly influencing sacroiliac and lumbar spine dysfunction.

The decision to treat tight ('tethered') hamstring should therefore take account of why it is tight, and consider that in some circumstances it is offering beneficial support to the SIJ, or that it is reducing low back stress.

Chain reactions and 'tight–loose' changes

Vleeming et al (1997) connect gravitational strain with changes of muscle function and structure, which lead predictably to observable postural modifications and functional limitations. 'Postural muscles, structurally adapted to resist prolonged gravitational stress, generally resist fatigue. When overly stressed, however, these same postural muscles become irritable, tight, shortened' (Janda 1986). The antagonists to these postural muscles

demonstrate inhibitory characteristics described as 'pseudoparesis' (a functional, non-organic weakness) or 'myofascial trigger points with weakness' when they are stressed.

Observable changes emerge through overuse, misuse and abuse of the postural system, demonstrating common dysfunctional postural patterns.

General treatment options

Ward (1997) has described methods for restoration of 'three-dimensionally patterned functional symmetry'.

Identification of patterns of ease–bind or loose–tight in a given body area, or the body as a whole, should emerge from sequential assessment of muscle shortness and restriction, or palpation, or any comprehensive evaluation of the status of the soft tissues of the body.

- Appropriate methods for release of areas identified as tight, restricted or tethered might usefully involve soft-tissue manipulation methods such as myofascial release (MFR), muscle energy techniques (MET), neuromuscular technique (NMT), positional release technique (PRT), singly or in combination, plus other effective manual approaches.
- If joints fail to respond adequately to soft-tissue mobilisation, the use of articulation/mobilisation or high-velocity thrust methods may be incorporated, as appropriate to the status (age, structural integrity, inflammatory status, pain levels, etc.) of the individual. It is suggested, however, that in sensitive or acute situations positional release methods offer a useful first line of treatment with little or no risk of exacerbating the condition.
- Identification and appropriate deactivation of myofascial trigger points contained within these structures.
- Reeducation and rehabilitation (including homework) of posture, breathing and patterns of use, in order to restore functional integrity and prevent recurrence, as far as is possible.

- Exercise (homework) has to be focused, time-efficient, and within the patient's easy comprehension and capabilities, if compliance is to be achieved.

The question of why tissues become 'functionally and structurally three-dimensionally asymmetrical' needs some consideration, since out of the reasons for the development of somatic dysfunction emerge possible therapeutic strategies.

MUSCULOSKELETAL–BIOMECHANICAL STRESSORS

(Basmajian 1974, Dvorak & Dvorak 1984, Janda 1983, Korr 1978, Lewit 1999, Travell & Simons 1992)

The many forms of stress affecting the body in the sort of sequential manner discussed below can be categorised as falling into general classifications of physiological, emotional, behavioural and/or structural.

These might include (Barlow 1959):

- Congenital factors such as short or long leg, small hemipelvis, fascial influences (e.g. cranial distortions involving the reciprocal tension membranes due to birthing difficulties such as forceps delivery)
- Overuse, misuse and abuse factors such as injury or inappropriate or repetitive patterns of use involved in work, sport or regular activities
- Immobilisation–disuse (irreversible changes can occur after just 8 weeks (Lederman 1997)
- Postural stress pattern which are often related to emotional states
- Inappropriate breathing patterns (Lewit 1980)
- Chronic negative emotional states such as depression, anxiety, etc.
- Reflexive influences (trigger points, facilitated spinal regions) – see later in this chapter for discussion of this important aspect of somatic dysfunction.

A biomechanical stress sequence

When the musculoskeletal system is 'stressed' (overused, used inappropriately, traumatised, underused, etc.) a sequence of events occurs which can be summarised as follows:

- 'Something' (see list above) occurs leading to increased muscular tone
- If this is anything but short-term, retention of metabolic wastes commences
- Increased tone simultaneously results in a degree of localised oxygen deficit resulting in relative ischaemia
- Ischaemia does not produce pain but an ischaemic muscle which contracts rapidly does (Lewis 1942, Liebenson 1996)
- Increased tone may lead to a degree of oedema
- Retention of wastes/ischaemia/oedema all contribute to discomfort or pain which in turn reinforces hypertonicity
- Inflammation or at least chronic irritation may evolve
- Neurological reporting stations in the distressed tissues will bombard the CNS with information regarding their status, resulting in neural sensitisation and the evolution of facilitation – a tendency to hyper-reactivity
- Macrophages are activated as is increased vascularity and fibroblastic activity
- Connective tissue production increases with cross-linkage leading to shortened fascia
- Chronic muscular stress (a combination of the load involved and the number of repetitions, or the degree of sustained influence) results in the gradual development of hysteresis in which collagen fibres and proteoglycans are rearranged to produce an altered structural pattern
- This results in tissues which are more easily fatigued than normal and more prone to damage if strained
- Since all fascia/connective tissue is continuous throughout the body, any distortions or contractions developing in one region can create fascial deformations elsewhere, so negatively influencing structures supported by, or attached to, the fascia, e.g. nerves, muscles, lymph structures, blood vessels
- Hypertonicity in muscles leads to inhibition of antagonist(s) and aberrant behaviour in synergist(s)

- Chain reactions evolve in which some muscles (postural) shorten while others (phasic) weaken
- Because of sustained increased muscle tension ischaemia in tendinous structures occurs, leading to the development of periosteal pain; and also in localised areas of muscles leading to myofascial trigger-point evolution. Ischaemic influences, and trigger points, are discussed later in this chapter
- Compensatory adaptations evolve leading to habitual, 'built-in', patterns of use emerging as the CNS learns to compensate for modifications in muscle strength, length and functional behaviour
- Abnormal biomechanics result, involving malcoordination of movement (for example erector spinae tighten while rectus abdominis is inhibited)
- The normal firing sequence of muscles involved in particular movements alters resulting in additional strain
- Joint biomechanics are directly influenced by the accumulated influences of such soft-tissue changes and can themselves become significant sources of referred and local pain, reinforcing soft-tissue dysfunctional patterns (Schiable 1993)
- Deconditioning of the soft tissues becomes progressive as a result of the combination of simultaneous events involved in soft-tissue pain: 'spasm' (guarding), joint stiffness, antagonist weakness, overactive synergists, etc.
- Progressive evolution of localised areas of neural hyper-reactivity occurs (facilitated areas) paraspinally, or within muscles (myofascial trigger points)
- Within these trigger points increased neurological activity occurs (for which there is EMG evidence) which is capable of influencing distant tissues adversely (Hubbard 1993, Simons 1993)
- Energy wastage due to unnecessarily sustained hypertonicity and excessively active musculature leads to generalised fatigue
- More widespread functional changes develop – for example affecting respiratory function and body posture – with repercussions on the total body economy
- In the presence of a constant neurological feedback of impulses to the CNS/brain from neural reporting stations indicating heightened arousal (a hypertonic muscle status is the alarm reaction of the flight/fight alarm response) there will be increased levels of psychological arousal and a reduction in the ability to relax, with consequent reinforcement of hypertonicity
- Functional patterns of use of a biologically unsustainable nature emerge
- At this stage restoration of normal function requires therapeutic input which addresses both the multiple changes which have occurred and the need for a re-education of the individual as to how to use their body, to breathe, carry and use themselves, in more sustainable ways.

The chronic adaptive changes which develop in such a scenario lead to the increased likelihood of future acute exacerbations as the increasingly chronic, less supple and resilient biomechanical structures attempt to cope with additional stress factors resulting from the normal demands of modern living.

In this sequence it is not difficult to see how any technique which offers the chance for enhanced circulation and drainage, more normal tonal balance and reduction of pain, would help to minimise dysfunctional tendencies. Positional release procedures achieve these effects, so reducing the negative sequelae of somatic dysfunction, while at the same time enhancing the adaptation potentials of the tissues involved.

At some point, if stresses are constant or mounting, all adaptation potentials reach a stage of exhaustion, as in an elastic band which snaps when stretched too far. How is the practitioner to know when an individual, or a particular region, joint or area, has reached that elastic limit?

Postural compensation patterns (Zink & Lawson 1979)

Fascial compensation is seen as a useful, beneficial and above all functional (i.e. no obvious symptoms result) response on the part of the musculoskeletal system, for example as a result of anomalies such as a short leg, or to overuse.

Decompensation describes the same phenomenon where adaptive changes are seen to be dysfunctional, to produce symptoms, evidencing a failure of homeostatic mechanisms (i.e. adaptation and self-repair). Zink and Lawson (1979) have described a model of postural patterning resulting from the progression towards fascial decompensation.

By testing the tissue 'preferences' (loose–tight) in different areas Zink maintains that it is possible to classify patterns in clinically useful ways:

- ideal patterns (minimal adaptive load transferred to other regions)
- compensated patterns, which alternate in direction from area to area (e.g. atlantooccipital–cervicothoracic–thoracolumbar–lumbosacral) and which are commonly adaptive in nature
- uncompensated patterns which do not alternate, and which are commonly the result of trauma.

It is well to keep in mind the previous discussion of 'tight–loose' assessments when these patterns are evaluated.

Zink has described four crossover sites where fascial tensions can be noted, occipitoatlantal (OA), cervicothoracic (CT), thoracolumbar (TL), lumbosacral (LS). These sites are tested for rotation and side-bending preference. Zink's research showed that most people display alternating patterns of rotatory preference with about 80% of people showing a common pattern of L-R-L-R (termed the 'common compensatory pattern' or CCP) (Fig. 2.2A). Zink observed that the 20% of people whose compensatory pattern did not alternate (Fig. 2.2B) had poor health histories. Treatment of either CCP, or uncompensated fascial patterns, has the objective of trying, as far as is possible, to create a symmetrical degree of rotatory motion at the key crossover sites. The methods used range from direct muscle energy approaches, to indirect positional release techniques.

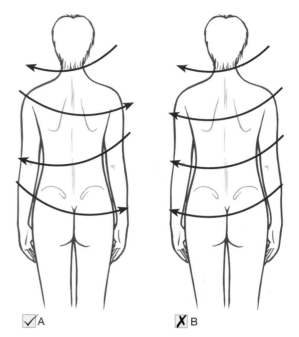

☑A   ☒B

Figure 2.2 (**A**) Compensated pattern of alternating crossover patterns indicates minimal adaptive load transferred to other regions. (**B**) Uncompensated patterns do not alternate and may be the result of trauma.

Assessment of tissue preference in Zink sequence

Occipitoatlantal area

- Patient is supine
- Operator sits at head, slightly to one side so that s/he is facing the corner of the table
- One hand (caudal hand) cradles the occiput with opposed index finger and thumb controlling the atlas
- The neck is flexed so that rotatory motion is focused into the upper cervical area only
- The other hand is placed on patient's forehead
- The contact on the occipitoatlantal joint evaluates the tissue preference as the area is slowly rotated left and right.

Cervicothoracic area

- Patient is supine in relaxed posture
- Practitioner sits at head of table and slides hands under the patient's scapulae

- Each hand independently assesses the area being palpated for its 'tightness–looseness' preferences by easing first one and then the other scapula area towards the ceiling
- By holding tissues in their 'loose' or ease, directions (or by holding tissues in their 'tight' or bind directions – and introducing isometric contractions), changes can be encouraged.

Thoracolumbar area

- Patient is supine, operator at waist level faces cephalad and places hands over lower thoracic structures, fingers along lower rib shafts laterally
- Treating the structure being palpated as a cylinder the hands test the preference this has to rotate around its central axis, one way and then the other. As an additional assessment, once this has been established, the preference to sidebend one way or the other is evaluated, so that combined ('stacked') positions of ease, or bind, can be established
- By holding tissues in their 'loose' or ease, positions – (or by holding tissues in their 'tight' or bind positions – and introducing isometric contractions, or by just waiting for a release), changes can be encouraged.

Lumbosacral area

- Patient is supine, operator stands below waist level facing cephalad and places hands on anterior pelvic structures, using the contact as a 'steering wheel' to evaluate tissue preference as the pelvis is rotated around its central axis seeking information as to its 'tightness–looseness' (see above) preferences. Once this has been established, the preference to sidebend one way or the other is evaluated, so that combined ('stacked') positions of ease, or bind, can be established
- By holding tissues in their 'loose' or ease, positions (or by holding tissues in their 'tight' or bind positions – and introducing isometric contractions, or by just waiting for a release), changes can be encouraged.

These general evaluation approaches, which seek evidence of compensation and of global adaptation patterns involving loose and tight tissues, offer a broad means of commencing rehabilitation, by altering structural features associated with dysfunction.

The discussion above has focused largely on gross, global patterns of adaptation, compensation and dysfunction. In the notes below a summary is provided of aspects of local dysfunction, much of it reflexogenically derived, involving, among other features, myofascial trigger points. This is a particularly rewarding therapeutic area, in which positional release methods have much to offer.

FACILITATION AND THE EVOLUTION OF TRIGGER POINTS

(Korr 1976, Patterson 1976)

Facilitation is the osteopathic term for what happens when neural sensitisation occurs. There are at least two forms of facilitation, spinal (or segmental) and local (e.g. trigger-point). Visceral dysfunction results in sensitisation and ultimately facilitation of paraspinal neural structures at the level of the nerve supply to that organ. In cardiac disease, for example, the muscles alongside the spine at the upper thoracic level, from which the heart derives its innervation, become hypertonic.

The area becomes facilitated, with the nerves of the area, including those passing to the heart, becoming hyperirritable. EMG readings of the upper thoracic paraspinal muscles show greater activity than surrounding tissues, as well as palpating as hypertonic and more painful to pressure.

Once facilitation occurs all additional stress impacting the individual, of any sort, whether emotional physical, chemical, climatic or mechanical, leads to an increase in neural activity in the facilitated segments, and not to the rest of the (unfacilitated) spinal structures.

Korr (1978) has called such an area a 'neurological lens', since it concentrates neural activity to the facilitated area, so creating more activity and also a local increase in muscle tone at that level of the spine. Similar segmental (spinal) facilitation occurs in response to any visceral disease, affecting the segments of the spine from which neural supply to that organ derive.

Other causes of segmental (spinal) facilitation can include biomechanical stress – injury, over-activity, repetitive patterns of use, poor posture or structural imbalance (short leg for example).

Korr tells us that when subjects who have had facilitated segments identified 'were exposed to physical, environmental and psychological stimuli similar to those encountered in daily life the sympathetic responses in those segments was exaggerated and prolonged. The disturbed segments behaved as though they were continually in or bordering on a state of "physiologic alarm"' (Korr 1978).

How to recognise a facilitated area

A number of observable and palpable signs indicate an area of segmental (spinal) facilitation. Beal (1983) tells us that such an area will usually involve two or more segments, unless traumatically induced, in which case single segments are possible. The paraspinal tissues will palpate as rigid or board-like.

With the patient supine and the palpating hands under the patient's paraspinal area to be tested (standing at the head of the table for example and reaching under the shoulders for the upper thoracic area) any ceilingward 'springing' attempt on these tissues will result in a distinct lack of elasticity, unlike more normal tissues above or below the facilitated area (Beal 1983).

Palpable or observable features

Gunn and Milbrandt (1978) and Grieve (1986), have all helped to define the palpable and visual signs which accompany facilitated areas:

- A gooseflesh appearance is observable in facilitated areas when the skin is exposed to cool air – as a result of a facilitated pilomotor response.
- A palpable sense of 'drag' is noticeable as a light touch contact is made across such areas,

due to increased sweat production due to facilitation of the sudomotor reflexes.

- There is likely to be cutaneous hyperaesthesia in the related dermatome, as the sensitivity (for example to a pinprick) is increased due to facilitation.
- An 'orange peel' appearance is noticeable in the subcutaneous tissues when the skin is rolled over the affected segment, due to subcutaneous trophoedema.
- There is commonly localised spasm of the muscles in a facilitated area, which is palpable segmentally as well as peripherally in the related myotome. This is likely to be accompanied by an enhanced myotatic reflex due to the process of facilitation.

Local (trigger point) facilitation in muscles

A process of local facilitation occurs when particularly vulnerable sites of muscle (origins and insertions for example) are overused, abused, misused or disused. Localised areas of hypertonicity develop, sometimes accompanied by oedema, sometimes with a stringy feel – but always with sensitivity to pressure.

Many of these palpably painful, tender, sensitive, localised, facilitated points are myofascial trigger points, which are not only painful themselves when pressed, but when active will also transmit or activate pain (and other) sensations some distance away from themselves, in 'target' tissues.

Melzack and Wall (1988) have stated that there are few if any chronic pain problems which do not have trigger-point activity as a major part of the picture, perhaps not always as a prime cause but almost always as a maintaining feature (Melzack & Wall 1988).

In the same manner as the facilitated areas alongside the spine, trigger points will become more active when stress, *of whatever type*, makes adaptive demands on the body as a whole, not just on the area in which they are found.

When not actively directing pain to a distant area, trigger points (locally tender or painful to applied pressure) are said to be 'latent'. The same signs as described for spinal, segmental facilitation can be observed and palpated in these localised areas.

Selective motor unit involvement

(Waersted et al 1993)

The effect of psychogenic influences on muscles may be more complex than a simplistic 'whole' muscle or region involvement. Researchers at the National Institute of Occupational Health in Oslo, Norway have demonstrated that a small number of motor units in particular muscles may display almost constant, or repeated, activity when influenced psychogenically (a normal individual performing a reaction-time task). Using the trapezius muscle as the focus of attention the researchers were able to demonstrate low amplitude levels of activity (using surface EMG) when individuals were inactive. They explain this phenomenon as follows:

In spite of low total activity level of the muscle, a small pool of low-threshold motor units may be under considerable load for prolonged periods of time. Such a recruitment pattern would be in agreement with the 'size principle' first proposed by Henneman (1957), saying that motor units are recruited according to their size. Motor units with Type 1 (postural) fibres are predominant among the small, low-threshold units. If tension-provoking factors are frequently present and the subject, as a result, repeatedly recruits the same motor units, the hypothesised overload may follow, possibly resulting in a metabolic crisis and the appearance of Type 1 fibres with abnormally large diameters, or 'ragged-red' fibres, which are interpreted as a sign of mitochondrial overload (Edwards 1988, Larsson 1990).

The researchers report that similar observations have been noted in a pilot study (Waersted et al 1992).

The implications of this information are profound, since they suggest that emotional stress can selectively involve postural fibres of muscles, which shorten over time when stressed (Janda 1983). The possible 'metabolic crisis' suggested by this research has strong parallels with the evolution of myofascial trigger points as suggested by Wolfe and Simons (1992).

Trigger points – the Travell and Simons' model

A great deal of research has been conducted since the first edition of *Myofascial Pain and Dysfunction: The Trigger Point Manual*, Volume 1 was published by Williams and Wilkins in 1983. In the second edition (Simons et al 1998), the authors have to a large extent validated their theories with research findings, and present evidence which suggests that what they term 'central' trigger points (those forming in the belly of the muscle) develop almost directly in the centre of the muscle's fibres, where the motor endplate innervates it, at the neuromuscular junction. They suggest the following:

- Dysfunctional endplate activity occurs, commonly associated with a strain, causing acetylcholine (ACh) to be excessively released at the synapse, along with stored calcium.
- The presence of high calcium levels apparently keeps the calcium-charged gates open, and the ACh continues to be released.
- The resulting ischaemia in the area creates an oxygen/nutrient deficit, which in turn leads to a local energy crisis.
- Without available ATP, the local tissue is unable to remove the calcium ions which are 'keeping the gates open' for ACh to keep escaping.
- Removing the superfluous calcium requires more energy than sustaining a contracture, so the contracture remains.
- The resulting muscle-fibre contracture (involuntary, without motor potentials) needs to be distinguished from a contraction (voluntary with motor potentials) and spasm (involuntary with motor potentials).
- The contracture is sustained by the chemistry at the innervation site, not by action potentials from the cord.
- As the endplate keeps producing ACh flow, the actin/myosin filaments attenuate to a fully shortened position (a weakened state) in the immediate area around the motor endplate (at the centre of the fibre).
- As the sarcomeres shorten, they begin to bunch and a contracture knot forms.

- This knot is the 'nodule' which is the palpable characteristic of a trigger point.
- As this process occurs the remainder of the sarcomeres (those not bunching) of that fibre are stretched, creating the taut band, which is usually palpable.

This model currently represents the most widely held understanding as to the aetiology of trigger points. There is further discussion of the trigger point phenomenon in Chapter 6, as well as of treatment options.

Positional release and trigger points

It is this localised, palpable, painful entity which can be used in positional release as a monitor, to guide the tissues towards a state of optimal ease or comfort, where tissues are least stressed. This is the objective of that aspect of positional release methodology known as strain/counterstrain, because in that 'ease' state, circulatory enhancement flushes previously congested and ischaemic tissues (see below), allowing neurological resetting to occur, and helping to restore some degree of normality to the functions of the region. This is discussed further in Chapter 3. Additionally, the trigger point deactivation approach known as integrated neuromuscular inhibition technique (INIT – briefly described in Chapter 1 and more fully explained in Chapter 6) involves a logical sequence which incorporates PRT, together with ischaemic compression, muscle energy technique and subsequent toning of weak antagonists.

Simons et al (1998) discuss a variety of what they term 'trigger point release' procedures, ranging from direct pressure to a range of stretching possibilities, and including PRT routines (such as SCS), which they refer to as 'indirect techniques'. They conclude that the most successful use of PRT in treating trigger points is likely to be for those points which are close to attachments, rather than the triggers found in the belly of muscles, which Simons and Travell suggest are likely to benefit from more robust treatment methods.

ISCHAEMIA AND MUSCLE PAIN

(Lewis 1931, Lewis 1941, Rodbard 1975)

When the blood supply to a muscle is inhibited, pain is not usually noted unless or until that muscle is asked to contract. In such a case, pain is likely to be noted within 60 seconds (as in intermittent claudication). The precise mechanisms are open to debate, but are thought to involve one or more of a number of processes, including lactate accumulation and potassium ion build-up.

Pain receptors are sensitised when under ischaemic conditions, it is thought due to bradykinin influence. This is confirmed by the use of drugs which inhibit bradykinin release, allowing an active ischaemic muscle to remain relatively painless for longer periods (Digiesi 1975).

Trigger point activity itself may induce relative ischaemia in target tissues and this suggests that any appropriate manual treatment, movement or exercise program which encourages normal circulatory function is likely to modulate these negative effects and reduce trigger point activity.

Ischaemia and trigger point evolution

Hypoxia (apoxia) can occur in a number of ways, most obviously in ischaemic sites, where circulation is impaired, possibly due to a sustained hypertonic state. If hypertonia is a major aetiological feature in the evolution of trigger points then those muscles which have the greatest propensity towards hypertonia – the postural Type 1 muscles – should receive closest attention (Jacobs & Falls 1997, Liebenson 1996).

Trigger points may therefore be used as monitors of improved oxygenation (possibly via breathing retraining), rather than being directly treated to deactivate them, leading to the following thoughts:

- As oxygenation improves trigger points are likely to become less reactive and painful.
- Enhanced breathing function represents a reduction in overall stress, reinforcing the concepts associated with facilitation: that as stress of whatever kind reduces, trigger points react less acutely.

- Direct deactivation tactics are not the only way to handle trigger points.
- Trigger points can be seen to be acting as 'alarm' signals, virtually quantifying the current levels of adaptive demand being imposed on the individual.

As will be noted in Chapter 3, one of the influences which derives from tissues being held in ease during PRT treatment is enhanced circulation, which is bound to reduce ischaemia.

Trigger point deactivation possibilities include (Chaitow 1996, Kuchera 1997):

- inhibitory soft-tissue techniques including neuromuscular therapy/massage
- chilling techniques (spray, ice)
- acupuncture, injection, etc.
- positional release methods
- muscle energy (stretch) techniques
- myofascial release methods
- correction of associated somatic dysfunction possibly involving HVT adjustments and/or osteopathic or chiropractic mobilisation methods
- education and correction of contributory and perpetuating factors (posture, diet, stress, habits, etc.)
- self-help strategies (stretching, etc.)
- combination sequences such as INIT (integrated neuromuscular inhibition technique – see Chapter 6).

REFERENCES

Barlow W 1959 Anxiety and muscle tension pain. British Journal of Clinical Practice 3(5)

Basmajian J 1974 Muscles alive. Williams & Wilkins, Baltimore

Beal M 1983 Palpatory testing of somatic dysfunction in patient's with cardiovascular disease. J American Osteopathic Association 82: 73–82

Chaitow L 1996 Modern Neuromuscular Techniques. Churchill Livingstone, Edinburgh

D'Ambrogio K, Roth G 1997 Positional Release Therapy. Mosby, St Louis

Digiesi V 1975 Effect of proteinase inhibitor on intermittent claudication. Pain 1: 385–389

DiGiovanna E 1991 Somatic Dysfunction. In: DiGiovanna E, Schiowitz S (eds) An Osteopathic Approach to Diagnosis and Treatment. Lippincott, Philadelphia: 6–12

Dvorak J, Dvorak V 1984 Manual Medicine – Diagnostics. Georg Thiem Verlag Thieme-Stratton, Stuttgart

Edwards R 1988 Hypotheses of peripheral and central mechanisms underlying occupational muscle pain and injury. European J Applied Physiology 57: 275–281

Gibbons P, Tehan P 2001 Spinal manipulation: indications, risks and benefits. J Bodywork and Movement Therapies, in press

Greenman P 1996 Principles of Manual Medicine, 2nd edn. Williams & Wilkins, Baltimore

Grieve G (ed) 1986 Modern Manual Therapy. Churchill Livingstone, Edinburgh

Gunn C, Milbrandt W 1978 Early and subtle signs in low back sprain. Spine 3: 267–281

Henneman E 1957 Relation between size of neurons and their susceptibility to discharge. Science 126: 1345–1347

Hubbard D 1993 Myofascial trigger points show spontaneous EMG activity. Spine 18: 1803

Jacobs A, Falls W 1997 Anatomy. In: Ward R (Ed) Foundations for Osteopathic Medicine. Williams & Wilkins, Baltimore

Janda V 1983 Muscle Function Testing. Butterworths, London

Janda V 1986 Muscle weakness and inhibition in back pain syndromes. In: Grieve G (ed) Modern Manual Therapy of the Vertebral Column. Churchill Livingstone, Edinburgh

Jones L 1981 Strain and counterstrain. Academy of Applied Osteopathy, Colorado Springs

Jull G, Bogduk N 1988 Accuracy of manual diagnosis for cervical zygapophysial joints. Medical J Australia 148: 233–236

Kaltenborn F 1985 Mobilization of the Extremity Joints. Olaf Norlis Bokhandel, Oslo, Norway

Korr I 1976 Spinal cord as organiser of disease process. Academy of Applied Osteopathy Yearbook

Korr I 1978 Neurologic mechanisms in manipulative therapy. Plenum Press, New York

Kuchera M 1997 Travell & Simons' myofascial trigger points. In: Ward R (ed) Foundations of Osteopathic Medicine. Williams & Wilkins, Baltimore

Kuchera M, Kuchera W 1997 General postural considerations. In: Ward R (ed) Foundations for Osteopathic Medicine. Williams & Wilkins, Baltimore

Larsson S-E 1990 Chronic trapezius myalgia – morphology and blood flow studied in 17 patients. Acta Orthop Scand 61: 394–398

Lederman E 1997 Fundamentals of Manual Therapy. Churchill Livingstone, Edinburgh

Lewis T 1931 Observations upon muscular pain in intermittent claudication. Heart 15: 359–383

Lewis T 1941 Pain. Macmillan, London

Lewit K 1980 Relation of faulty respiration to posture. J American Osteopathic Association 79(8): 525–529

Lewit K 1999 Manipulative Therapy in Rehabilitation of the Locomotor System, 3rd edn. Butterworths, London

Liebenson C 1996 Rehabilitation of the Spine. Williams & Wilkins, Baltimore

Lord S, Bogduk N 1996 In: Allen M (ed) Musculoskeletal Pain Emanating from Head and Neck. Haworth Medical Press, New York

McPartland J, Goodridge J 1997 Counterstrain and traditional osteopathic examination of the cervical spine compared. J Bodywork and Movement Therapies 1(3): 173–178

Melzack R, Wall P 1988 The Challenge of Pain. Penguin, London

Moss M 1962 The functional matrix. In: Kraus B (ed) Vistas in Orthodontics. Lea & Febiger, Philadelphia

Murphy D 2000 Conservative management of cervical syndromes. McGraw Hill, New York

Patterson M 1976 Model Mechanism for Spinal Segmental Facilitation. Academy of Applied Osteopathy Yearbook, Colorado Springs

Rodbard S 1975 Pain associated with muscular activity. American Heart J 90: 84–92

Schiable H 1993 Afferent and spinal mechanisms of joint pain. Pain 55: 5

Simons D 1993 Myofascial pain and dysfunction: review. J Musculoskeletal Pain 1(2): 131

Simons D, Travell J, Simons L 1998 Myofascial Pain and Dysfunction: The Trigger Point Manual 2nd edn. Williams & Wilkins, Baltimore

Travell J, Simons D 1983 Myofascial Pain and Dysfunction Vols. 1 and 2. Williams & Wilkins, Baltimore

van Wingerden J-P 1997 The role of the hamstrings in pelvic and spinal function. In: Vleeming A et al (eds) Movement, Stability and Low Back Pain. Churchill Livingstone, Edinburgh

Vleeming A 1989 Load application to the sacrotuberous ligament: influences on sacroiliac joint mechanics. Clinical Biomechanics 4: 204–209

Vleeming A et al (eds) 1997 Movement, Stability and Low Back Pain. Churchill Livingstone, Edinburgh

Ward R 1997 Foundations for Osteopathic Medicine. Williams & Wilkins, Baltimore

Waersted M, Eken T, Westgaard R 1992 Single motor unit activity in psychogenic trapezius muscle tension. Arbete och Halsa 17: 319–321

Waersted M, Eken T, Westgaard R 1993 Psychogenic motor unit activity – a possible muscle injury mechanism studied in a healthy subject. J Musculoskeletal Pain 1(3/4): 185–190

Wolfe F, Simons D 1992 Fibromyalgia and myofascial pain syndromes. J Rheumatology 19(6): 944–951

Zink G, Lawson W 1979 Osteopathic structural examination and functional interpretation of the soma. Osteopathic Annals 7(12): 433–440

3

Modified strain/counterstrain technique

The best known of the variations which utilise positional release techniques (PRT) is that derived from the clinical research of Laurence Jones, whose pioneering work evolved into a method of treatment of joint and soft-tissue dysfunction of supreme gentleness, to which he gave the name strain/counterstrain (SCS) (Jones 1981). Modifications (by the author) of Jones counterstrain methods will be described in this chapter, as will a further variant, known as positional release therapy (D'Ambrogio & Roth 1997).

HOW DOES SCS WORK?

It is important to state at the outset that the various theories as to how positional release achieves its effects remain largely unproven, conjectural, tentative assumptions. The basic scientific research has as yet not been performed to validate the hypotheses, which are discussed below. The reader is advised to adopt a robustly critical frame of mind, while attempting to evaluate the mechanisms described which *might* be functioning. Some of the assumptions made are based on animal models. Others are deduced and assumed from clinical evidence and experience. Very little concrete certainty exists, apart from the reality that positional release methods are safe and effective. How they achieve their benefits remains for future research.

Jones' concept as to how SCS works is based on the predictable physiological responses of muscles in particular situations, most notably in relation to acute or chronic strains. He describes how, in a balanced state, the proprioceptive functions of the various muscles supporting a joint will be feeding a flow of information, derived from the neural receptors in those muscles and their tendons, to the higher centres. For example, the Golgi tendon organs will be reporting on tone while the various receptors in the spindles will be firing a constant stream of information (slowly or rapidly depending upon the demands being placed on the tissues) regarding their resting length (and any changes which might be occurring in that length). In a dysfunctional state (see descriptions below under Neurological Concepts) inappropriately excessive degrees of tone may be sustained, leading to chronic imbalances between agonists, antagonists and associated muscles. In some instances the excessive tone may relate to some degree of segmental or local (i.e. trigger point) facilitation (see Chapter 2).

D'Ambrogio and Roth (1997) state that:

Positional release therapy appears to have a damping influence on the general level of excitability within the facilitated [see chapter 2] segment. Weiselfish (1993) has found that this characteristic of PRT is unique in its effectiveness and has utilized this feature to successfully treat severe neurologic patients, even though the source of the primary dysfunction arose from the supraspinal level.

It is the dampening, calming, influence on the neurological features of hyper-reactive and stressed tissues, which seems to characterise the results observed following appropriate use of PRT. Circulatory and fascial influences are also considered possible mechanisms for PRT's benefits.

NEUROLOGICAL CONCEPTS

1. The proprioceptive hypothesis

(Korr 1947, 1975, Mathews 1981)

Jones first observed the phenomenon of spontaneous release when he 'accidentally' placed a patient who was in considerable pain and some degree of compensatory distortion, into a position of comfort (ease) on a treatment table (Jones 1964).

Despite no other treatment being given, after just 20 minutes resting in a position of relative ease, the patient was able to stand upright and was free of pain. The pain-free position of ease into which Jones had helped the patient was one which exaggerated the degree of distortion in which his body was being held. He had taken the patient into the direction of 'ease' (as opposed to 'bind'), since any attempt to correct or straighten the body would have been met by both resistance and pain. In contrast, moving the body further into distortion was acceptable and easy, and seemed to allow the physiological processes involved in resolution of spasm, etc., to operate. This position of ease is the key element in what later came to be known as strain/counterstrain.

Example

The events which occur at the moment of strain may provide the key to understanding the mechanisms of neurologically induced positional release. Take, for example, an all too common example of someone bending forwards from the waist. At this time the flexor muscles would be short of their resting length, and the neural reporting structures (muscle spindles) in these muscles would be firing slowly, indicating little or no activity and no change of length taking place.

At the same time, the opposite group of muscles – the spinal erector group in this example – would be stretched or stretching and firing rapidly. Any stretch affecting a muscle (and therefore its spindles) will increase the rate of reporting, which will reflexively induce further contraction (myotatic stretch reflex) and an increase in tone in that muscle and an instant inhibition (reciprocal) of the functional antagonists to it, so further reducing the already limited degree of reporting from their spindles.

This feedback link with the central nervous system is the primary muscle spindle afferent response, and it is thought to be modulated by an additional muscle spindle function which involves the gamma-efferent system, which is controlled from higher (brain) centres. In simple terms, the gamma-efferent system influences the primary afferent system: for example, when a muscle is in a quiescent state, when it is relaxed and short with little information coming from the primary receptors, the gamma-efferent system might fine-tune and increase ('turn up') the sensitivity of the primary afferents to ensure a continued information flow (Mathews 1981). It is important to acknowledge that these neurological concepts are largely based on animal studies, and that definitive basic science studies to validate them have not yet been performed in humans.

Crisis

Now imagine an emergency situation arising (the person loses their footing while stooping, or the load they are lifting shifts), which creates immediate demands for stabilisation being made on both sets of muscles (the short, relatively 'quiet' flexors and the stretched, relatively actively firing extensors), even though they are in quite different states of preparedness for action. The flexors would be 'unloaded', relaxed and providing minimal feedback to the control centres, while the spinal extensors would be at stretch, providing a rapid outflow of spindle-derived information, some of which ensures that the relaxed flexor muscles remain relaxed, due to inhibitory activity.

The central nervous system would at this time be receiving minimal information as to the status of the relaxed flexors and at the moment that the crisis demand for stabilisation occurred, these shortened/relaxed flexors would be obliged to stretch quickly to a length which would balance the already stretched extensors – which would most probably be contracting rapidly. As this happened, the annulospiral receptors in the short (flexor) muscles would respond to the sudden stretch demand by contracting even more – the stretch reflex. The neural reporting stations in these shortened muscles would be firing impulses as if the muscles were being stretched, even when the muscle remained well short of its normal resting length. At the same time, the extensor muscles, which had been at stretch and which, in the alarm situation, were obliged to rapidly shorten, would remain longer than their normal resting length as they attempt to stabilise the situation (Korr 1976).

Korr has described what he believes happens in the abdominal muscles (flexors) in such a situation. He says that because of their relaxed status, short of their resting length, there occurs in these muscles a silencing of the spindles; however, due to the demand for information from the higher centres, gamma gain is increased reflexively, and as the muscle contracts rapidly to stabilise the alarm demands, the central nervous system would receive information that the muscle, which is actually short of its neutral resting length, was being stretched.

In effect, the muscles would have adopted a restricted position as a result of inappropriate proprioceptive reporting. As DiGiovanna explains (Jones 1964):

With trauma or muscle effort against a sudden change in resistance, or with muscle strain incurred by resisting the effects of gravity for a period of time, one muscle at a joint is strained and its antagonist is hyper-shortened. When the shortened muscle is suddenly stretched the annulospiral receptors in that muscle are stimulated causing a reflex contraction of the already shortened muscle. The proprioceptors in the short muscle now fire impulses as if the shortened muscle were being stretched. Since this inappropriate proprioceptor response can be maintained indefinitely a somatic dysfunction has been created.

In effect, the two opposing sets of muscles would have adopted a stabilising posture to protect the threatened structures, and in doing so would have become locked into positions of imbalance in relation to their normal function. One would be shorter and one longer than their normal resting length (Fig. 3.1).

At this time, any attempt to extend the area/joint(s) would be strongly resisted by the tonically shortened flexor group. The individual would be locked into a forward-bending distortion (in our example).

The joint(s) involved would not have been taken beyond their normal physiological range and yet the normal range would be unavailable, due to the shortened status of the flexor group (in this particular example). Going further into flexion, however, would present no problems or pain.

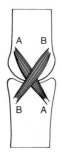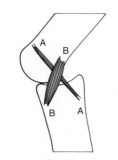

Figure 3.1A Normal unstrained joint in normal position with muscles A and B in a non-stressed state.

Figure 3.1B Normal joint in an extreme position in which stress occurs which will result in strain, as illustrated in Figure 3.1C.

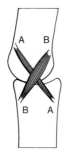

Figure 3.1C Joint in a strained state in which muscle A, which had been excessively stretched, is splinted/contracted and resists movement, and muscle B, short at the time of the stress, is slightly stretched and is neither splinted nor contracted. Any attempt at returning to the situation as illustrated in Figure 3.1A would meet with resistance, while a return to the position of stress, 3.1B, would be easily and painlessly achieved and could allow for a spontaneous positional release of the hypertonicity and splinting in muscle A.

Walther (1988) summarises the situation as follows:

When proprioceptors send conflicting information there may be simultaneous contraction of the antagonists ... without antagonist muscle inhibition, joint and other strain results [and in this manner] a reflex pattern develops which causes muscle or other tissue to maintain this continuing strain. It [strain dysfunction] often relates to the inappropriate signalling from muscle proprioceptors that have been strained from rapid change that does not allow proper adaptation.

This situation would be unlikely to resolve itself spontaneously and is the 'strain' position in

Jones' strain/counterstrain method. We can recognise it in an acute setting in torticollis, as well as in acute lumbago. It is also recognisable as a feature of many types of chronic somatic dysfunction in which joints remain restricted due to muscular imbalances of this type, occurring as part of an adaptive process.

This is a time of intense neurological and proprioceptive confusion. This is the moment of 'strain'. SCS offers a means of quietening the neurological confusion and excessive, or unbalanced, tone.

2. The nociceptive hypothesis
(Bailey & Dick 1992, Van Buskirk 1990)

In order to appreciate a second possible neurological influence involved in strain we need a different example. Let us consider someone involved in a simple whiplash-like neck stress as their car came to an unexpected halt. The neck would be thrown backwards into hyperextension, provoking all of the factors described above involving the flexor group of muscles in the forward-bending strain.

The extensor group would be rapidly shortened and the various proprioceptive changes leading to strain and reflexive shortening would operate. At the time of the sudden braking of the car, there would occur hyperextension of the flexors of the neck, scalenes etc., which would be violently stretched, inducing actual tissue damage. Nociceptive responses would occur (which are more powerful than proprioceptive influences) and these multisegmental reflexes would produce a flexor withdrawal, dramatically increasing tone in the flexor group. The neck would now display hypertonicity of both the extensors and the flexors; pain, guarding and stiffness would be apparent and the role of clinician would be to remove these restricting influences layer by layer.

Where pain is a factor in strain this has to be considered as producing an overriding influence over whatever other more 'normal' reflexes are operating.

In the simple example of neck strain described, it is obvious that, in real life, matters are likely to be even more complicated, since a true whiplash would introduce both rapid hyperextension and hyperflexion and a multitude of layers of dysfunction.

More complex than described

The proprioceptive and nociceptive reflexes which might be involved in the production of strain are also likely to involve other factors, including chemically mediated changes. D'Ambrogio and Roth (1997) elucidate:

Free nerve endings are distributed throughout all of the connective tissues of the body with the exception of the stroma of the brain. These receptors are stimulated by neuropeptides produced by noxious influences, including trauma ... Impulses generated in these neurons spread centrally and also peripherally along the numerous branches of each neuron. At the terminus of the axons, peptide neurotransmitters such as substance P are released. The response of the musculoskeletal system to these painful stimuli may thus play a central role in the development [and maintenance] of somatic dysfunction.

As Bailey and Dick (1992) explain:

Probably few dysfunctional states result from a purely proprioceptive or nociceptive response. Additional factors such as autonomic responses, other reflexive activities, joint receptor responses, [biochemical features] or emotional states must also be accounted for.

It is at the level of our basic neurological awareness that understanding of the complexity of these problems commences.

Safe solution

Fortunately, the methodology of positional release does not demand a complete understanding of what is going on neurologically, since what Jones and his followers, and those clinicians who have evolved the art of strain/counterstrain to newer levels of simplicity, have shown, is that by a slow, painless return to the position of strain, aberrant neurological activity currently locked into place in the strained tissues can resolve itself, irrespective of the mechanisms involved.

Making sense of garbled information
(DiGiovanna 1991, Jones 1964, 1966)

The reaction of the body to this confusing and stressed situation apparently varies with the time available to it. Should a deliberate and controlled response be possible, allowing the stretched muscles to slowly return to normal, then resolution of the potential problem might take place with no dysfunction arising.

This can happen only if a controlled and not a panic return towards the neutral position is achieved. All too often, however, the situation is one of an almost-panic response, as the body makes a rapid attempt to restore stability to the region and finds the neural reporting information incoherent (one moment the abdominals are saying, 'all is well, we are relaxed and short', and the next they are firing rapidly and lengthening, while there is a sudden stretch imposed on already stretched spinal extensors, which are trying to shorten at the same time in order to produce balance).

Restriction

The result is likely to involve the shortened muscles being 'fixed' in a position short of their normal resting length, from which they cannot easily be lengthened without pain (Fig. 3.2).

The person bending, as described in our earlier example, would be locked in flexion with an acute low back pain. The resulting spasm in tissues 'fixed' by this or other similar neurologically induced 'strains' causes the fixation of associated joint(s), and prevents any attempt to return to neutral. Any attempt to force the distorted spine (in this example) towards its anatomically correct position, would be strongly resisted by the shortened fibres. It would, however, not be difficult or painful to take the joint(s) further towards the position in which the strain occurred, effectively shortening the fibres, now in spasm even further, and so reducing tension on affected tissues, causing a reduction in excessive proprioceptive reporting. It is also possible that enhanced vascular and interstitial circulatory function, in previously tense tissues

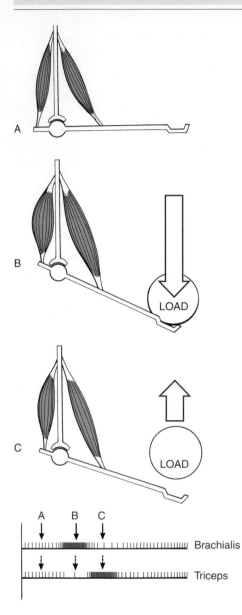

Figure 3.2 A The arm flexor (brachialis) and extensor (triceps brachii) muscles in an easy, normal position, as shown by the rate of firing indicated on the scale for each muscle.

Figure 3.2B A sudden force is applied which results in the flexors (A) being stretched while the extensors (B) protect the joint by rapidly shortening. The firing rate relating to hyperextension and hypershortening is indicated on the scale.

Figure 3.2C Flexor stretch receptors have been excited by this sudden demand and these continue to fire as though stretch were continuing even though a relatively normal position has been achieved. The rate of firing of both flexors and extensors continues to be maintained at an inappropriately high rate. This is the situation in a strained joint. DiGiovanna (1991) explains: The joint is restricted within its physiological range of motion [and is prevented] from achieving its full range of motion. It is therefore an active process rather than a static injury usually associated with a strain.

when held at 'ease', would moderate the activity of inflammation-enhancing chemical mediators.

Towards 'ease'

Jones found that by taking the joint/area close to the position in which the original strain took place an interesting phenomenon was observed, in which the proprioceptive functions were given an opportunity to reset themselves, to become coherent again, during which time pain in the area lessened. This is the 'counterstrain' element of the system. If the position of ease were held for a period (Jones suggests 90 seconds) the spasm in hypertonic, shortened tissues commonly resolves, following which it is usually possible to return the joint/area to a more normal resting position, if this action is performed extremely slowly. The muscles which had been overstretched might remain sensitive for some days, but for all practical considerations the joint would be normal again.

Jones has found that by carefully positioning the joint, whether this be a small extremity joint, or a spinal region, into a position of neutral or 'ease' (which is frequently an exaggeration of the distorted position in which the body is holding the area or a close replica of the position in which the original strain took place) a resolution of spasm/hypertonia takes place.

Since the position during Jones' therapeutic methods is the same as that of the original strain, the shortened muscles are repositioned in such a manner as to allow the dysfunctioning proprioceptors to cease their activity. Korr's explanation for the physiological normalisation of tissues brought about through positional release (Korr 1976) is that:

The shortened spindle nevertheless continues to fire, despite the slackening of the main muscle, and the CNS is gradually able to turn down the gamma discharge and, in turn enables the muscles to return to 'easy neutral', at its resting length. In effect, the physician has led the patient through a repetition of the lesioning process with, however, two essential differences. First it is done in slow motion, with gentle muscular forces, and second there have been no surprises for the CNS; the spindle has continued to report throughout.

CIRCULATORY CONCEPTS

There exists yet another mechanism which positional release can usefully modify in strained tissues – circulatory embarrassment. We know from the research of Travell and Simons that in stressed soft tissues there are likely to be localised areas of relative ischaemia – lack of oxygen – and that this can be a key factor in production of pain and altered tissue status which leads to the evolution of myofascial trigger points (Travell & Simons 1983).

Studies on cadavers have shown that when a radiopaque dye is injected into muscles, this is more likely to spread into the vessels of the muscle when a 'counterstrain' position of ease is adopted than when the muscle is in a neutral position.

Rathbun and Macnab (1970) demonstrated this by injecting a suspension into the arm of a cadaver while the arm was maintained at the side. No filling of blood vessels occurred. When, on the other arm, following injection of a radiopaque suspension, the arm was placed in a position of flexion, abduction and external rotation (position of 'ease' for the supraspinatus muscle), there was almost complete filling of the blood vessels as a result.

Jacobson and colleagues (1989) suggest that, 'unopposed arterial filling may be the same mechanism that occurs in living tissue during the 90 second counterstrain treatment.'

CONNECTIVE TISSUE AND FASCIAL CONCEPTS

Fascia offers a unifying medium, a structure which literally 'ties everything together', from the soles of the feet to the meninges which surround the brain. This ubiquitous material offers support, separation and structure to all other soft tissues and because of this produces distant effects whenever dysfunction occurs in it. Levin (1986) has described fascia as comprising innumerable building blocks, shaped as icosyhedrons (20-sided structures) which produce, in effect, kinetic chains in which tensions are transmitted everywhere in the body, partly by hydrostatic pressure.

Dean Juhan (1987) expands on this:

Besides this hydrostatic pressure (which is exerted by every fascial compartment, not just the outer wrapping), the connective tissue framework – in conjunction with active muscles – provides another kind of tensional force that is crucial to the upright structure of the skeleton. We are not made up of stacks of building blocks resting securely upon one another, but rather of poles and guy-wires, whose stability relies not upon flat-stacked surfaces but upon proper angles of the poles and balanced tensions on the wires. Buckminister Fuller coined the term 'tensegrity' to describe this principle of structure, and his inventive experiments with it have clarified it as one of nature's favorite devices for achieving a maximum of stability with a minimum of materials.

Juhan continues:

This principle of tensegrity describes precisely the relationship between the connective tissues, the muscles, and the skeleton. There is not a single horizontal surface anywhere in the skeleton that

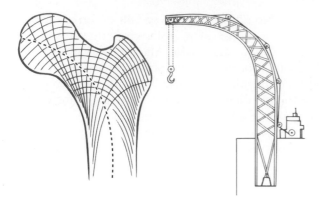

Figure 3.3 The head of the femur and a crane are both tensegrity structures, as they employ both compression and tension-resisting elements.

provides a stable base for anything to be stacked upon it. Our design was not conceived by a stonemason. Weight applied to any bone would cause it to slide right off its joints if it were not for the tensional balances that hold it in place and control its pivoting. Like the beams in a simple tensegrity structure, our bones act more as spacers than as compressional members; more weight is actually borne by the connective system of cables than by the bony beams.

With these models in mind, of stacked and packed icosyhedrons, as well as tensegrity structures (Fig. 3.3) which easily comply with compressive and tension forces, and the unique plastic and elastic properties of connective tissue, we have the possibility of visualising a structure capable of absorbing and accommodating to a variety of forces and adaptations. The beneficial effects of holding tissues at ease when stressed also emerges. As D'Ambrogio and Roth (1997) explain:

A perceived condition in one area of the body may have its origin in another area and therapeutic action at the source will have an immediate effect on all secondary areas, including the site of symptom manifestation. It may also account for some of the physiologic effects that produce the [spontaneous] release phenomenon.

Anatomy trains

Myers (1997) has described a number of clinically useful sets of myofascial chains – the connections between different structures ('long functional continuities') which he terms 'anatomy trains'.

These are not distinct from tensegrity features, but are more specific linkages, which may be seen to be connected when some positional release methods are performed. In particular, strain/counterstrain methods for normalising rib restrictions can involve some bizarre positioning of the entire body, with remarkable effects. If the 'trains' which Myers describes (see below) are considered, these 'positions of ease' will be seen to be quite logical.

The five major fascial chains
(Myers 1997)

The superficial back line (Fig. 3.4) involves a chain which starts with:

- plantar fascia, linking the plantar surface of the toes to the calcaneus
- gastrocnemius, linking calcaneus to the femoral condyles
- hamstrings, linking the femoral condyles to the ischial tuberosities
- sacrotuberous ligament, linking the ischial tuberosities to the sacrum
- lumbosacral fascia, erector spinae and nuchal ligament, linking the sacrum to the occiput
- scalp fascia, linking the occiput to the brow ridge.

The superficial front line (Fig. 3.5) involves a chain which starts with:

- the anterior compartment and the periostium of the tibia, linking the dorsal surface of the toes to the tibial tuberosity
- rectus femoris, linking the tibial tuberosity to the anterior inferior iliac spine and pubic tubercle
- rectus abdominis as well as pectoralis and sternalis fascia, linking the pubic tubercle and the anterior inferior iliac spine with the manubrium
- sternocleidomastoid, linking the manubrium with the mastoid process of the temporal bone.

The lateral line (Fig. 3.6) involves a chain which starts with:

- peroneal muscles, linking the first and fifth metatarsal bases with the fibular head

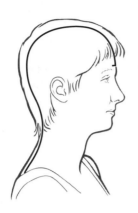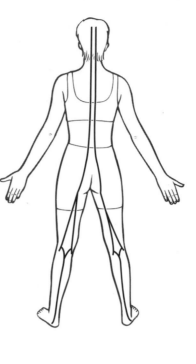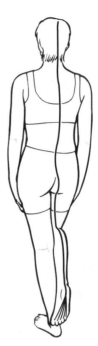

Figure 3.4   The superficial back line.

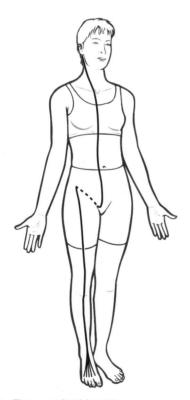

Figure 3.5   The superficial front line.

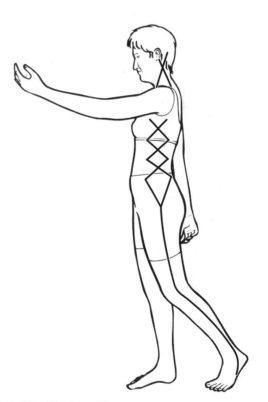

Figure 3.6   The lateral line.

- ilio tibial tract, tensor fascia latae and gluteus maximus, linking the fibular head with the iliac crest
- external obliques, internal obliques and (deeper) quadratus lumborum, linking the iliac crest with the lower ribs
- external intercostals and internal intercostals, linking the lower ribs with the remaining ribs
- splenius cervicis, iliocostalis cervicis, sternocleidomastoid and (deeper) scalenes, linking the ribs with the mastoid process of the temporal bone.

The spiral lines (Fig. 3.7) involve a chain which starts with:

- splenius capitis, which wraps across from one side to the other, linking the occipital ridge (say on the right) with the spinous processes of the lower cervical and upper thoracic spine on the left
- continuing in this direction the rhomboids (on the left) link via the medial border of the scapula with serratus anterior and the ribs (still on the left), wrapping around the trunk via the external obliques and the abdominal aponeurosis on the left, to connect with the internal obliques on the right and then to a strong anchor point on the anterior superior iliac spine (right side)
- from the ASIS, the tensor fascia latae and the iliotibial tract link to the lateral tibial condyle
- tibialis anterior links the lateral tibial condyle with the first metatarsal and cuneiform
- from this apparent end-point of the chain (first metatarsal and cuneiform), peroneus longus rises to link with the fibular head
- biceps femoris connects the fibular head to the ischial tuberosity
- the sacrotuberous ligament links the ischial tuberosity to the sacrum
- the sacral fascia and the erector spinae link the sacrum to the occipital ridge.

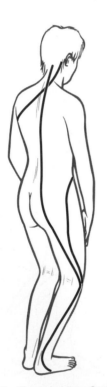
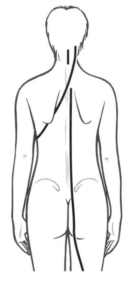
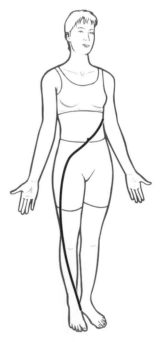

Figure 3.7 The spiral line. Outlines taken from Calais-Germain (1993).

The deep front line describes several alternative chains involving the structures anterior to the spine (internally, for example):

- the anterior longitudinal ligament, diaphragm, pericardium, mediastinum, parietal pleura, fascia prevertebralis and the scalene fascia, which connect the lumbar spine (bodies and transverse processes) to the cervical transverse processes, and via longus capitis to the basilar portion of the occiput
- other links in this chain might involve a connection between the posterior manubrium and the hyoid bone via the subhyoid muscles, and
- the fascia pretrachealis between the hyoid and the cranium/mandible, involving the suprahyoid muscles
- the muscles of the jaw linking the mandible to the face and cranium.

Myers includes in his chain description structures of the lower limbs which connect the tarsum of the foot to the lower lumbar spine, making the linkage complete. Additional smaller chains involving the arms are described as follows.

Back-of-the-arm lines (Fig. 3.8):

- the broad sweep of trapezius links the occipital ridge and the cervical spinous processes to the spine of the scapula and the clavicle
- the deltoid, together with the lateral intermuscular septum, connects the scapula and clavicle with the lateral epicondyle
- the lateral epicondyle is joined to the hand and fingers by the common extensor tendon
- another track on the back of the arm can arise from the rhomboids, which link the thoracic transverse processes to the medial border of the scapula
- the scapula in turn is linked to the olecranon of the ulna by infraspinatus and the triceps
- The olecranon of the ulna connects to the small finger via the periosteum of the ulna
- a 'stabilisation' feature in the back of the arm involves latissimus dorsi and the thoracolumbar fascia, which connects the arm

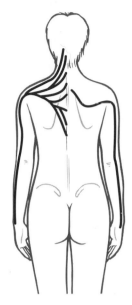

Figure 3.8   The back-of-the-arm lines.

with the spinous processes, the contralateral sacral fascia and gluteus maximus, which in turn attaches to the shaft of the femur
- vastus lateralis connects the femur shaft to the tibial tuberosity and (via this) to the periosteum of the tibia

Front-of-the-arm lines (Fig. 3.9)

- latissimus dorsi, teres major and pectoralis major attach to the humerus close to the medial intramuscular septum, connecting it to the back of the trunk
- the medial intramuscular septum connects the humerus to the medial epicondyle which connects with the palmar hand and fingers by means of the common flexor tendon
- an additional line on the front of the arm involves pectoralis minor, the costocoracoid ligament, the brachial neurovascular bundle and the fascia clavipectoralis, which attach to the coracoid process
- the coracoid process also provides the attachment for biceps brachii (or brachialis) linking this to the radius and the thumb via the flexor compartment of the forearm
- a 'stabilisation' line on the front of the arm involves pectoralis major attaching to the ribs, as do the external obliques, which then run to

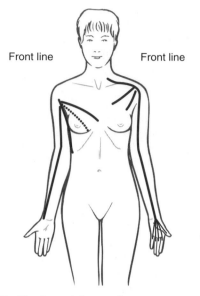

Front line   Front line

Figure 3.9   The front-of-the-arm lines.

the pubic tubercle, where a connection is made to the contralateral adductor longus, gracilis, pes anserinus, and the tibial periosteum.

It is likely that in taking a distressed, strained (chronic or acute) muscle or joint painlessly into a position which allows for a reduction in tone in the tissues involved, some modification takes place of neural reporting, as well as local circulation being improved. D'Ambrogio and Roth (1997) summarise what is thought to happen to the fascia during PRT thus 'it is hypothesised that PRT, by reducing the tension on the myofascial system, also engages the fascial components of dysfunction. The reduction in tension on the collagenous cross-linkages appears to induce a disengagement of the electrochemical bonds and a conversion back [from the gel-like] to the sol [solate] state'.

The end-result of such positioning, if painless, slowly performed and held for an appropriate length of time, is a reduction in hyper-reactivity of the neural structures, a resetting of these to painlessly allow a more normal resting length of muscle to be achieved, reduction in fascial (di)stress, as well as enhanced circulation.

Variations on this theme are the focus of this book. In this and subsequent chapters some of the many methods for using this therapeutic

approach will be examined. The focus of this chapter is Jones' strain/counterstain, and how to use it. In order to do so the phenomenon of the 'tender point' needs to be thoroughly grasped.

TENDER POINTS AND THE POSITION OF EASE

Jones' discovery that almost all somatic dysfunction has associated areas of palpable tenderness, often only tender when palpated or probed, led to the realisation that when the joint or area is suitably positioned to ease the tenderness in these points, associated hypertonia or spasm, usually diminished. He called these points 'tender points'. Describing his methods he states: 'Finding the myofascial tender point, and the correct position of release, will probably take a few minutes at first. Watching a skilled physician find a tender point, in a few seconds, and a position of release in a few seconds more, may give a false impression of simplicity to the beginner'.

It may take longer than a few minutes to locate tender points initially; however, accurate palpation methods, such as the 'drag' method (see Chapter 4), can usually be rapidly learned if practiced regularly. Once found, the tense tender point is palpated, with just less than sufficient pressure to cause pain in normal tissue. The pain sensitivity should be apparent to both the physician and the patient. By careful guiding of the joint (or other tissue) while constantly palpating the tender point (or by intermittently probing it), a monitoring of progress towards the ideal neutral (reduced or no pain in the palpated point) position is eventually achieved.

The practitioner senses and evaluates reducing (desirable) or increasing (undesirable) levels of muscle tension in the palpated tissues, as well as the patient's report of either increasing or diminishing levels of sensitivity/pain in the palpated point. These indicators are used to guide the operator to the position where eventually there is a feeling of relative ease in the soft tissues, together with markedly reduced pain in the tender point. An absence of 'bind' and also, most importantly, the patient's report that pain has significantly lowered, are the desired indicators.

Jones states, 'The point of maximum relaxation accompanied by an abrupt increase in joint mobility, within a very small arc, is the mobile point'. This term designates the ideal position of comfort to the patient. After holding this for 90 seconds the operator slowly returns the area to its neutral position.

What are the tender points?

Jones equates them with trigger points (Travell & Simons 1983, 1992) and Chapman's neurolymphatic reflexes (Owens 1982). However, this comparison cannot be strictly accurate despite an inevitable degree of overlap in all reflexively active points on the body surface. There are differences in the nature, if not in the feel, of these different point systems (Kuchera & McPartland 1997). For example, myofascial trigger points will refer sensitivity, pain or other symptoms to a target area when pressed, which is not usually the case with Chapman's reflex points (neurolymphatic points) which are found in pairs and not singly, as are Jones' tender points and most trigger points.

Osteopathic physician Eileen DiGiovanna (1991) states, 'Today many physicians believe there is a relationship among trigger points, acupuncture points and Chapman's reflexes. Precisely what the relationship may be is unknown'. She quotes from a prestigious osteopathic pioneer, George Northrup, who stated as far back as 1941, 'One cannot escape the feeling that all of the seemingly diverse observations [regarding reflex patterns of surface 'points'] are but views of the same iceberg, the tip of which we are beginning to see, without understanding either its magnitude or its depth of importance' (Northrup 1941).

Felix Mann, one of the pioneers of acupuncture in the West, has entered the controversy as to the existence, or otherwise, of acupuncture meridians (and indeed acupuncture points). In an effort to alter the emphasis which traditional acupuncture places on the specific charted positions of points, he stated (Mann 1983):

McBurney's point, in appendicitis, has a defined position. In reality it may be 10 cm higher, lower, to the left or right. It may be 1 cm in diameter, or occupy the whole of the abdomen, or not occur at all. Acupuncture points are often the same, and hence it is pointless to speak of acupuncture points in the classical traditional way. Carefully performed electrical resistance measurements do not show alterations in the skin resistance to electricity corresponding with classical acupuncture points. There are so many acupuncture points mentioned in some modern books, that there is no skin left which is not an acupuncture point. In cardiac disease, pain and tenderness may occur in the arm; however, this does not occur more frequently along the course of the heart meridian than anywhere else in the arm.

Hence, Mann concludes, meridians do not exist, or – more confusingly perhaps – that the whole body is an acupuncture point! Leaving aside the validity of Mann's comment, it is true to say that if all the multitude of points described in acupuncture, traditional and modern, together with those points described by Travell and colleagues, Chapman and Jones were to be placed together on one map of the body surface, we would soon come to the conclusion that the entire body surface is a potential acupuncture point.

The discussion in Chapter 2 on the evolution of soft-tissue dysfunction in general (along with the tight–loose concept), and trigger points in particular, offers a representation in which some areas are seen to become short, tight and bunched, while others become lax, stretched or distended. If the broad guideline of 'exaggerating the distortion' (see Chapter 1) is brought into consideration in such situations, this suggests that whatever is short, tight and bunched is likely to benefit by having these characteristics amplified, reinforced and held. Using a tender point (whether or not it is also a trigger point, or plays some other role in relation to reflex activity) to guide the tissues towards the precisely balanced degree of crowding, folding, and compression, describes SCS methodology simplistically but accurately.

Are Ah Shi points and tender points the same?

It is worth remembering that, in acupuncture, there exists a phenomenon known as the 'spontaneously sensitive point'. These arise in response to trauma, or joint dysfunction, and are regarded, for the duration of their existence, as 'honorary' acupuncture points.

Most acupuncture points which receive treatment via needling, heat, pressure, lasers, etc., are clearly defined and mapped. The only exception to this rule relates to these spontaneously arising (Ah Shi) points, associated with joint problems, which become available for treatment for the duration of their sensitivity.

In an earlier text (Chaitow 1991) I make the following comment: 'Local tender points in an area of discomfort may be considered as spontaneous acupuncture points. The Chinese term these Ah Shi points, and use them in the same way as classical points, when treating painful conditions'. It is worth recalling that in Chinese medicine, as well as use of acupuncture, acupressure of Ah Shi points is also considered an appropriate form of treatment. It would seem that Jones' points are in many ways the same, if not identical, to Ah Shi points (Chaitow 1991).

Positioning to find ease

As we have seen, Jones discovered a further use for tender points, apart from pressing or puncturing them. Maintaining a sufficient degree of pressure on such a point allows the patient to be able to report on the level of pain being produced as the joint is positioned. It becomes a monitor and guide for the practitioner. The disappearance, or at least marked diminution of pain noted on pressure, after holding the joint in the position of ease for the prescribed period, is instant evidence as to the success of the procedure.

The holding, or periodic probing, of the point during the 90-second period recommended by Jones leads to a further question, one which Jones acknowledges as being asked of him quite frequently. This queries whether the pressure on the tender point is not in itself therapeutic? Jones answers, 'The question is asked whether the repeated probing of the tender point is therapeutic, as in acupressure, or Rolfing techniques [or ischaemic compression as used in neuromuscular technique]. It is not intentionally therapeutic, but is used solely for diagnosis and evidence of accuracy of treatment'.

This answer could be thought of as being equivocal for it does not address the possibility of a therapeutic end-result from the use of pressure on the tender point, but states only the intention of such pressure. It may be assumed that some therapeutic effect does derive from sustained inhibitory (also known as 'ischaemic') pressure, on such a spontaneously arising tender point, for several reasons:

- ischaemia is reversed when pressure is released (Simons & Travell 1998)
- neurological 'inhibition' results from sustained efferent barrage (Ward 1997)
- mechanical stretching occurs as 'creep' of connective tissue commences (Cantu & Grodin 1992)
- piezolectric effects modify hardened 'gel tissues, towards a softer more 'sol-like' state (Barnes 1997)
- mechanoreceptor impulses interfere with pain messages ('gate theory') (Melzack & Wall 1988)
- analgesic endorphin and enkephalins are released in local tissues and the brain (Baldry 1993)
- 'Taut bands' associated with trigger points, release due to local biochemical modifications (Simons & Travell 1998)
- Traditional Chinese medicine concepts associate digital pressure with altered energy flow
- In the use of acupuncture there is clear evidence of a pain-reducing effect when pressure methods are applied to acupuncture points.

Since acupuncture authorities both in China and the West include spontaneously tender (Ah Shi) points (which seem to be in every way the same as Jones' points) as being suitable for needling or pressure techniques, the avoidance of a clear answer on this point by Jones may be taken to indicate that he has not really addressed himself to this possibility. That his method has other mechanisms which achieve release of pain and spasm in injured joints is beyond doubt. The total effect of strain/counterstain would seem to derive from a combination of the positioning of the joint in a neutral position, and the pressure on the tender point.

The positioning is similar, but not identical, to that described in functional technique by Harold Hoover (see Ch. 8). Hoover's methods involved the positioning of a joint or tissues which display a limited range of motion in what he called a 'dynamic neutral' position. He sought a position in which there was a balance of tensions, fairly near the anatomical neutral position of the joint. Jones also aims at a position of ease, but he relates more to the identical position in which the original strain occurred, or by exaggeration of existing distortions. By combining the position of ease, in which the shortened muscle(s) are able to release themselves, while simultaneously applying pressure (which, despite Jones' doubts, appears to almost certainly involve a therapeutic effect) dramatic improvements in severe and painful conditions are possible.

Jones came to a number of conclusions as a result of his work, which may be summarised as follows:

- The pain in joint dysfunction is related very much to the position in which the joint is placed – varying from acute pain in some positions, to a pain-free position which would be almost directly opposite the position of maximum pain.
- The dysfunction in a joint which has been strained is the result of something which occurs in response to the strain – a reaction to it. The palpable evidence of this is found by searching not in the tissues which were placed under strain, but by searching for tenderness in the (usually shortened) antagonists of these overstretched tissues.
- These painful structures in joint problems are usually not those which were stretched at the time of the injury, but which were in fact shortened, and which have remained so. In these shortened tissues the tender points will be found.

Jones' technique

Jones describes the use of the points as follows:

A physician skilled in palpation techniques will perceive tenseness and/or oedema as well as tenderness. The tenderness, often a few times greater than that for normal tissue, is for the beginner the most valuable sign.

He tends to maintain his palpating finger over the tender point, to monitor expected changes in tenderness. With the other hand he positions the patient into a posture of comfort and relaxation. He may proceed successfully just by questioning the patient as to comfort, reduction in pain, etc, as he probes intermittently, while moving towards the position of ease.

If he is correct in the positioning he is engineering, the patient reports diminished tenderness in the tender area. By intermittent deep palpation, as he fine-tunes the positioning, he monitors the tender point, seeking the ideal position at which there is at least a two-thirds reduction in tenderness. (This degree of pressure stimulus, similar to that applied in the treatment of similar tender points by acupressure or Tsubo techniques, and as explained above, must have some therapeutic implications.)

The key to successful normalisation via these methods is the achievement of the position of maximum ease of the joint, in which the tender point becomes markedly less sensitive to palpation pressure. Most importantly, the subsequent return to the neutral resting position, after the maintenance of the joint in this position of ease for not less than 90 seconds, is very slowly accomplished. Without this slow repositioning, the likelihood exists of a sudden return to a shortened state of the previously disturbed structures.

THE GEOGRAPHY OF SCS

Tender points, relating to acute and chronic strain, can be found in almost all soft-tissue locations which have come under adaptation stress. Although Simons and Travell (1998) indicate that trigger points close to attachments are the ones most likely to benefit from positional release methods (see previous chapter), D'Ambrogio and Roth (1997) state:

Tender points are found throughout the body, anteriorly, posteriorly, medially, and laterally … on muscle origins or insertions, within the muscle belly, over ligaments, tendons, fascia and bone.

Jones has identified a large number of conditions which are related to predictable tender points and from his vast clinical experience, and a lengthy process of trial and error, he has concluded that when tender points are found on the anterior surface of the body they are (with a few exceptions) indicative of the associated joint requiring a degree of forward-bending during its treatment. The location (in this case on the anterior aspect of the body) also indicates that the joint was probably initially injured in a forward-bending position.

Thus, information as to the original injury position (or observation of the direction in which adaptation is directing distortion) helps to direct the search for the tender points to the likeliest aspect of the body. The exception to this rule is that the tender point related to the fourth cervical vertebra, when injured in flexion, is not necessarily treated with the neck in flexion, but may require side-bending and rotation, away from the side affected. Reduction in pain from the tender point during positioning and fine-tuning will produce the guide to the best position.

Tender points found on the posterior aspect of the body indicate joint dysfunction which calls for some degree of backward-bending in the treatment. There are also exceptions to this rule, notably involving the piriformis muscle, and the third and fifth cervical vertebrae. These exceptions may involve a degree of flexion on treatment.

Figs 3.10A, 3.10B and 3.10C will guide the reader to the most common tender-point positions, as noted by Jones. A limited number of specific descriptions as to technique are given in this text, since, as indicated, the positioning of the joint will depend upon the nature of the injury which befell it.

Proprioceptive skills, and the use of careful palpation, will enable the required technique to be acquired. Reading of Jones' (1981) book, or that of D'Ambrogio and Roth (1997) is suggested, for greater detail and understanding of his approach for those who wish to work in this structured manner.

The examples which follow are adapted from Jones' text (Jones 1981) and are not recommenda-

---

Box 3.1 Ideal settings for application of SCS/PR

- For reduction of stiffness (hypertonia) in pre- and post-operative patients
- In cases involving muscle spasm – where more direct methods would not be tolerated
- Where contraction is a feature – reducing tone before stretching tissues after use of muscle energy or other techniques
- In cases of acute and multiple strain – whiplash for example
- As part of any treatment of chronic soft-tissue dysfunction
- As part of a sequence (INIT) of treating trigger points – after NMT and before MET
- In treatment of sensitive, frail, delicate individuals or sites
- In treatment of joint dysfunction where hypertonia is the prime restricting factor.

---

tions but are for general information only. Settings in which SCS/positional release might ideally be applied are given in Box 3.1.

The suggested positions of ease relate to the findings of Jones and his followers over many years, and while they are largely accurate the author is critical of formulae which prescribe a set protocol for any given joint or muscular strain and encourages the use of 'Goodheart's guidelines', which are in Chapter 4, as well as the development of palpation skills which allow for sensing of ease in the tissues, rather than reliance on verbal feedback from the patient as to the current level of discomfort as tissues are being positioned and repositioned.

Notes on positioning

When positioning/fine-tuning the body as a whole or just the part in question (arm, leg, etc.) it is normally found that tender points on the anterior aspect of the body require flexion, and those on the posterior aspect require extension as a first part of the process of easing pain or excessive tone.

The more lateral the point is from the midline the greater the degree of side-bending and/or rotation required to achieve ease.

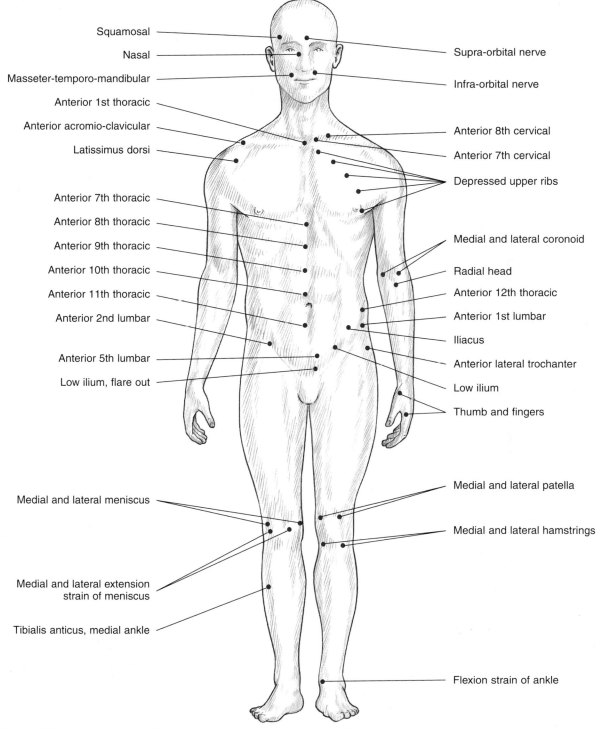

Squamosal

Nasal

Masseter-temporo-mandibular

Anterior 1st thoracic

Anterior acromio-clavicular

Latissimus dorsi

Anterior 7th thoracic

Anterior 8th thoracic

Anterior 9th thoracic

Anterior 10th thoracic

Anterior 11th thoracic

Anterior 2nd lumbar

Anterior 5th lumbar

Low ilium, flare out

Medial and lateral meniscus

Medial and lateral extension
strain of meniscus

Tibialis anticus, medial ankle

Supra-orbital nerve

Infra-orbital nerve

Anterior 8th cervical

Anterior 7th cervical

Depressed upper ribs

Medial and lateral coronoid

Radial head

Anterior 12th thoracic

Anterior 1st lumbar

Iliacus

Anterior lateral trochanter

Low ilium

Thumb and fingers

Medial and lateral patella

Medial and lateral hamstrings

Flexion strain of ankle

Figure 3.10A   Jones' points on the anterior body surface, commonly relating to flexion strains.

Figure 3.10   Location of Jones' tender points, which are bilateral in response to specific strain (acute or chronic) but are shown on only one side of the body in these illustrations. The point locations are approximate and will vary within the indicated area, depending upon the specific mechanics and tissues associated with the particular trauma or strain.

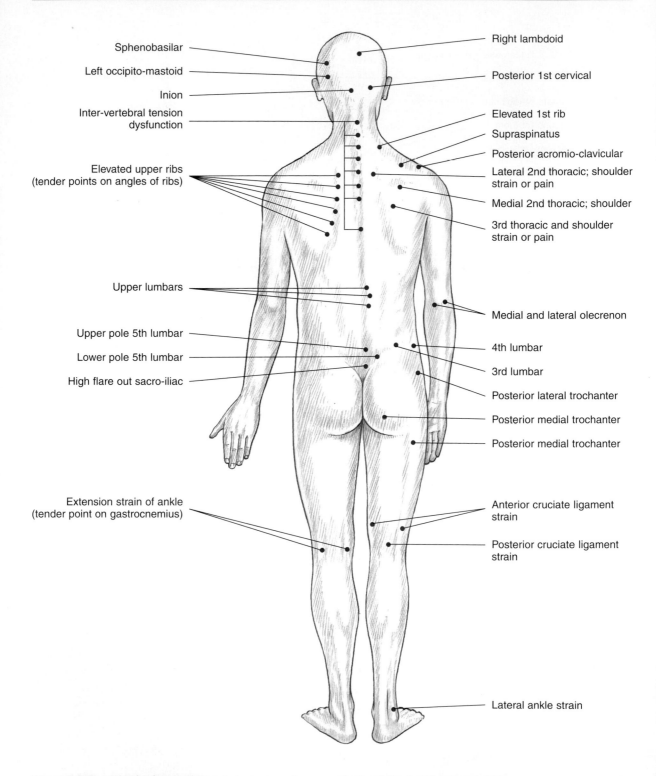

Sphenobasilar

Left occipito-mastoid

Inion

Inter-vertebral tension dysfunction

Elevated upper ribs (tender points on angles of ribs)

Upper lumbars

Upper pole 5th lumbar

Lower pole 5th lumbar

High flare out sacro-iliac

Extension strain of ankle (tender point on gastrocnemius)

Right lambdoid

Posterior 1st cervical

Elevated 1st rib

Supraspinatus

Posterior acromio-clavicular

Lateral 2nd thoracic; shoulder strain or pain

Medial 2nd thoracic; shoulder

3rd thoracic and shoulder strain or pain

Medial and lateral olecrenon

4th lumbar

3rd lumbar

Posterior lateral trochanter

Posterior medial trochanter

Posterior medial trochanter

Anterior cruciate ligament strain

Posterior cruciate ligament strain

Lateral ankle strain

Figure 3.10B   Jones' points on the posterior body surface, commonly relating to extension strains.

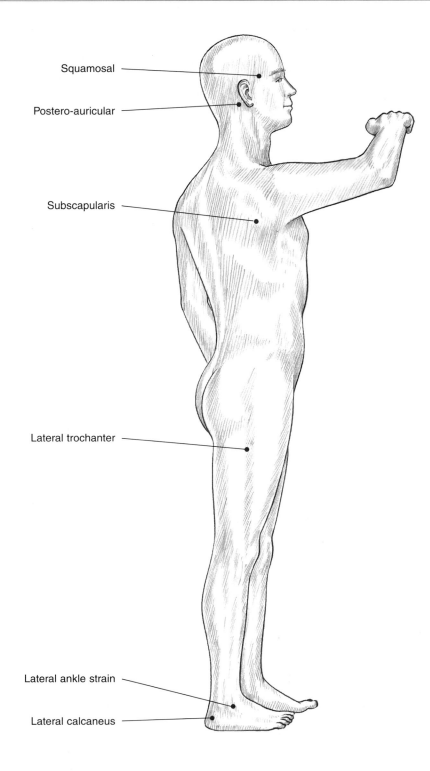

Squamosal

Postero-auricular

Subscapularis

Lateral trochanter

Lateral ankle strain

Lateral calcaneus

Figure 3.10C   Jones' points on the lateral body surface, commonly relating to strains involving side-bending or rotation.

Notes on prioritising points for treatment

When selecting a tender point for use as a monitor in SCS treatment there are often a confusing number of possibilities. The consensus among clinicians (McPartland & Klofat 1995) experienced in use of SCS is that choice should be based on treating:

- First, the most sensitive point found in the area with the largest accretion of tender points
- If there are a number of similarly tender points, the most proximal and/or medial of these should be chosen, and
- If there exists an apparent 'line' of points choose one close to the centre of the chain to 'represent' the others
- Clinical experience suggests that no more than five points should be treated at any one session to avoid adaptive overload, and that one treatment weekly is usually adequate.

These 'rules' are based on experience rather than research. An example might be where tender points of similar intensity are noted in the low back as well as the hip region. The low back point would receive primary attention (i.e. the most proximal point treated first). However, if tender points were found in the low back and hip, but the hip point was more sensitive, this would receive primary attention (i.e. most sensitive point treated first). If a row of points was noted between the low back and the hip and these were equally sensitive, the most central point in the row would receive primary attention (i.e. treat middle of a line of points first).

Notes on feedback

In order to have instant feedback as to the degree of pain/sensitivity/discomfort being felt as the tender point is palpated, it is useful to ask the patient to 'grade' the pain out of 10 (0 = no pain) and to give frequent reports as to the 'value' of the pain being noted during the process of fine-tuning. A reduction to a score of 2 or 3 (approximately 70% reduction in pain) is regarded as adequate to achieve the release required. (In the

USA a method commonly suggested is to say to the patient, 'The amount of pain you feel when I press this point is a dollar's worth. I want you to tell me when there is only 30 cents worth of pain.')

Whichever approach is chosen it is important to instruct the patient that a conversation is not what is needed, but simple indications as to the benefits or otherwise, in terms of pain felt in the point being palpated and monitored, of the various changes in position which are being made.

Notes on fine-tuning the ease position

A crowding of the tissues to induce slackness in the affected tissues is a usual final aspect of the 'fine-tuning' once initial pain reduction has been achieved. Additional ease can often be achieved by asking the patient to fully inhale or exhale to evaluate which phase of the breathing cycle reduces pain (or which reduces increased tone) the most.

Eye movements can also be used in this way – always allowing the patient's report of pain levels and/or your palpation of a sense of ease in the tissues, to guide you towards the 'comfort zone'.

Tips and comments about positioning into ease

1. There should be NO increase in pain elsewhere in the body during the treatment process.
2. It is not necessary to maintain possibly painful pressure on the tender point throughout, although this almost certainly has an 'acupressure' effect (ischaemic compression/inhibition/endorphin release, etc.).
   Intermittent pressure applied periodically, to evaluate the effects of a change in position in order to ascertain the degree of sensitivity still present, is the preferred Jones method.

For how long is the ease position held?

How long the position of ease is held is a matter of some debate. Jones has suggested that 90 seconds is optimal. Schiowitz (1990) (see facilitated positional release discussion in Chapter 9) suggests that just 5 seconds is adequate.

D'Ambrogio and Roth (1997), and Weiselfish (1993) indicate that in order to treat neurological conditions a 3-minute hold may be required, and that fascial responses may take up to 20 minutes. In truth, sensitivity to the changes occurring in the tissues informs the practitioner as to when there has been a 'spontaneous release' in response to positioning. The patient will also usually be aware of the altered sensation which takes place with release.

Following the position of ease

- It is necessary for a slow return to be made to the neutral start position, in order to avoid ballistic proprioceptors firing, and restoring the dysfunctional pattern which has just released.
- The patient should be advised to avoid strenuous activity over the following days.
- Reassessment of the tender point should indicate that a reduction in previous sensitivity of at least 70% has taken place.
- Post-treatment soreness is a common phenomenon and the patient should be warned that this may occur and that it should pass over the next 48 hours or so without further attention.

Why is this chapter titled 'modified' SCS?

Jones laid down strict instructions and guidelines. Tender points in relation to most permutations of each joint's possible directions of strain were identified and located according to Jones' findings, and their respective positions of ease were described in detail. Nothing was left for the operator except to find the point relating to this or that joint's strain and to follow instructions. The author has found that this method of 'treatment by rote' is often inappropriate, in as much as in a significant number of instances it fails to meet the needs of the particular patient being treated.

The praiseworthy efforts of Jones and his followers to provide the answers left the operator floundering when the information provided failed to coincide with the needs of individuals whose strain patterns differed in some way and therefore required an approach which varied from that laid down by Jones' rules.

In an earlier text (Chaitow 1983) the author described his own modifications of Jones' work as 'strain/counterstrain' and was reprimanded by letter by Jones (1985), who pointed out that what was being presented differed significantly from his methodology, asking that this be made clear in the text if legal action was to be avoided! The change which satisfied Jones in subsequent editions was confined to the addition of the word 'modified' to the chapter heading on SCS.

The listings which follow (p. 53 onwards) describe the main sites, as identified by Jones, and also give the most usual directions of ease as presented in his writings and teachings.

The author suggests that these should not be taken as absolute, for the reasons explained above, and should be used as a starting point in guiding the operator towards the desired position of ease. If ease (pain reduction in the palpated tender point) is not achieved in the position suggested by Jones, then that which emerges by careful fine-tuning is the 'correct' position. The body, in other words, is being 'consulted' during the positioning phase, and its answer comes in the form of a reduction in pain in the palpated point.

As will become clear in the chapters which present functional technique and facilitated positional release (Chapters 8 and 9), the use of pain in a point as a guide to the state of 'ease' is not the only manner of arriving at the point of tissue balance – palpated reduction in 'bind' can be used as an equally clear message from the tissues to indicate that 'ease' is being approached.

Another modification to Jones' original approach which the author suggests as being useful involves the maintenance of pressure on the tender point throughout the repositioning process, rather than the intermittent probing urged by Jones. Ischaemic compression which is sustained equates with acupressure methodology, producing endorphin release as well as localised reduction in hypertonicity. The only drawback to sustained compression involves patient sensitivity and this approach is therefore more appropriate for patients who are not frail and sensitive.

It is suggested that both sustained compression and intermittent probing be tried (and indeed that both are useful in different settings) so that readers can come to their own conclusion as to which approach they prefer and which presents the most useful outcome.

A final variation which the author feels worthy of restating involves having, where convenient, the patient apply pressure to the tender point sufficient to register pain. In many instances, especially in intercostal areas, this has proved very useful, allowing freedom of movement for the operator as the positioning process is carried out and, in some instances more significantly, allowing pressure to be applied to areas of extreme sensitivity by the patient themselves when they were unable to tolerate operator application of pressure.

It is for these various reasons that the approach to the methodology of Jones is termed 'modified', and that the directions below (p. 53) are termed 'simplified'.

SCS: contraindications and cautions

- Particular care should be taken in application of SCS in cases of malignancy, aneurysm and acute inflammatory conditions.
- Skin conditions may make application of pressure to the tender point undesirable.
- Protective spasm should not be treated unless the underlying conditions are well considered (osteoporosis, bone secondaries, disc herniation, fractures, etc.).
- Recent major trauma or surgery precludes anything other than gentle superficial positional release methods (see Chapter 7 concerning SCS in hospital settings).
- Infectious conditions call for caution and care.
- Any increase in pain during the process of positioning shows that an undesirable direction, movement or position is being employed. Sensations such as numbness or aching may

arise during the holding of the position of ease, and as long as this is moderate and not severe the patient should be encouraged to relax and view the sensation as transient and part of the desirable changes taking place.
- Caution should be exercised when placing the neck into extension. It is as well to maintain verbal communication with the patient at all times and to ask them to keep the eyes open so that any signs of nystagmus are observable.

Indications for SCS (alone or in combination with other modalities)

NOTE: The fact that conditions are included in the partial listing, below, is not meant to suggest that SCS/PRT could do other than offer symptomatic relief. Alleviation of pain, enhanced mobility and, in some instances, resolution of the actual dysfunctional condition, may be anticipated following appropriate use of SCS. See also the list of contraindications, above.

- Painful and restricted muscles and joints, irrespective of cause
- Degenerative spinal and joint conditions, including arthritis
- Post-surgical pain and dysfunction
- Osteoporosis
- Post-traumatic pain and dysfunction, such as sporting injuries, whiplash, ankle sprain, etc.
- Repetitive strain conditions
- Fibromyalgia pain (see Chapter 6)
- Headache
- Paediatric conditions such as torticollis
- Respiratory conditions which might benefit from normalization of primary and accessory breathing muscles, ribs and thoracic spinal restrictions
- Neurological conditions such as dysfunction following cerebral vascular accidents (stroke), spinal or brain injury or degenerative neural conditions such as MS (Weiselfish 1993).

The concept of scanning before treating

Where should treatment commence? What should be treated first? Is there a way of prioritising areas of dysfunction and choosing 'key' locations for primary attention?

The notes on selecting and prioritising points for treatment earlier in this chapter, as well as the discussion on soft-tissue dysfunction in Chapter 2, should offer some general guidelines as to how and when dysfunctional tissues should be selected for treatment. The author, to a large extent, works with a model of care which attempts to achieve one of two objectives (and sometimes both) when treating general or local (e.g. soft-tissue) dysfunction. It can be argued that all potentially beneficial therapeutic interventions depend for the manifestation of that benefit on the response of the body and tissues being treated. In other words the treatment (involving any technique whatsoever) has a catalytic influence, but is of itself not capable of 'curing' anything.

The objectives, relating to the two areas of influence within which all therapeutic interventions operate, can be summarised as follows:

- Reduction of the adaptive load to which the organism as a whole, or the local tissues, are adapting (or failing to adapt), i.e. 'lighten the load'
- Enhancement of the ability of the organism as a whole, or of the local tissues, to adapt to whatever stress load is being coped with, i.e. 'enhance homeostatic functions'.

An additional awareness needs to be, 'don't make matters worse', by overloading adaptive functions even more. Therefore the decision as to which, and how many, points to treat at a given time, using PRT methods, as well as whether to combine this with other methods of treatment, depends on individual characteristics including age, vulnerability, the chronicity or acuteness of the condition, as well as the specific objectives in the case, with all these considerations being related to assessment findings and therapeutic objectives.

Clinicians such as D'Ambrogio and Roth (1997) argue for a 'scanning evaluation' (SE) which records tender points, as well as their severity, when the entire body is evaluated. Just as a postural evaluation will provide a number of pointers which might relate to the patient's

symptoms, or the palpation and eliciting of active trigger points might show patterns which explain the pain being experienced by the patient, or testing for shortness, weakness or malcoordination in muscles might correlate with somatic dysfunction, so might a grid, or map, of areas of tenderness ('tender points') and their severity be seen to contribute to the formulation of a plan of therapeutic action. A major element in this mapping approach is identification of dominant tender points (DTP), the deactivation of which can lead to a chain reaction in which lesser tender areas will normalize. This concept is not dissimilar to that of Simons and Travell (who maintain that chains of active trigger points can be 'switched off' in much the same manner). As D'Ambrogio and Roth (1997) explain, 'several patients may have the same complaint (e.g. knee pain, shoulder pain, or low back pain) but the source of the condition, as revealed by the SE [and the DTP], may be different for each ... By identifying the location of key dysfunctions and treating restrictive muscular and fascial barriers, the pain may begin to subside'. For details of the complex mapping and charting exercise, as recommended by D'Ambrogio and Roth the reader is referred to their book.

The main author of this text suggests that the mapping and charting exercise is a useful procedure, albeit time-consuming, and that for busy therapists the guidelines offered earlier in this chapter (see p. 50) will suffice and should provide good clinical results.

SUMMARY OF SIMPLIFIED STRAIN/ COUNTERSTRAIN TECHNIQUE

Cervical flexion strains

Anterior strain of C1. The tender point is found in a groove between the styloid process and angle of the jaw. Treatment is usually by rotation of the head of the supine patient away from the side of dysfunction, either maintaining pressure or repetitively probing Jones' point (Fig. 3.11). Fine-tune is usually by side-bending away from the painful side.

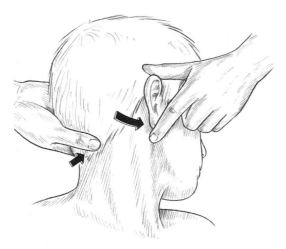

Figure 3.11 First cervical flexion strain tender point lies between the styloid process and the angle of the jaw. A likely position of ease is as illustrated. However, alternative positions of ease could involve movement of the head and neck in different directions.

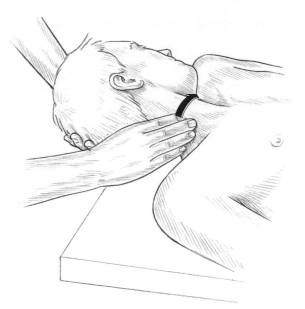

Figure 3.12 Flexion strain of a lower cervical vertebra with the tender point as illustrated (palpated by right middle finger). The position of ease is often as illustrated but might involve alternative positioning (see text).

An alternative or second point for C1 flexion strain is ½ inch anterior to the angle of the mandible. Treat by flexion and rotation, approximately 45° away from the side of pain as a rule.

Remaining cervical anterior strain tender points are on or about the tips of the transverse processes of the involved vertebrae (Fig. 3.12). Treat (usually) by forward-bending and rotation to remove pain from the tender point. In general, the higher the palpated tender point the more rotation away from it is needed in fine-tuning. The lower the point the more flexion, and the less rotation, may be required.

Whenever the information is provided that Jones suggests rotation towards the point, this is the likeliest beneficial direction towards which to move, however, should this fail to achieve results, it may be found that rotation away from the side of pain provides greater ease.

Cervical side-flexion strains

Tender points are relocated as follows:

- for C1 side-flexion restriction – tip of transverse process of C1
- for C2–6 side-flexion restriction – on the lateral aspects of the articular processes (Fig. 3.13).

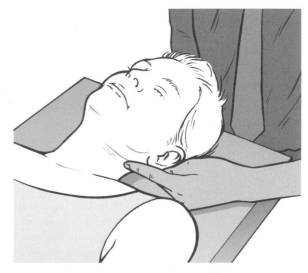

Figure 3.13 Treatment for C2–6 side-flexion strain.

- Treatment involves pressure being applied to the tender point and side-flexion towards or away from the side being treated, depending on the tissue response and patient reports as to pain levels. Fine-tuning might involve slight increase in flexion, extension or rotation.

Suboccipital strains

The tender points associated with upper cervical/ suboccipital strains are located on the occiput or in the muscles attaching to it, such as rectus capitis anterior, obliquus capitis superior and rectus capitis posterior major and minor. Treatment involves either localising cranial flexion or cranial extension to the C1 area and applying precisely focused flexion or extension procedures, which markedly reduces the tenderness from the palpated tender point. For example:

● If a tender point is located on rectus capitis anterior, just medial to the insertion of semi-spinalis capitis, inferior to the posterior occipital protuberance, it is said by Jones (1981) to relate to flexion strain of the region. The ease position involves localised flexion of the suboccipital region. The patient is supine with the practitioner seated or standing at the head of the table. One hand palpates the tender point while simultaneously applying light distraction of the occiput, in a cephalad direction. The other hand rests on the frontal bone and applies light caudad pressure, inducing upper cervical flexion, bringing the chin close to the trachea (Fig. 3.14), until an appropriate tissue response is noted, accompanied by a reduction in perceived tenderness. Fine-tuning may also be required, possibly involving rotation towards and side-flexion away from the treated side.

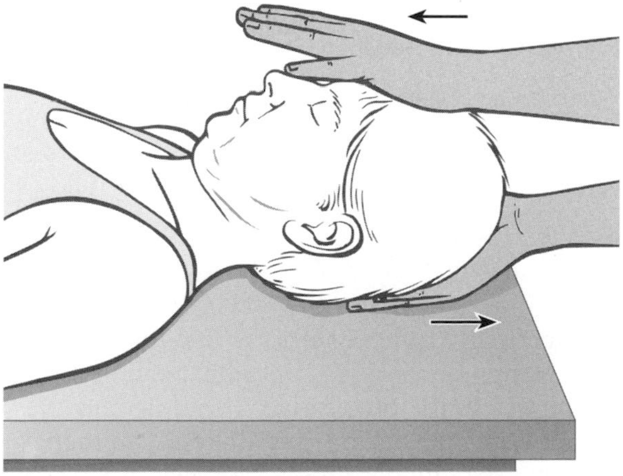

● If a tender point is located on obliquus capitis superior, approximately 1.5 cm medial to the mastoid process, it is said by Jones (1981) to relate to an extension strain of the region. The ease position involves localised extension of the tissues. The patient is supine and the practitioner is at the head of the table with one hand supporting the head, and with one finger of that hand localising the tender point. The other hand is on the crown of the head and applies light pressure to induce upper cervical extension (occiput extends on C1). This position, together with fine-tuning involving side-flexion and/or rotation, should establish the position of ease (Fig. 3.15).

● If a tender point is located on the occiput (using cephalad and medial pressure), just lateral to the insertion of semispinalis capitis, or on the superior surface of the second cervical transverse process, the dysfunctional tissues may involve rectus capitis posterior major or minor (commonly traumatised through whiplash injuries or stressed through a forward-head posture). The ease positions for either point involve upper

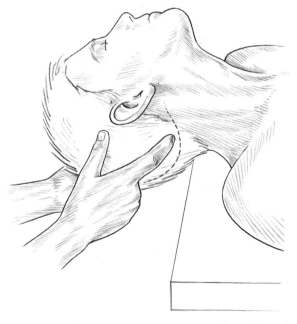

Figure 3.15   First cervical extension strain. The position of ease requires extension of the neck and (usually) rotation away from the side of pain.

Figure 3.14   Treatment for first cervical flexion strain.

cervical extension. The treatment position is almost identical to that suggested in the previous description, or the practitioner uses the heel of the hand, which is supporting the patient's head, to induce extension.

Other cervical extension strains

These tender points are found on or about the spinous processes, and treatment should commence by introduction of increased extension. Extension strains in the lower cervical area are usually treated by taking the pain out of the palpated Jones point, via extension of the head on the neck. In a bed-bound patient the patient lies on the side with the painful side uppermost, so that fine-tuning can be accomplished via slight side-bending and rotation towards the side of the lesion.

Exceptions include C3/4 extension strains, which can usually be treated in either flexion or extension. C8 extension strain may also need to be treated in slight extension, with marked side-bending and rotation away from, rather than towards, the side of strain (C8 point lies on the transverse process of C7).

Extension strains of the lower cervical and upper thoracic spine

The patient should be prone. Jones states:

The head is supported by the doctor's left hand holding the chin. The operator's left forearm is held along the right side of the patient's head for better support. The right hand monitors tender points on the right side of the spinous processes. The forces applied are mostly extension, with slight sidebending and rotation left [Fig. 3.16].

The tender points of the posterior thorax are located interspinally, paraspinally and at the rib angles, when there exist extension dysfunctions of intervertebral joints, side-bending dysfunction, and ribs that are more comfortable when elevated.

The simplicity of Jones' methods is obvious. The shortened fibres relate to the areas where tender points are to be found, and the positioning is such as to increase the shortening already existent, while palpating the tender points. 90 seconds

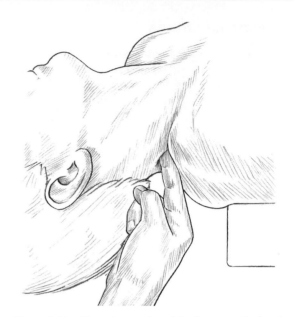

Figure 3.16 Extension strains of the lower cervical and upper thoracic spine usually require extension and slight side-bending, and rotation away from the painful side.

of holding the position of ease is all that there is to the method. The skill required lies in localising the tender points, and identifying and duplicating the nature of the original strain or injury.

There are few exceptions to Jones' directions in this region, for extension strains. However, the reader should constantly be aware of the need to use other positions to achieve ease if the directions given by Jones fail to produce ease and relief from pain.

Rib dysfunction

Assessment of elevated first rib

Among the commonest rib dysfunctions that of an elevated first rib. Assessment of this is as follows:

- Patient is seated and practitioner stands behind (Fig. 3.17)
- The practitioner places his hands so that the fingers can draw posteriorly the upper trapezius fibres lying superior to the first rib
- The tips of the practitioner's middle and index, or middle and ring fingers, can then most easily be placed on the superior surface of the posterior shaft of the first rib

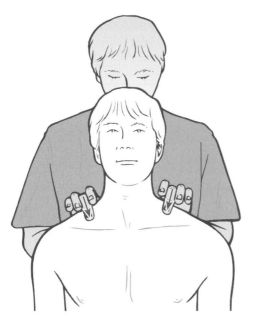

Figure 3.17   Position for assessment of elevated first rib.

- Symmetry is evaluated as the patient breathes lightly
- The commonest dysfunction is for one of the pair of first ribs to be 'locked' in an elevated position ('exhalation restriction')
- The superior aspect of this rib will palpate as tender and attached scalene structures are likely to be short and tight (Greenman 1996).

  or

- Patient is seated and practitioner stands behind
- The practitioner places his hands so that the fingers can draw posteriorly the upper trapezius fibres lying superior to the first rib
- The tips of the practitioners middle and index, or middle and ring, fingers can then most easily be placed on the superior surface of the posterior shaft of the first rib
- The patient exhales and shrugs his shoulders and the palpated first ribs behave asymmetrically (one moves superiorly more than the other), or
- The patient inhales fully and the palpated first ribs behave asymmetrically (one moves inferiorly more than the other)

- The commonest restriction of the first rib is into elevation and the likeliest soft-tissue involvement is of anterior and medial scalenes (Goodridge & Kuchera 1997).

Treatment of elevated first rib

The patient is seated and the practitioner stands behind with his contralateral foot on the table, patient's arm draped over practitioner's knee (Fig. 3.18). The practitioner's ipsilateral hand palpates the tender point on the superior surface of the first rib.

Using body positioning, the practitioner induces a side-shift (translation) of the patient away from the treated side. At the same time, using his contralateral hand, the practitioner eases the patient's head into slight extension, side-flexion away from and rotation towards, the tender point, in order to fine-tune until tenderness reduces by 70%. This is held for not less than 90 seconds.

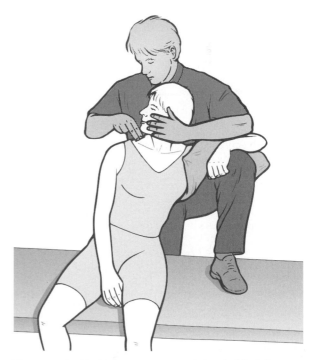

Figure 3.18   Position for treatment of elevated first rib.

Elevated and depressed rib assessment and treatment

Identification of rib dysfunction is not difficult. Restrictions in the ability of a given rib to move fully (as compared with its pair) during inhalation indicates a depressed status while an inability to move fully (as compared with its pair) into exhalation indicates an elevated status (Fig. 3.19).

Assessment of rib status – ribs 2 to 10:

- Patient is supine, practitioner stands at waist level facing the patient's head, with a single finger contact on superior aspect of one pair of ribs.
- The practitioner's dominant eye determines the side of the table from which he is approaching the observation of rib function – right eye dominant calls for standing on the patient's right side.
- The fingers are observed as the patient inhales and exhales fully (eye focus is on an area between the palpating fingers so that peripheral vision assesses symmetry of movement).
- If one of a pair of ribs fails to rise as far as its pair on inhalation it is described as a

depressed rib, unable to move fully to its end of range on inhalation ('exhalation restriction').
- If one of a pair of ribs fails to fall as far as its pair on exhalation it is described as an elevated rib, unable to move fully to its end of range on exhalation ('inhalation restriction').

Assessment of rib status – ribs 11 and 12

- Assessment of eleventh and twelfth ribs is usually performed with the patient prone, with a hand contact on the posterior shafts to evaluate full inhalation and exhalation motions (Fig. 3.20).
- The eleventh and twelfth ribs usually operate as a pair, so that if any sense of reduction in posterior motion is noted on one side or the other, on inhalation, the pair are regarded as depressed, unable to fully inhale ('exhalation restriction').
- If any sense of reduction in anterior motion is noted on one side or the other, on exhalation, the pair are regarded as elevated, unable to fully exhale ('inhalation restriction').

Depressed rib strains produce points of tenderness on the anterior thorax, commonly close to the anterior axillary line.

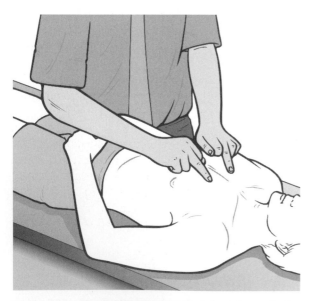

Figure 3.19 Position for assessment of rib status – ribs 2 to 10.

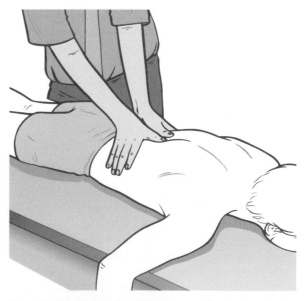

Figure 3.20 Position for assessment of rib status – ribs 11 and 12.

Elevated ribs relate to tender points on the posterior thorax, commonly in the intercostal space above or below the affected rib, at the angle of the ribs posteriorly. In order to gain access, the scapula requires distraction or lifting to allow for palpation of these points relating to those ribs lying under it. This is done by the arm of the affected side of the patient being pulled across the chest, or the shoulder being raised by a pillow, with the patient supine (see Fig. 3.21A). The operator stands on the side of the disorder, and palpation of the tender point, once identified, is continuous, as positional change is engineered.

The patient's knees should be in a flexed position during treatment of elevated ribs, and then be allowed to move to the side of the dysfunction. If this fails to achieve ease (perceived either as palpated change or resulting from reported pain reduction in tender point), the knees are allowed to move towards the opposite side to evaluate the effect on palpated pain. As a rule, pain will reduce by around 50% as the knees fall to one side or the other. The head may be turned towards or away from the affected side to further fine-tune and release the stress in the palpated tissues. Additional fine-tuning for elevated ribs may then be accomplished by raising the arm or shoulder cephalad, in effect exaggerating the positional deformity. The influence of respiratory function may also be used to evaluate which stage of the cycle reduces discomfort (in the tender point) most. If identified the patient is asked to maintain that phase for as long as is comfortable.

The tender point for a depressed rib, lying as it does in the intercostal space above or below the affected rib on the anterior axillary line, is easily palpated by the patient.

For treatment of depressed ribs, the patient may be supine or in a partially seated, recumbent position. If supine the knees are flexed and falling to one side or the other (see Fig. 3.21B), whichever produces better release in the tissues being palpated at the anterior axillary line. The head may be turned towards or away from the affected side to further fine-tune and release the stress in the palpated tissues. For additional fine-tuning, the operator stands on the side of dysfunction and draws the patient's arm, on the side of dysfunction, caudad until release is noted. In some cases the other arm may need to be elevated and even have traction applied, to enhance release of tender-point discomfort.

Alternatively, the patient may be seated (see Fig. 3.22) and resting against the support offered by the practitioner's flexed leg (foot on table) and trunk. The practitioner palpates the tender point with one hand and uses the other to support the head and guide it into rotation for fine-tuning, as a combination of flexion and side-flexion/rotation is encouraged by modification of the position of the supporting leg. Once the tender point being monitored reduces in intensity by 70% or more this is held for not less than 90 seconds.

A notable improvement in respiratory function is commonly noted after this simple treatment

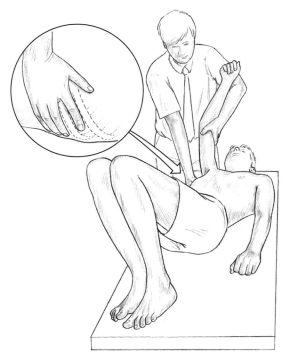

Figure 3.21A Positional release of an elevated rib involves the monitoring of a tender point on the posterior surface close to the angle of the ribs in an interspace above or below the affected rib. Ease is achieved by means of taking the flexed knees to one side or the other, with fine-tuning involving positioning of the head, neck and/or the arms. Assessment of the influence of respiratory function on the tender point pain may also be used.

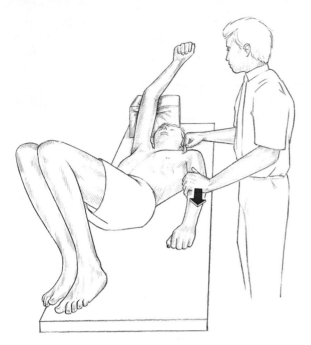

Figure 3.21B   Positional release of a depressed rib involves the monitoring of a tender point on the anterior axillary line, in an interspace above or below the affected rib. Ease is achieved by positioning of flexed legs, head and/or arms, as well as use of the respiratory cycle, until a position is found in which the palpated pain eases markedly or vanishes from the tender point.

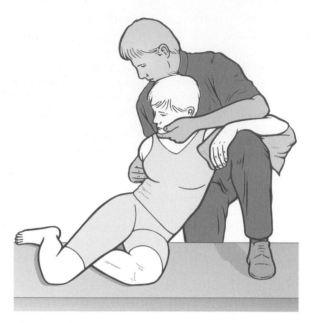

Figure 3.22   Alternative position for treatment of depressed ribs (see text).

method, with an obvious increase in the excursion of the thoracic cage and subjective feelings of 'ease of breathing' being reported.

Interspace dysfunction

Tender points for strains of these tissues lie between the insertions of the contiguous ribs into the cartilages of the sternum. Ribs may be noted to be overapproximated, and the pain reported when the tender points are palpated may be very strong. The more recent the strain the more painful the points; oedema and induration will usually be palpable.

In chronic conditions, pressure on these soft tissues will produce a reactivation of the extreme tenderness noted in more recent strains. These strains are found in costochondritis, the persistent pain noted in cardiac patients. They are implicated in respiratory dysfunction and their release

assists in normalisation. They are common in people with asthma and following bronchitis, as well as the all-too-common pattern of upper chest breathing relating to patent or incipient hyperventilation, which produces major stress of the intercostal structures and the likelihood of such tender points being located on palpation.

Treatment involves placing the patient supine while the tender point is contacted by the operator or the patient (Fig. 3.23). The operator should be on the side of dysfunction with his caudad hand providing contact on the point, unless the patient is performing this function. The cephalad hand cradles the patient's head/neck and flexes this and draws it towards the side of dysfunction at an angle of approximately 45° towards the foot of the bed.

If fine-tuning is adequate, the pain on palpation will ease after some 30 seconds and the position should be further maintained for the full 90-second period.

This same procedure for release of interspace dysfunction tender points can be achieved in a seated position, and can be taught as a home-treatment to the patient. The point is located and the patient on her own, or with guidance, is

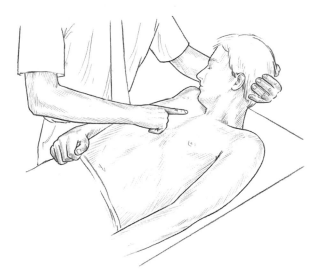

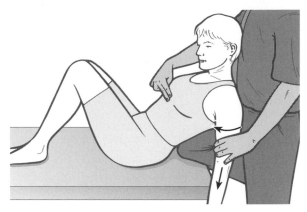

Figure 3.24   Position for assessment and treatment of T2 to T6 flexion strain.

Figure 3.23   Interspace dysfunction involves flexion of the head and neck and usually the thoracic spine towards the palpated tender point, which lies close to the sternum. A seated position (not illustrated) offers an alternative for achieving this positioning.

flexed gently towards the pain side until it vanishes. This position is held for 90 seconds and another point located and treated. It is hard to envisage a simpler protocol.

Additional rib techniques are described in Chapter 7, especially where thoracic function has been disturbed by surgical procedures.

 Flexion strains of the thoracic spine

In a rotation strain of the mid-thoracic region, it is possible for there to coexist both extension and flexion strains, say flexion (anterior) strain on the left and extension (posterior) strain on the right.

According to Jones, T1 anterior (flexion) strain is located on the superior surface of the manubrium on the midline. T2 to T6 flexion strains lie on the sternum approximately $\frac{1}{2}$ to $\frac{3}{4}$ of an inch apart (Fig. 3.24).

Anterior T7 point lies close to the midline, bilaterally under the xyphoid. Other anterior T7 tender points are found on the costal margin close to the xyphoid.

T8 to T11 anterior (flexion strain) dysfunction produces tender points which lie in the abdom-

inal wall, approximately 1 inch lateral to the midline (Fig. 3.10A).

A horizontal line $\frac{1}{2}$ inch below the umbilicus locates the 10th thoracic anterior (flexion) strain tender point.

1 and 3 inches above T10 lie the points for T9 and T8 respectively. $1\frac{1}{2}$ inches below the T10 point is T11; and the T12 point lies on the crest of the ilium at the mid-axillary line.

Treatment for anterior strains T1 to T6 usually involves the head of the supine patient being flexed to the chest while the tender point is contacted as a monitor of adequate ease.

Fine-tuning is usually by slight rotation of the chin towards or away from the side of dysfunction. The head may be supported in flexion by the operator's thigh for the necessary 90 seconds of release time.

For lower thoracic flexion strains (Fig. 3.25), a pillow should be placed under the supine patient's buttocks, allowing the lower spine to fall into flexion. The patient's knees should be flexed and supported by the operator (hand or thigh for support), who stands at waist-level facing the patient and palpating the tender point. Fine-tuning is by movement into side-bending and/or rotation, one way or the other, using the patient's legs as a lever (T8).

T9 to T12 flexion strains involve the same position (head and buttocks on a pillow, the patient's flexed knees supported by the operator's thigh, operator's foot on the table). The operator is

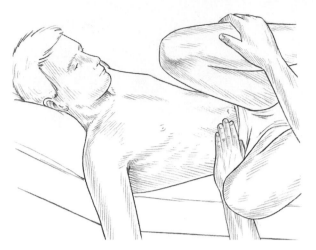

Figure 3.25 Lower thoracic flexion strains involve positioning the supine patient into flexion while the tender point on the abdominal wall is palpated.

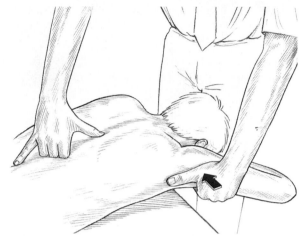

Figure 3.26 Position of ease for tender points relating to extension strains of the thoracic region of the spine. A seated position (not illustrated) provides a useful alternative for achieving this.

standing on the side of the strain and, having crossed the patient's ankles, fine-tuning is via a movement which introduces slight side-bending, or which slightly alters the degree of flexion. The tender point should be constantly monitored.

T12 treatment requires more side-bending than other thoracic strains. Jones's method for dealing with flexion strain of the upper thoracics in non-bedbound patients involves the patient seated on a couch and leaning back onto the operator's chest/abdomen so that forced flexion of the upper body may be achieved. A variety of changes in the position of the patient's arms may then be used as part of the 'fine-tuning' process in order to introduce 'ease' into different thoracic segments.

Extension strains of the thoracic spine

These are treated in a similar manner to that used for extension strains of the cervical spine. Points are usually found on, or close to, the spinous processes, bilaterally, or in the lateral paravertebral muscle mass (Fig. 3.26). It is usual to find that the lower the strain, the closer is the tender point to the transverse process. Direct extension (backwards-bending) is the usual method employed, with the patient side-lying, seated, supine or prone. If side-lying, the arms should be placed so as to avoid rotation of the spine, resting on a pillow.

For the T5 to T8 levels the arms are usually held slightly above head level, to increase extension.

For T9 to T12 the patient may be treated lying supine with the operator on the side of the lesion. The operator's cephalad hand is inserted under the spine to palpate the point, while the caudad hand grasps the patient's contralateral hand, and draws this towards himself, so that the opposite shoulder lifts by 30–45°. In this position, fine-tuning is accomplished. The pull on the arm on the side opposite to the lesion/tender point causes extension and rotation in the region of the strain. Once the tender point is noted to ease in sensitivity, or tissue alteration is felt to be adequate, the fine-tuning is complete and the position is held for 90 seconds.

Flexion strains from ninth thoracic to first lumbar vertebrae

Jones explains:

This one procedure is usually effective for any of this group. To permit the supine to flex at the thoracolumbar region, a table capable of being raised at one end is desirable [see Fig. 3.25]. A flat table may be used if a large pillow is placed under the patient's hips, raising them enough to permit flexion to reach the desired level of the spine. With the patient supine, the physician raises the patient's knees and places his own thigh below those of the patient. By applying cephalad pressure on the patient's thighs, he produces marked flexion of the patient's thoracolumbar spine. Usually, the best results come from rotation of the knees moderately towards the side of tenderness. These joint dysfunctions account for many low-back pains that are not associated with tenderness of the vertebrae posteriorly. The pain is referred from the anterior dysfunction, into the low lumbar, sacral and gluteal areas. Treatment directed to the posterior pain sites of these dysfunctions, rather than to the origins of the pain, has been disappointing.

Treatment for flexion strain from ninth thoracic to first lumbar level is usually achieved by placing the patient supine in flexion, using a cushion for the upper back and flexing the knees and hips, which are usually rotated towards the side of dysfunction. The tender point will be found on the abdominal midline, or slightly to one side, and should be palpated during this manoeuvre. The operator's cephalad hand palpates the tender point while the patient's position is modified until the point no longer palpates as tender. This position is held for 90 seconds, after which a slow return is made to a neutral position. A flexion strain would produce a tender point anteriorly and calls for a flexed position for release to occur.

The position involves marked flexion through the joint, as well as appropriate side-bending and rotation, resulting in reduction of sensitivity in the tender points on the anterior body surface. Once this is achieved, the position is held for 90 seconds.

Flexion strains of the lumbar spine

Gross positioning is as for thoracic strains, taking the patient into flexion.

L1 has two tender points: one is at the tip of the anterior superior iliac spine and the other on the medial surface of the ilium just medial to the anterior superior iliac spine (ASIS) (see Fig. 3.27).

The tender point for second lumbar anterior strain is found lateral to the anterior inferior iliac spine (AIIS).

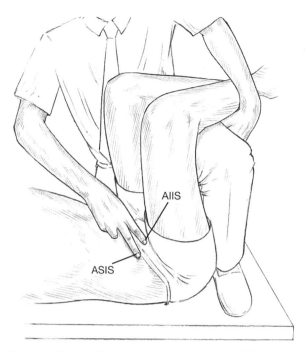

Figure 3.27 Position of ease for flexion strain of T9 to lower lumbar regions involves flexion, side-bending and rotation until ease is achieved in monitored tender point on the lower abdominal wall or the ASIS area.

The tender point for L3 is not easy to find but lies on the lateral surface of the AIIS, pressing medially.

L4 tender point is found at the insertion of the inguinal ligament on the ilium.

L5 points are on the body of the pubes, just to the side of the symphysis. Treatment for these points is similar to that used for thoracic flexion strains except that the patient's knees are placed together (ankles are usually kept crossed in treatment of thoracic strains) (Fig. 3.10A).

In bilateral strains both sides must be treated. L3 and L4 usually require greater side-bending in fine-tuning.

Extension strains of the lumbar spine

L1 and L2 sensitive points are found over the tips of the transverse processes of the respective vertebrae. They may be treated with the patient prone or side-lying. If prone, the operator stands on the side opposite the strain, grasping the leg of

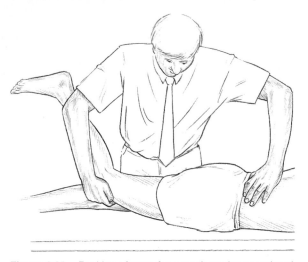

Figure 3.28 Position of ease for a tender point associated with an extension strain of the lumbar spine involves use of the legs of the prone patient as means of achieving extension and fine-tuning.

the side of the lesion, just above the knee, bringing it up and towards the operator in a scissor-like movement (see Fig. 3.28).

Similarly, if the patient is side-lying, with the side of dysfunction uppermost, the upper leg can be extended to introduce backward-bending into the region of the strain. When this is done and the palpated tender point is less painful, or when a tissue change is noted, fine-tuning is accomplished by slightly raising or lowering the leg.

The tender point for extension strain of L3 is found about 3 inches lateral to the post-superior iliac spine, just below the superior iliac spine. L4 tender point lies an inch or two lateral to this following the contour of the crest.

Treatment of L3 and 4 extension strains is accomplished with patient prone, operator on side of dysfunction. The operator's knee or thigh can be usefully placed under the raised thigh of the patient to hold it in extension while fine-tuning it, accomplished usually via abduction and external rotation of the foot. This procedure can also be performed with the patient side-lying, dysfunction side uppermost. The operator's foot should be placed on the bed behind the patient's lower leg. The patient's uppermost leg is raised and the extended thigh of this leg can then be supported on the operator's thigh.

Rotation of the foot and positioning of the patient's leg in a more anterior or posterior plane, always in a degree of extension, is the fine-tuning mechanism to reduce or remove pain from the palpated tender point during this process.

There are three L5 tender points for extension strain. The first, known as the upper pole L5 strain, is found bilaterally between the spinous process of L5 and the spinous process of S1 (Fig. 3.10B). This is treated as in extension strains of L1 and L2 (using scissor-like extension of the prone patient's leg on the side of the lesion and fine-tuning by variation in position).

The middle pole L5 point is found in the superior sulcus of the sacrum and relates to strain which is treated with the patient lying on the unaffected side. Jones suggests that the lower arm of the patient is extended over the edge of the bed hanging towards the floor. The operator stands in front of and facing the patient. The knee of the patient's upper leg (affected side) is flexed and rests on the operator's thigh or abdomen. The fine-tuning of the area is achieved by slight movement which takes the flexed leg caudad or cephalad, or which elevates or depresses it while the tender point is being monitored for ease and reduction of pressure-induced pain.

The lower pole of L5 extension strain lies on the body of the sacrum, centrally. Treatment is via the same position and method as in L1 and L2 and upper pole L5.

Sacral foramen tender points and low back pain

In 1989 osteopathic physicians Jerry Hamen and Leonard Worth, together with a then osteopathic medical student, Maurice Ramirez, identified a series of 'new' tender points, collectively known as medial sacral tender points (to differentiate them from Jones' lateral border tender points previously identified by him and described in his main text). These new points were found to relate directly to low back and pelvic dysfunction and were found to be amenable to very simple SCS methods of release (Ramirez et al 1989).

Since the original presentation of the evidence of the value of these 'new' points, Ramirez, together with osteopathic physicians Susan Cislo and Harold Schwartz, have described additional sacral foramen tender points which relate to sacral torsion. They too have provided clear guidelines as to the usefulness of these in treatment of low back pain associated with sacral torsion, using counterstrain methods (Cislo et al 1991).

The original finding of the 'new' medial sacral points occurred when a patient with chronic low back pain and pelvic hypermobility was being treated. Use of counterstrain methods was found to be efficient using anterior and posterior lumbar tender points; however, despite relative comfort, the patient was left with 'tender points in the middle of the sacrum, associated with no problems'. These were originally ignored but when the patient's back pain recurred, the sacral points were re-evaluated and a number of release positions were attempted. Recognising that the usual 'crowding' or 'folding' of tissue to induce ease in tender points was impossible in the mid-sacral area, the researchers then experimented with application of pressure to various areas of the sacrum.

They explain their progress from then on:

In the 3 weeks following this initial encounter with the unnamed sacral tender points, 14 patients with the presenting complaint of low back (sacral or lumbar, with or without radicular) pain demonstrated tenderness at one or more of the new sacral tender points. Ultimately we found six new tender points, all of which were relieved by positional release techniques to the sacrum.

 Location of the new sacral medial points

Collectively known as the 'medial sacral tender points' (see Fig. 3.29) these are located as follows:

- The cephalad two are just lateral to the midline (but medial to points previously described by Jones) approximately 1.5 cm medial to the inferior aspect of the PSIS bilaterally, and they are known as PS1 (for posterior sacrum).
- The caudad two points are known as PS5 and are found approximately 1 cm medial and 1 cm

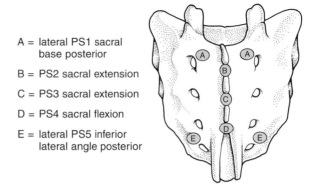

A = lateral PS1 sacral
       base posterior

B = PS2 sacral extension

C = PS3 sacral extension

D = PS4 sacral flexion

E = lateral PS5 inferior
       lateral angle posterior

Figure 3.29   Positions of tender points relating to sacral dysfunction.

superior to the inferior lateral angles of the sacrum bilaterally.
- The remaining two points are on the midline: one (PS2) lies between the first and second spinous tubercles of the sacrum, identified as being involved in sacral extension, and the other (PS4) on the cephalad border of the sacral hiatus, which is identified as a sacral flexion point.
- Schwartz has identified a seventh point lying between the second and third sacral tubercles (PS3), which relates to sacral extension.

Identification of medial sacral tender points

The authors (Cislo et al 1991) note that when they started trying to identify the precise locations of the sacral tender points they used the skin evaluation methods as described above. However, they state: 'We have found that when these tender points occur in groups the associated sudomotor change is frequently confluent over the mid-sacrum. For this reason, we have begun to check all six points on all patients with low back pain, even in the absence of sudomotor changes'.

They report that this process of localisation can be rapid if the bony landmarks are used during normal structural examination.

 Treatment of medial sacral tender points

With the patient prone, pressure on the sacrum is applied according to the tender point being treated. The pressure is always straight downwards, in order to induce rotation around either a perceived transverse or oblique axis of the sacrum.

The PS1 points require pressure at the corner of the sacrum opposite the quadrant in which the tender point lies (left PS1 requires pressure at the right inferior lateral angle).

The PS5 points require pressure near the sacral base on the contralateral side (a right PS5 point requires downward – to the floor – pressure on the left sacral base just medial to the SI joint).

The release of PS2 (sacral extension) tender point requires downwards pressure (to the floor) to the apex of the sacrum in the midline.

The lower PS4 (sacral flexion) tender point requires pressure to the midline of the sacral base.

Schwartz tender point PS3 (sacral extension) requires the same treatment as for PS2 described above.

In all of these examples it is easy to see that the pressure is attempting to exaggerate the existing presumed distortion pattern relating to the point, which is in line with the concepts of SCS and positional release as explained earlier in this and the previous chapter.

Problems when medial sacral points are too sensitive

From time to time pressure on the sacrum itself was found to be too painful for particular patients, and a refinement of the techniques of SCS was therefore devised for the medial points (not the midline ones). The patient should be placed on a table, prone, with head and legs elevated (an adaptable McManus-type table can achieve this, as can appropriately-sited pillows and bolsters), inducing extension of the spine, which usually relieves the palpated pain by approximately 40%.

Different degrees of extension (and sometimes flexion) should be attempted to find the position which reduces sensitivity in the point(s) most effectively. When this has been achieved, side-bending the upper body or the legs away from the trunk should be carefully introduced, to assess the effects of this on the palpated pain. The final position is held for 90 seconds once pain has been reduced by at least 75% in the tender point(s).

Sacral foramen tender points

Once again it was treatment of a 'difficult' patient which led to the discovery of these additional tender points.

A patient with low back pain, with a recurrent sacral torsion, was being treated using SCS methods with poor results. When muscle energy procedures were also inadequate, a detailed survey was made of the region, and an area of sensitivity which had previously been ignored was identified in one of the sacral foramina.

Experimentation with various release positions for this tender point resulted in benefits and also in the examination of this region in other patients with low back pain and evidence of sacral torsion. 'All the patients [who were examined] demonstrated tenderness at one of the sacral foramina, ipsilateral to the engaged oblique axis [of the sacrum].'

Sacral torsion

Mitchell et al (1979) have given simple guidelines as to the identification of sacral torsion. In summary they state that:

- Sacral torsions derive their names from the direction taken by the anterior aspect of the sacral base as it rotates around an oblique axis.
- If the sacrum rotates left on a left oblique axis it is given the name of a 'left on left sacral torsion'. This would be considered to be a forward torsion (as would a 'right on right sacral torsion').
- If the sacrum rotates right on a left oblique axis it is called a 'right on left sacral torsion' and (along with a 'left on right torsion') is considered a backward torsion.
- Application of a 'spring test' to the prone patient's lumbosacral junction can be used to confirm the backward or forward torsion finding.

- If the spring test produces no anterior movement (positive test) at the junction, this confirms a backward torsion, whereas if springing allows anterior movement at the junction, the test is considered negative and the torsion is said to be a forward one.'

The discoverers of these points have named them according to their anatomic position and differentiate them from sacral border tender points previously identified by Jones and from the medial tender points discussed above.

The researchers give the following information regarding their location (see also Fig. 3.30):

Clinically, these tender points are located by their positions relative to the posterior superior iliac spines. The most cephalad of the points [SF1 – sacral foramen tender point 1] is 1.5 cm directly medial to the apex of the PSIS. Each successively numbered sacral foramen tender point [SF2, SF3, SF4] lies approximately 1 cm below the preceding tender point location.

Locatinwg and treating sacral foramen tender points

Evaluation of the sacral foramina should be a fairly rapid process. Once a sacral torsion has been identified, the foramina on the ipsilateral side are examined by palpation and the most sensitive of these is treated. A left torsion (forward or backward) would therefore involve the foramen on the left side being assessed.

Alternatively, palpation of the foramina using the skin-drag method for rapid evaluation (see

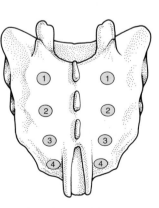

1 = sacral foramen SF1

2 = sacral foramen SF2

3 = sacral foramen SF3

4 = sacral foramen SF4

Figure 3.30   Sacral foramen tender points as described in the text.

Chapter 4) would reveal dysfunction, even if the precise nature of that dysfunction remained unclear. If there was obvious skin-drag over a foramen, and if compression of that foramen was unduly painful, some degree of sacral torsion would be probable on the same side as the tender foramen.

The patient lies prone with the operator on the side of the patient contralateral to the foramen tender point to be treated. The operator would therefore be seated or standing on the right of the prone patient when a left torsion was being treated.

The leg on the side in which the practitioner is working (contralateral to the tender point side, therefore the right leg in this example) is abducted to about 30°, with slight flexion at the hip allowing the patient's leg to be supported on the operator's lap, knee in extension if he is seated, or supported over the edge of the table if practitioner is standing.

The operator, while applying pressure to the sensitive foramen with his caudad hand, applies pressure to the ilium on the right (on the side on which he is seated or standing), directed anteromedially, using his right forearm or hand (in this example). The point of arm or hand contact should be approximately 1 inch lateral to the patient's right PSIS.

The degree of relief of sensitivity initiated in the palpated sacral foramen tender point by the leg abduction, hip flexion and the forearm pressure on the ilium should be approximately 70%.

With the operator maintaining finger contact but not pressure on the palpated point, the position of ease is held for 90 seconds before a slow return to neutral (leg back to the table, contact released) is passively brought about.

Whether the sacral torsion is on a forward or backward axis it should respond to the same treatment protocol as described.

NOTE: Despite the extreme gentleness of the methods involved in the application of all positional release in general and strain/counterstrain in particular there is, in about a third of patients, a reaction in which soreness, fatigue, etc., may be noted, just as in more strenuous therapeutic measures. This reaction is considered to be the result of the homeostatic adaptation process which the organism is obliged to go through in response to the treatment, and which is a feature of many apparently very light forms of treatment. Since the philosophical basis for much bodywork involves the concept of the treatment itself acting as a catalyst, with the normalisation or healing process being the prerogative of the body itself, the reaction described above is an anticipated part of the process.

Other areas

This summary of SCS tender-point locations and suggested positions of ease is not comprehensive. A thorough reading of Jones's (1981) text is recommended, along with attendance at postgraduate lectures, seminars and workshops which teach the essence and detail of the method.

In the next chapter, which offers guidence as to how to start using SCS, 'exercises' are described involving the upper and lower limbs, while in Chapter 6, PRT methods for use in treating muscular conditions and trigger points are described. With the information in this and subsequent chapters, and using the basic principle of identifying areas of tenderness in shortened structures, and easing these by positioning, it should be possible for the reader to become familiar with the clinical possibilities offered by PRT in general and SCS in particular, without becoming bound by rigid formulaic procedures.

At its simplest SCS suggests that if something is restricted or painful, with some tissues 'tight', and others 'loose':

- Consider the tight structures as primary sites for tender points
- Locate the most tender point
- Monitor this point while positioning the tissues to reduce the perceived pain by not less than 70%
- Hold the position of comfort/ease for not less than 90 seconds
- Slowly return to neutral, and reassess.

Hopefully the detailed explanations in this chapter will have produced sufficient awareness to allow experimentation with the principles involved, in clinical settings, of both the areas presented and others.

As long as the guiding principles of producing no additional pain and relieving pain from the palpated tender point during the positioning and fine-tuning are adhered to, no damage can possibly be done, and a profound degree of pain-relief and functional improvement is possible.

REFERENCES

Bailey M, Dick L 1992 Nociceptive considerations in treating with counterstrain. J American Osteopathic Association 92: 334–341

Baldry P 1993 Acupuncture, Trigger Points and Musculoskeletal Pain. Churchill Livingstone, Edinburgh

Barnes M 1997 The basic science of myofascial release. J Bodywork and Movement Therapies 1(4): 231–238

Calais-Germain B 1993 Anatomy of Movement. Eastland Press, Seattle

Cantu R, Grodin A 1992 Myofascial Manipulation. Aspen Publications, Gaithersburg, Maryland

Chaitow L 1983 Soft tissue manipulation. Thorsons/HarperCollins, London (USA: Healing Arts Press, Vermont)

Chaitow L 1991 Acupuncture treatment of pain. Healing Arts Press, Vermont

Cislo S, Ramirez M, Schwartz H 1991 Low back pain: treatment of forward and backward sacral torsion using counterstrain technique. J American Osteopathic Association 91(3): 255–259

D'Ambrogio K, Roth G 1997 Positional Release Therapy. Mosby, St Louis

DiGiovanna E 1991 An osteopathic approach to diagnosis and treatment. Lippincott, Philadelphia

Goodridge J, Kuchera W 1997 Muscle energy techniques for specific areas. In: Ward R (ed) Foundations for Osteopathic Medicine. Williams and Wilkins, Baltimore

Greenman P 1996 Principles of Manual Medicine, 2nd edn. Williams and Wilkins, Baltimore

Jacobson E et al 1989 Shoulder pain and repetition strain injury. J American Osteopathic Association 89: 1037–1045

Jones L 1964 Spontaneous release by positioning. The Doctor of Osteopathy 4: 109–116

Jones L 1966 Missed anterior spinal lesions – a preliminary report. The Doctor of Osteopathy 6: 75–79

Jones L 1981 Strain and counterstrain. Academy of Applied Osteopathy, Colorado Springs

Jones L 1985 Personal communication.

Juhan D 1998 Job's Body, 2nd edn. Station Hill Press, Barrytown, New York

Korr I 1947 The neural basis of the osteopathic lesion. J American Osteopathic Association 48: 191–198

Korr I 1975 Proprioceptors and somatic dysfunction. J American Osteopathic Association 74: 638–650

Korr I 1976 Collected papers of I M Korr. American Academy of Osteopathy, New York, Ohio

Kuchera M L, McPartland J M 1997 Myofascial trigger points: an introduction. In: Word R (ed) Foundations for Osteopathic Medicine. Williams & Wilkins, Baltimore, MD

Levin S 1986 The icosohedron as the three-dimensional finite element in biomechanical support. Proceedings of the Society of General Systems Research on Mental Images, Values and Reality, May 1986. Society of Systems Research, Philadelphia

McPartland J M, Klofat I 1995 Strain and Counterstrain. Technik Kursunterlagen. Landesverbände der Deutschen Gesellschaft für Manuelle Medizin, Baden

Mann F 1983 International Conference of Acupuncture and Chronic Pain. September, 1983

Mathews P 1981 Muscle spindles – their messages and their fusimotor supply. In: Brookes V (ed) Handbook of Physiology. American Physiological Society, Bethesda

Melzack R, Wall P 1988 The Challenge of Pain, 2nd edn. Penguin, London

Mitchell F, Moran P, Pruzzo H 1979 Evaluation and treatment manual of osteopathic muscle energy procedures. Valley Park

Myers T 1997 Anatomy Trains. J Bodywork & Movement Therapies 1(2): 134–135; and 1(3): 99–101

Northrup T 1941 Role of the reflexes in manipulative therapy. J American Osteopathic Association 40: 521–524

Owens C 1982 An endocrine interpretation of Chapman's reflexes. Academy of Applied Osteopathy, Colorado Springs

Ramirez M, Hamen J, Worth L 1989 Low back pain: diagnosis by six newly discovered sacral tender points and treatment with counterstrain. J American Osteopathic Association 89(7): 905–913

Rathbun J, Macnab I 1970 Microvascular pattern at the rotator cuff. J Bone and Joint Surgery 52: 540–553

Schiowitz S 1990 Facilitated positional release. American Osteopathic Association 90(2): 145–156

Simons D Travell J 1998 Myofascial Pain and Dysfunction: The Trigger Point Manual Vol 1, 2nd edn. Williams and Wilkins, Baltimore

Travell J, Simons D 1983 Myofascial Pain and Dysfunction, Vol 1. Williams and Wilkins, Baltimore

Travell J, Simons D 1992 Myofascial Pain and Dysfunction, Vol 2. Williams and Wilkins, Baltimore

Van Buskirk R 1990 Nociceptive reflexes and somatic dysfunction. J American Osteopathic Association 90: 792–809

Walther D 1988 Applied Kinesiology. SDC Systems, Pueblo

Ward R C 1997 Foundations of Osteopathic Medicine. Williams and Wilkins, Baltimore

Weiselfish S 1993 Manual therapy for the orthopedic and neurologic patient. Regional Physical Therapy, Hertford, Connecticut

4

Learning SCS

KEY ELEMENTS OF SCS

The elements which need to be kept in mind as SCS methods are learned, and which are major points of emphasis in programmes which teach it (Jones 1981), are summarised in Box 4.1.

CONVENTIONAL SCS TRAINING

The usual method for learning SCS methodology involves learning the locations, and practicing the finding, of tender points, followed by practice of the positioning of the body/associated area, in order to take the pain away from the palpated tender point.

Box 4.1   SCS guidelines

The four keys which allow anyone to apply SCS efficiently are:
1. An ability to localise by palpation soft tissue changes related to particular strain dysfunctions, acute or chronic
2. An ability to sense tissue change as it moves into a state of ease, comfort, relaxation and reduced resistance
3. The ability to guide the patient as a whole, or the affected body part, towards a state of ease with minimal force
4. The ability to apply minimal palpation force as the changes in the tissues are evaluated.

The guidelines which should therefore be remembered and applied are:
1. Locate and palpate the appropriate tender point
2. Use minimal force
3. Use minimal monitoring pressure
4. Achieve maximum ease/comfort
5. Produce no additional pain anywhere else.

Finding tender points depends upon palpation skills which can be learned and which practice can refine into a practical ability which allows for the very rapid location of areas of localised soft tissue dysfunction.

Most researchers into positional release and SCS who discuss tender point characteristics speak of sudomotor changes as a primary feature, usually associated with increased or decreased temperature as compared with surrounding tissues. Phenomena such as blanching, erythema and sweating of the skin which overlies tense, tender and often oedematous tender points, are all used as a means of identification when manual palpation is used (Jones 1964, Jones 1981, Schwartz 1986).

The simplest method of palpation involves a light passage across the skin of one digit, which seeks a sense of 'drag' in which the elevated sympathetic, sudomotor activity becomes apparent, as the finger or thumb feels a momentarily retarded passage over the skin, due to increased hydrosis.

Pressure applied into the tissues below such localised skin changes (described as 'hyperalgesic skin zones' by Dr Karel Lewit (1991)) usually evinces an increased degree of sensitivity or pain. Whether this or some other form of soft tissue evaluation is used, the tender points, which Jones has catalogued, need to be identified. They frequently differ from myofascial trigger points inasmuch as Jones' tender points *may* refer pain elsewhere when compressed, whereas active trigger points *always* refer pain elsewhere. They lie (see Ch. 3) in tissues which were shortened at the time of strain, or which are chronically shortened in response to chronic strain, and are seldom in areas in which the patient was previously aware of pain.

SCS guidelines

The general guidelines which Jones gives for relief of the dysfunction with which such tender points are related involves directing the movement of these tissues towards ease, which commonly involves the following elements:

- For tender points on the anterior surface of the body, flexion, side-bending and rotation is most commonly towards the side of the palpated point, followed by fine-tuning to reduce sensitivity by at least 70%.
- For tender points on the posterior surface of the body, extension, side-bending and rotation is most commonly away from the side of the palpated point, followed by fine-tuning to reduce sensitivity by at least 70%.
- The closer the tender point is to the midline the less side-bending and rotation is usually required, and the further from the midline the more side-bending and rotation may be required, in order to effect ease and comfort in the tender point (without any additional pain or discomfort being produced anywhere else).
- The direction towards which side-bending is introduced when attempting to find a position of ease often needs to be away from the side of the palpated pain point, especially in relation to tender points found on the posterior aspect of the body.
- Despite the previous comment, there are many instances in which ease will be noted when side-bending towards the direction of the painful point. These guidelines therefore offer a suggestion as to the likeliest directions of ease and not 'rules'. Individual tissue characteristics will ultimately determine the ideal directions which will achieve comfort/ease for the point being monitored.

Suggestions regarding the length of time positions of ease should be maintained will be found in Box 4.2.

Using these guidelines, it is possible to begin to practice the use of SCS on a model, fellow student, a willing volunteer, or even oneself.

Further clinical guidelines

As discussed in Chapter 3 there has emerged out of the clinical experience of thousands of practitioners over the past 40 years a number of simple yet effective ways of selecting which of many areas of discomfort and 'tenderness' should receive primary attention (McPartland & Klofat 1195).

The advice can be summarised as follows:

- Choose the most painful, the most medial and the most proximal tender points for primary attention, within the area of the body which demonstrates the greatest aggregation of tender points.

- If a chain, or line, of tender points is identified, treat the most central of these.
- No more than five tender points should receive attention at any one treatment session, if a relatively robust individual is involved.
- The more dysfunctional, ill, pain-ridden and/or fatigued the patient, the fewer the number of tender points that should be treated at any one session (between one and three in such cases).

Where to look for tender points

- Use of Jones' (or D'Ambrogio & Roth 1997) 'maps' offers one way of deciding where to palpate for a tender point.
- If the patient can identify a movement in which tissues were strained, the concept of 'replicating the position of strain' (see Chapter 1) may be used, with the tender point likely to be located in tissues short at the time of strain.
- If the patient displays obvious distortion, or a marked imbalance in terms of 'loose–tight' tissues, the tender points most likely to be useful as monitors will be found in the tight (i.e. short) tissues and the ease position is likely to be an exaggeration of the presenting

distortion (see notes in Chapter 1), as tissues which are short are shortened even more during the positioning process.

- If the patient demonstrates a movement which is painful, or which is restricted, then Goodheart's guidelines (see Chapter 1) suggest that the tender points most useful for monitoring will be located in the muscles or soft tissues which would perform the opposite movement to that which is painful or restricted.
- Any area of local tenderness probably represents a response to some degree of imbalance, chronic strain or adaptive change. Using such a point as a monitor while local or general positioning is introduced to remove the sensitivity from it will almost certainly help to modify whatever stress pattern is causing or maintaining it.

SCS EXERCISES

1. The SCS 'box' exercise
(Woolbright 1991)

Colonel Jimmie Woolbright (1991), Chief of Aeromedical Services at Maxwell Airforce Base, Alabama, has devised a teaching tool which enables SCS skills to be acquired and polished.[1]

'Box' exercise guidelines

- As the head and neck are positioned (see Figs 4.1A and 4.1B) no force at all should be used.
- Each position adopted is not the furthest the tissues can be taken in any given direction but rather that in which the first sign of resistance is noted. Thus, a direction to take the patient/model's head and neck into side-bending and rotation to the right would involve the very lightest of guidance towards that position, with no force and no effort, and no strain or pain being noted by the patient.

---

[1] This is not a treatment protocol but is a means of learning how to acquire a sense of ease in palpated tissues while using minimal effort in guiding the patient towards that state.

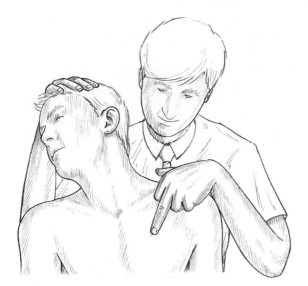

Figure 4.1A   The second head/neck position of the 'box' exercise as pain and tissue tension is palpated and monitored (in this instance in the left upper pectoral area).

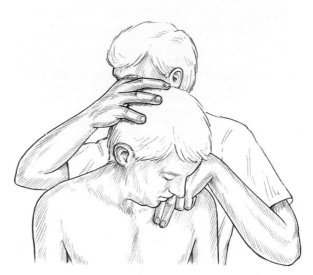

Figure 4.1B   The fourth and final head/neck position of the 'box' exercise as pain and tissue tension is palpated and monitored.

● As each position described below in this 'box exercise' is achieved three key elements require consideration:

– Is the patient comfortable and unstressed by this position? If not, too much effort is being used, or they are not relaxed.

– In this position, are the palpated tissues (in this exercise those on the upper left thoracic area) less sensitive to compression pressure?

– In this position, are the palpated tissues reducing in tone, feeling more at 'ease', with less evidence of 'bind'?

The information derived by the palpating hand (left in this example) should, at the end of the exercise, allow the operator to judge which of the various head/neck positions offered the most 'ease' to the palpated tissues (see Fig. 4.2).

It will be found that while only one position of the head and neck (in this particular application of the exercise) offers the greatest reduction in palpated tension or reported pain, there are other secondary positions which also offer some reduction in these two key elements (pain and hypertonicity), just as a number of the positions adopted during application of the 'box' exercise will demonstrably increase tension and/or pain.

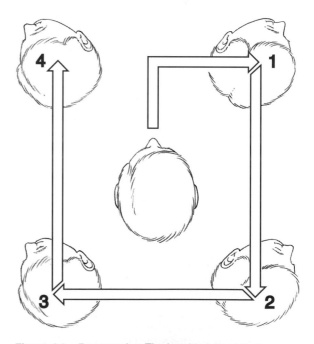

Figure 4.2   Box exercise. The head is taken into four positions: flexion with side-bending and rotation right (1), extension with side-bending and rotation right (2), extension with side-bending and rotation left (3), flexion with side-bending and rotation left (4). As these positions are gently adopted, tenderness and/or tissue tension is monitored.

Woolbright (1991) notes that there are what he terms 'mirror-image' points which are 'directly diagonally across from the anticipated position of release', and that these may at times offer a better position of ease than that designated as the likeliest by virtue of Jones' research.

Method[2]

● The patient/model is seated with the operator standing behind.

● The operator's right hand rests very lightly on the crown of the patient's head (palm on head, fingertips touching forehead, or the hand can be transversely placed on the head so that the heel of the hand is on one side and the fingertips on the other) while the left hand/fingertips palpate an area of tenderness and tension a little below the patient's left clavicle, in the pectoral muscles.

● As the patient exhales, the head is guided with minimal effort into flexion and it is gently side-bent and rotated to the right to go to position 1.

● Pausing momentarily to assess changes in the palpated tissues and/or to obtain feedback as to reduction or otherwise in sensitivity, the operator then takes the head out of right rotation (while maintaining a slight right side-bend) and as the patient inhales, the operator introduces a slight pressure on the brow which allows the head to 'float' up out of flexion and into extension. When the easy limit of extension is reached, rotation to the right is again introduced (position 2) (Fig. 4.1A).

● After a brief pause for evaluation, the head is then moved gently to the left, losing the right side-bending/rotation as the head crosses the midline. First side-bending and finally some rotation to the left, to an easy end-point, is introduced as the head comes to rest in position 3, still in extension.

● The head/neck is then, after a momentary pause, eased out of rotation and into flexion (during an exhalation) while left side-bending is maintained. Rotation to the left is again introduced as the head/neck comes to rest in flexion, as in position 4 (Fig. 4.1B).

● Taking the head back to the right and losing the side-bending/rotation at the midline returns it to the starting, neutral, position.

● Continuation to the right past the midline, again introducing flexion side-bending and subsequent rotation to the right takes it back to position 1.

● The head and neck are moved around the box (as described above) a number of times in order to assess for any additional relaxation (or increased bind) in the tissues under the palpating and monitoring hand.

● It is useful to try to note whether additional assistance to the process can be gained by having the patient/model, with eyes closed, 'look' up or down or sideways in the direction in which the head is moving, as it moves. Very often, experimenting with eye movements in this way allows for increased ease to be achieved, if the direction in which the eyes are looking is synchronised with the direction of movement.

● It is suggested that the operator can make the process of moving the model/patient around the box more fluid by duplicating the movements of the patient's eyes and breathing, as well as by leaning in the direction, and at the speed, of the movement that the patient is being directed to follow by the hand on the head.

● The whole exercise should be repeated a number of times (with different people) until the operator feels comfortable in using the 'box' approach to palpation of a specific tender point – noting the changes in tissue texture and reported

---

[2] All through this process, as the head/neck follows the pathway around the 'box', the momentary pauses held in each described position are designed to enhance the opportunity for evaluation of the palpated tissues. Woolbright says: 'Movement through the box should be fluidlike. A momentary hesitation should be made with each change in direction of movement as one moves serially from movement to movement and position to position.' The primary objective of the exercise is to allow the palpating hand to note which positions offer the most reduction in hypertonicity and/or which position(s) of the head/neck result in the greatest reduction in sensitivity, if the palpating fingers are applying compression to these tissues. It is a part of the training process for there to be a constant vigilance relating to the ever-changing feel of the tissues as they move from ease to bind and back again during the movements of the head/neck around the box.

pain under the listening/monitoring/palpating hand/finger.

● When palpating a posterior (extension) tender point, the box should be entered from neutral by first going into extension (on inhalation) with the addition of side-bending and rotation towards the side of the tender point followed by progressing around the box.

● When palpating an anterior (flexion) tender point, the box should be entered from neutral by flexing the head/neck (on exhalation) and then side-bending and rotating away from the side being palpated before progressing around the box.

● If, as the head and neck are being guided around the circuit of the box there seems to be a resistance to release of the tissues, a light muscle energy approach (a weak isometric contraction held for 7–10 seconds) can be usefully introduced to involve whichever tissues seem restricted and resistant, followed by a continuation of the movement through the box until a position of maximum ease is identified and held for 90 seconds.

2. SCS cervical flexion exercise

● The patient/model is supine and the operator sits or stands at the head of the table.

● An area of local dysfunction is sought using an appropriate form of palpation such as a 'feather-light', single-finger, stroking touch on the skin areas overlying the tips of the transverse processes of the cervical spine. Using this method, a feeling of 'drag' is being sought, which indicates increased sudomotor (sympathetic) activity and therefore a likely site of dysfunction, local or reflexively induced (Lewit 1991).

● When drag is noted, light compression is introduced to identify and establish a point of sensitivity, a tender point, which in this area represents (based on Jones' findings) an anterior (forward-bending) strain site.

● The patient is instructed in the method required for reporting a reduction in pain during the positioning sequence which follows. The author's approach is to say, 'I want you to score the pain caused by my pressure, before we start moving your head (in this example) as a "10" and

to not speak apart from giving me the present score (out of 10) whenever I ask for it'. The aim is to achieve a reported score of 3 or less before ceasing the positioning process. A commonly used American approach is to have the operator say to the patient, 'The pain when I press is a dollar's worth and I want you to tell me when the pain caused by my pressure is only worth 30 cents'.

● The head/neck is then taken lightly into flexion (see Fig. 4.3) until some degree of ease (based on the score, or the 'value', reported by the patient) is reported in the tender point, which is either being constantly compressed at this stage (this is the author's preference, if discomfort is not too great) (Chaitow 1991) or, intermittently probed (which is Jones' preference).

● When a reduction of pain by around 50% is achieved, fine-tuning is commenced, introducing a very small degree of additional positioning in order to find the position of maximum ease, at which time the reported 'score' should be reduced by at least 70%.

● At this time the patient may be asked to inhale fully and exhale fully, while observing for themselves changes in the palpated pain point, in

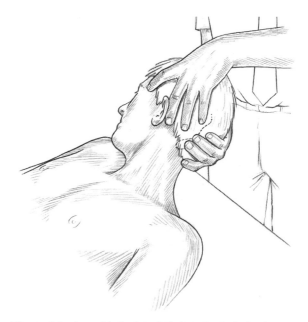

Figure 4.3 Learning to use strain/counterstrain for the treatment of a cervical flexion strain.

order to evaluate which phase of the cycle reduces it still more. That phase of the breathing cycle in which they sense the greatest reduction in sensitivity is maintained for a period which is tolerable to the patient (holding the breath in or out or at some point between the two extremes), while the overall position of ease continues to be maintained and the tender/tense area monitored.

● This position of ease is held for 90 seconds in Jones' methodology, although there exist mechanisms for reducing this, which will be explained in the next chapter. During the holding of the position of ease, the direct compression can be reduced to a mere touching of the point, along with a periodic probing to establish that the position of ease has been maintained.

● After 90 seconds, the neck/head is very slowly returned to the neutral starting position. This slow return to neutral is a vital component of SCS, since the neural receptors (muscle spindles) may be provoked into a return to their previously dysfunctional state if a rapid movement is made at the end of the procedure.

● The tender point/area may be retested for sensitivity at this time and should be found to be considerably less hypertonic.

3. SCS cervical extension exercise

● With the patient/model in the supine position but with the head clear of the end of the table and fully supported by the operator, areas of localised tenderness are sought by light palpation alongside or over the tips of the spinous processes of the cervical spine.

● Having located a tender point, compression is applied to elicit a degree of sensitivity or pain which the model/patient notes as representing a score of '10'.

● The head/neck is then taken into light extension along with side-bending and rotation, as in Fig. 4.4 (usually away from the side of the pain if this is not central), until a reduction of at least 50% is achieved in the reported sensitivity.

● The compression can be constant or intermittent, with the latter being preferable, if sensitivity is great.

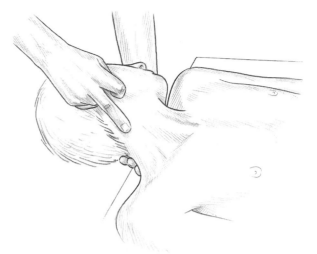

Figure 4.4 Learning to use strain/counterstrain for the treatment of a cervical extension strain.

● Once a reduction in sensitivity of at least 70% is achieved, inhalation and exhalation are monitored by the patient/model to see which reduces sensitivity even more, and this phase of the cycle is maintained for a comfortable period (Jones recommends 90 seconds).

● If intermittent compression of the point is being used this needs to be applied periodically during the 90-second holding period, in order to ensure that the position of ease has been maintained.

● After 90 seconds, a very slow and deliberate return to neutral is performed and the patient is rested for several minutes.

● The tender point should be repalpated for sensitivity, which may have reduced markedly, as should any sense of hypertonicity in the surrounding tissues.

4. SCS 'tissue tension' exercise
(Chaitow 1990)

SCS exercises 2 and 3 should be performed again; however, this time, instead of relying on feedback from the patient as to the degree of sensitivity being experienced in the tender point and using this feedback as the guide which takes the operator towards the ideal position of ease, the operator's own palpation of the tissues and their movement towards ease becomes the guide.

A light contact is maintained in the same place as pain/sensitivity was elicited from the tender point, while positioning of the head and neck is carried out, to achieve maximum `ease'.

A final position should be achieved which closely approximates the position in which reduction of the pain was achieved in the previous exercises.

This is an exercise which begins a process of palpatory skill acquisition and enhancement, which will be carried further in exercises involving functional technique described later in Chapter 8.

5. SCS exercise involving compression

Exercises 1, 2 and 3 should be performed again, but this time when pain/sensitivity and/or hypertonicity has reduced by 70% via positioning, and after the breathing element has been carried out to aid this process, a light degree of 'crowding' or compression is introduced by means of pressure onto the crown of the head through the long axis of the spine. No more than 1 lb (0.5 kg) of pressure should be involved. This can be achieved by use of pressure from the operator's abdomen, or from the hands which are holding and supporting the neck and head themselves.

This additional element of crowding/slackening the tissues should not increase either the sensitivity from the palpated point or cause pain anywhere else. If it does, crowding should be abandoned.

The more usual response is for the patient to report an even greater degree of pain relief and for the operator to sense greater ease in the palpated tissues.

This addition of crowding to the procedures reduces the time required during which the position of ease needs to be held, and mimics a major feature of a more recently introduced variation on the theme of positional release methodology, facilitated positional release (FPR – see Chapter 9). The time-scale for SCS when crowding is a feature is commonly given as 5–20 seconds.

6. SCS low back/lower limb exercise

With the patient prone, one of the lower limbs can be used as a 'handle' with which to modify tone and tension in the low back, as an area of this is palpated (Fig. 4.5).

The practitioner palpates an area of the lumbar musculature as a systematic evaluation is carried out of the effects of moving the ipsilateral or contralateral limb into (easy) extension, adduction and internal rotation, followed (having removed the rotation) by abduction and external rotation, while still in extension. This could be followed (after removing the rotation) by taking the abducted limb into flexion (over the edge of the table) and then external rotation, and finally, while still in flexion, removing the rotation by taking the limb into adduction and at its easy end-of-range introducing internal rotation. In this way an approximation of a 'box' movement will have been created while a low back area is palpated for changes in perceived pain or modifications of tone.

Assess which positions offer the greatest ease in low back areas as this sequence is repeated several times.

Evaluate whether greater influence is noted in the tissues being palpated when the ipsilateral or contralateral leg is employed as a lever.

According to SCS theory and clinical experience the likeliest positions of ease will be noted

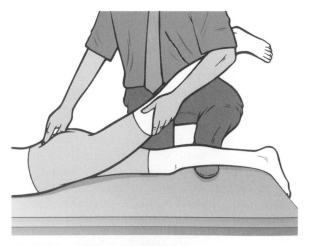

Figure 4.5 SCS lower limb exercise.

with the contralateral leg in extension. Other variables will influence which parts of the low back eases most when the limb is adducted or abducted and internally or externally rotated.

7. SCS upper limb exercise

Similarly, an arm can be used to introduce a series of movements while palpating tenderness and tension in the lateral epicondyle area. The patient is supine and one hand palpates the area of the lateral epicondyle. The other hand holds the wrist as the elbow is placed into extension with side-bending and rotation towards the side of the palpated tender point (i.e. externally).

Assess changes of palpated tone and reported pain with the arm in this position, and then introduce side-bending and rotation internally (still in extension) before introducing flexion, and while in flexion assessing the changes in palpated tone and reported discomfort. Introduce either internal or external rotation with side-bending to assess changes (Fig. 4.6).

The most probable position of ease for an anterior lateral epicondyle tender point is flexion with side-bending and external rotation. However, as in all tender points, the particular mechanisms involved in the dysfunctional strain

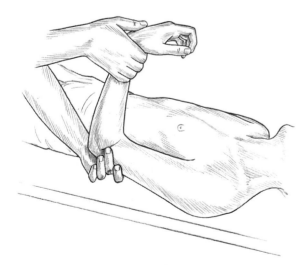

Figure 4.6 The lateral epicondyle is palpated as various positions of the lower arm (flexion, extension, rotation) are introduced to evaluate their influence on the palpated tissues.

pattern can make such predictions meaningless. In the end it is the position which achieves the maximum degree of ease, which produces the most beneficial effects.

These exercises offer a useful starting point for anyone new to SCS.

8. The Spencer shoulder sequence exercise

Note: Although described in this chapter as an 'exercise' the Spencer sequence is extremely useful clinically as an assessment and treatment approach. It should be obvious that instead of positional release methods, as described in the 'exercise' below, muscle energy techniques or other modalities could also be usefully employed.

The Spencer sequence, which derives from osteopathic medicine in the early years of the 20th century (Spencer 1916), is taught at all osteopathic colleges in the USA. Over the years it has been modified to include treatment elements other than the original articulation, mobilisation intent. The sequences can be transformed from an assessment/articulatory technique into a muscle energy approach or into a positional release method.

When used for assessment and treatment, the scapula is fixed firmly to the thoracic wall to focus on involvement of the glenohumeral joint, as a variety of movements are introduced, one at a time.

In all Spencer assessment and treatment sequences, the patient is side-lying, with the side to be assessed uppermost, arm lying at the side with the elbow (usually) flexed, with the practitioner facing slightly cephalad, at chest level (Patriquin 1992) (Fig. 4.7).

Assessment and PRT treatment of shoulder extension restriction

● The practitioner's cephalad hand cups the shoulder, firmly compressing the scapula and clavicle to the thorax while the patient's flexed elbow is held by the practitioner's caudad hand, as the arm is taken into passive extension towards the optimal 90°.

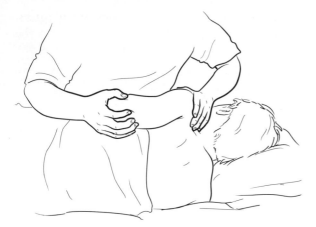

Figure 4.7 Spencer sequence treatment of shoulder extension restriction.

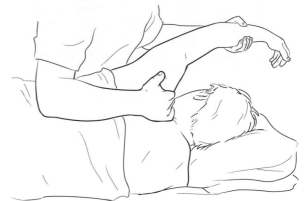

Figure 4.8 Spencer sequence treatment of shoulder flexion restriction.

- Any restriction in range of motion is noted, ceasing movement at the first indication of resistance.
- If restriction is noted during movement towards extension, the soft tissues implicated in maintaining this dysfunction would be the shoulder flexors – anterior deltoid, coracobrachialis and the clavicular head of pectoralis major.
- Palpation of these should reveal areas of marked tenderness.
- The most painful tender point (painful to digital pressure) elicited by palpation is used as a monitoring point as the arm is moved into a position which will reduce that pain by not less than 70%.
- This position of ease usually involves some degree of flexion and fine-tuning to slacken the muscle housing the tender point.
- This ease state should be held for 90 seconds, before a slow return to neutral and a subsequent re-evaluation of the range of motion.

Assessment and PRT treatment of shoulder flexion restriction

- Patient and practitioner have the same starting position as in the previous test (Fig. 4.7).
- The practitioner's non-table-side hand grasps the patient's forearm while the table-side hand holds the clavicle and scapula firmly to the chest wall.

- The practitioner slowly introduces passive shoulder flexion in the horizontal plane, as range of motion to 180° is assessed, by which time the elbow is fully extended (Fig. 4.8).
- At the very first indication of restriction in movement the movement into flexion ceases.
- If there is a restriction towards flexion, the soft tissues implicated in maintaining this dysfunction would be the shoulder extensors – posterior deltoid, teres major, latissimus dorsi, and possibly infraspinatus, teres minor and long head of triceps.
- Palpation of these should reveal areas of marked tenderness.
- The most painful tender point (painful to digital pressure) elicited by palpation should be used as a monitoring point, as the arm is moved into a position which will reduce that pain by not less than 70%.
- This position of ease will probably involve some degree of extension and fine-tuning to slacken the muscle housing the tender point.
- This ease state should be held for 90 seconds before a slow return to neutral and a subsequent re-evaluation of range of motion.

Shoulder articulation and assessment of circumduction capability with compression

- The patient is side-lying with elbow flexed while the practitioner's cephalad hand cups the

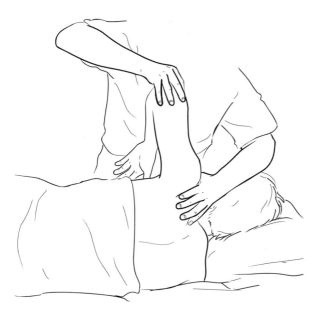

Figure 4.9 Spencer sequence assessment of circumduction capability with compression.

shoulder firmly, compressing the scapula and clavicle to the thorax (Fig. 4.9).

• The practitioner's caudad hand grasps the elbow and takes the shoulder through a slow clockwise (and subsequently an anti-clockwise) circumduction, while adding compression through the long axis of the humerus.

• Subsequently the same assessment is made with light traction being applied.

• If restriction or pain is noted in either of the circumduction sequences (clockwise and anti-clockwise, utilising compression or traction), evaluate which muscles would be active if precisely the opposite movement were undertaken.

• For example, if on compression and clockwise rotation, a particular part of the circumduction range involves either restriction or discomfort/pain, cease the movement and evaluate which muscles would be required to contract in order to produce an active reversal of that movement (Chaitow 1996, Jones 1981, Walther 1988).

• In these antagonist muscles, palpate for the most 'tender' point and use this as a monitoring point as the structures are taken to a position of ease which reduces the perceived pain by at least 70%.

• This is held for 90 seconds before a slow return to neutral, and retesting.

 Assessment and PRT treatment of shoulder abduction restriction

• The patient is side-lying as the practitioner cups the shoulder and compresses the scapula and clavicle to thorax with his cephalad hand, while cupping the flexed elbow with his caudad hand.

• The patient's hand is supported on the practitioner's cephalad forearm/wrist to stabilise the arm (Fig. 4.10).

• The elbow is abducted towards the patient's head as range of motion is assessed.

• Some degree of external rotation is also involved in this abduction.

• Pain-free easy abduction should be close to 180°.

• Note any restriction in range of motion.

• At the position of very first indication of resistance, the movement is stopped.

• If there is a restriction towards abduction the soft tissues implicated in maintaining this dysfunction would be the shoulder adductors – pectoralis major, teres major, latissimus dorsi,

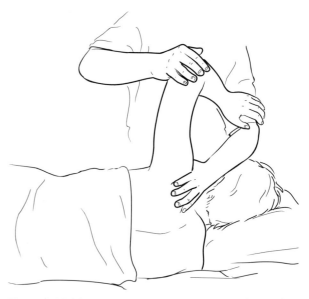

Figure 4.10 Spencer sequence assessment and treatment of shoulder abduction restriction.

and possibly the long head of triceps, coraco-brachialis, short head of biceps brachii.
- Since external rotation is also occurring in this movement there might be involvement of internal rotators in any restriction or pain.
- Palpation of these muscles should reveal areas of marked tenderness.
- The most painful tender point (painful to digital pressure) elicited by this palpation should be used as a monitoring point, as the arm is moved and fine-tuned into a position which reduces that pain by not less than 70%.
- This position of ease will probably involve some degree of adduction and external rotation, to slacken the muscle housing the tender point.
- This ease state should be held for 90 seconds, before a slow return to neutral and a subsequent re-evaluation of range of motion.

Assessment and PRT treatment of shoulder adduction restriction

- The patient is side-lying and the practitioner cups the shoulder and compresses the scapula and clavicle to the thorax with his cephalad hand, while cupping the elbow with his caudad hand.
- The patient's hand is supported on the practitioner's cephalad forearm/wrist to stabilise the arm.
- The elbow is taken in an arc forward of the chest so that the elbow moves both cephalad and medially as the shoulder adducts and externally rotates.
- The action is performed slowly and any signs of resistance are noted.
- If there is a restriction towards adduction the soft tissues implicated in maintaining this dysfunction would be the shoulder abductors – deltoid, supraspinatus.
- Since external rotation is also involved, other muscles implicated in restriction or pain may include internal rotators such as subscapularis, pectoralis major, latissimus dorsi and teres major.
- Palpation of these should reveal areas of marked tenderness.
- The most painful tender point (painful to digital pressure) elicited by palpation should be

used as a monitoring point as the arm is moved into a position which will reduce that pain by not less than 70%.
- This position of ease will probably involve some degree of abduction together with fine-tuning involving internal rotation, to slacken the muscle housing the tender point.
- This ease state should be held for 90 seconds before a slow return to neutral and a subsequent re-evaluation of range of motion.

Assessment and MET treatment of internal rotation restriction

- The patient is side-lying and her flexed arm is placed behind her back to evaluate whether the dorsum of the hand can be painlessly placed against the dorsal surface of the ipsilateral lumbar area (Fig. 4.11).
- This arm position is maintained throughout the procedure.
- The practitioner cups the shoulder and compresses the scapula and clavicle to the thorax with his cephalad hand while cupping the flexed elbow with the caudad hand.
- The practitioner slowly brings the elbow (ventrally) towards his body and notes any sign of restriction as this movement, which increases internal rotation, proceeds.

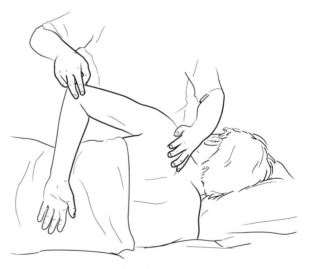

Figure 4.11 Spencer sequence assessment and treatment of internal rotation restriction.

- At the position of very first indication of resistance, movement is stopped.
- If there is a restriction towards internal rotation the soft tissues implicated in maintaining this dysfunction would be the shoulder external rotators – infraspinatus and teres minor – with posterior deltoid also possibly being involved.
- Palpation of these should reveal areas of marked tenderness.
- The most painful tender point (painful to digital pressure) elicited by palpation should be used as a monitoring point as the arm is moved into a position which will reduce that pain by not less than 70%.
- This position of ease will probably involve some degree of external rotation to slacken the muscle housing the tender point.
- This ease state should be held for 90 seconds before a slow return to neutral and a subsequent re-evaluation of range of motion.

Note: All Spencer assessments are performed passively in a controlled, slow, manner.

REFERENCES

Chaitow L 1990 Palpatory Literacy. Thorsons/Harper Collins, London

Chaitow L 1991 Modified strain/counterstrain. In: Soft Tissue Manipulation. Healing Arts Press, Rochester

Chaitow L 1996 Palpation Skills. Churchill Livingstone, Edinburgh

D'Ambrogio K, Roth G 1997 Positional Release Therapy. Mosby, St Louis

Jones L 1964 Spontaneous release by positioning. The Doctor of Osteopathy 4: 109–116

Jones L 1981 Strain and Counterstrain. Academy of Applied Osteopathy, Colorado Springs

Lewit K 1991 Manipulative Therapy in Rehabilitation of the Locomotor System. Butterworths, London

McPartland J M, Klofat I 1995 Strain und Counterstrain-Technik Kursunterlagen. Landesverbände der Deutschen Gesellschaft für Manuelle Medizin, Baden

Patriquin D 1992 Evolution of osteopathic manipulative technique: the Spencer technique. American Osteopathic Association 92: 1134–1146

Schiowitz S 1990 Facilitated positional release. J American Osteopathic Association 90(2): 145 156

Schwartz H 1986 The use of counterstrain in an acutely ill in-hospital population. J American Osteopathic Association 86(7): 433–442

Spencer H 1916 Shoulder technique. J American Osteopathic Association 15: 2118–2220

Walther D 1988 Applied Kinesiology. SDC Systems, Pueblo

Weiselfish S 1993 Manual Therapy for the Orthopedic and Neurologic Patient. Regional Physical Therapy, Hertford, Connecticut

Woolbright J 1991 An alternative method of teaching strain/counterstrain manipulation. J American Osteopathic Association 91(4): 370–376

5

Goodheart and Morrison's positional release variations and 'lift' techniques

GOODHEART'S PR VARIATIONS

George Goodheart (1984) has adapted Jones' original work in ways which make it more accessible, reducing the need for the constant reference to, or memorising of, lists and illustrations of the positions of hundreds of specifically sited tender points which Jones described in his years of research.

As briefly outlined in Chapter 1 (p. 6), Goodheart suggests that a suitable tender point be sought in the tissues antagonistic to those which are active when pain or restriction is observed or reported. In such circumstances, the antagonist muscles to those operating at the time pain is noted (or restriction observed or felt) will be those that house the tender point(s), and these are identified by palpation. Another way of understanding this concept is to consider that tender points will usually be found in tissues which have shortened. Take for example a situation in which:

- Turning the head to the right is either painful or restricted.
- The muscles operating to produce that action would be the muscles on the right of the neck, as well as the left sternocleidomastoid muscle.
- Restriction might well involve shortening of the muscles on the left.
- According to Goodheart's guidelines ('seek tender point in antagonist muscle to those active when pain or restriction is noted'), it is in these shortened structures that a tender point should be sought, and used as a monitor during SCS positioning.

- It is very important to avoid confusion which can derive from seeking a tender point in the tissues opposite the *site of pain* on movement. It is in the tissues opposite (antagonists to) those *which are active* in producing the painful or restricted movement that house the appropriate tender point.

Goodheart also suggests a simple test to identify a tender point's need for application of SCS, stating that if the muscle with which it is associated tests as weak following a maximal 3-second contraction, after first testing strong, it will benefit from positional release (Walther 1988).

Finally, he has shown that when the positional release treatment is successful the muscle will no longer weaken after a short, strong isometric contraction.

Whereas Jones' use of SCS is largely focused towards treatment of painful conditions, that of Goodheart has a different target. He has found that the neuromuscular function of muscles can be improved using SCS, even if no pain is present.

Goodheart's associate, David Walther, notes that:

Neuromuscular dysfunction that responds to strain/counterstrain technique may be from recent trauma, or be buried in the patient's history.

Goodheart and Walther agree with the interpretation of the role of neurological imbalance, which Jones and Korr (Korr 1975) have described as a key factor leading to many forms of soft tissue and joint dysfunction (see Ch. 3 p. 32), in which antagonistic muscles have failed to return to neurological equilibrium following acute or chronic strain. When this happens, an abnormal neuromuscular pattern will have been established which can benefit from positional release treatment. The muscles shortened in the process of strain, and not those stretched, and where pain is commonly sited, are the tissues which are utilised in the process of rebalancing. 'Understanding that the cause of the continued pain one suffers in a strain/counterstrain condition is usually not at the location of pain but in an antagonistic muscle is the most important step in solving the problem', says Walther. The tender point might lie in muscle, tendon, or ligament

and the perpetuating factor is the imbalance in the spindle cell mechanisms.

Since the patient can usually easily describe which movements increase their pain (or which are restricted) the search sites for tender areas are easily decided. It is necessary to seek tender points in tissues antagonistic to those involved in the active movement which hurts or is restricted. The tender points related to any such dysfunction pain or functional imbalance will lie in the shortened rather than the stretched tissues and fibres.

As stated above, Goodheart adds one more test to muscles which appear to require SCS treatment: he tests them for strength and if they are not weak, he has the muscle maximally contract for 3 seconds, after which, if it tests as weak, it is classified as suitable for SCS attention.

Goodheart's approach can usually be taught to patients for self-help or first-aid use. If taught appropriately, simple stiffness and discomfort can be self-treated. The patient may have an explanation offered, such as:

- If you wake with a stiff neck, test to see which direction of movement is stiffest, or hurts most.
- From that position, take your head back to its comfortable resting position, and as you do so feel to see which muscles are working to get you there.
- In these muscles, opposite those working when the painful or restricted movement is made, feel around for a very tender point.
- Once you have found this, gently position your head to take the pain away from the point you are lightly pressing – without creating any new pain.
- Once you have done this stay in that 'ease' position for several minutes then slowly return to normal, and see if the stiffness or pain has reduced. It will usually be much better.

Reducing the time the position of ease is held

Additionally, Goodheart has found that it is possible to reduce the length of time for which the position of ease is held, without losing the therapeutic benefits derived from the neurological and/or circulatory effects (see Ch. 3, p. 37) which are offered by that position's being maintained for 90 seconds, as in Jones' approach.

There are two elements to Goodheart's innovation:

1. When the position of ease has been found, a 'respiration assist' is added. The nature of the respiratory strategy used depends upon the location of the tender point: if it lies on the anterior surface of the body inhalation is used, and if on the posterior aspect, exhalation is used. This phase of breathing is held for as long as is comfortable, during which time the practitioner adds the second element.
2. A stretching of the tissues being palpated (the tender point) is introduced by means of the practitioner's fingers being spread over the tissues (Fig. 5.1).

Walther reports on Goodheart's approach as follows:

The patient takes a deep breath [the inhalation or exhalation phase being held, depending on anterior or posterior location of point] and holds it while the physician spreads his fingers over the previously tender point. The patient is maintained in the 'fine-tuned' position with the physician's fingers spreading the point and respiration assist for 30 seconds, as opposed to 90 seconds required without the assisting factors. On completion the patient is slowly and passively returned to a neutral position.

Effects of respiration

Is Goodheart's breathing instruction too simplistic?

It is necessary to look a little beyond the fact that clinical experience often supports Goodheart's breathing guidelines in application of SCS, in order to gain an understanding of what might be happening physiologically.

Cummings and Howell (1990) have demonstrated the effects of respiration on myofascial tension, showing that there is a mechanical effect of respiration on resting myofascial tissue (using the elbow flexors as the tissue being evaluated). They quote the work of Kisselkova and Georgiev (1976), who reported that resting EMG activity of

the biceps brachii, quadriceps femoris and gastrocnemius muscles, for example, 'cycled with respiration following bicycle ergonometer exercise, thus demonstrating that non-respiratory muscles receive input from the respiratory centres'.

They concluded that, 'these studies document both a mechanically and a neurologically mediated influence on the tension produced by myofascial tissues, which gives objective verification of the clinically observed influence of respiration on the musculoskeletal system and validation of its potential role in manipulative therapy'. But what is that role?

Lewit has helped to create subdivisions in the simplistic picture of 'breathing in enhances effort' and 'breathing out enhances movement', and a detailed reading of his book, *Manipulative Therapy in Rehabilitation of the Locomotor System* (Lewit 1991) is recommended for those who wish to understand the complexities of the mechanisms involved.

Among the simpler relationships which he has identified are:

- Movement into flexion of the lumbar and cervical spines is assisted by exhalation; and
- Movement into extension of the lumbar and cervical spine is assisted by inhalation; whereas
- Movement into extension of the thoracic spine is assisted by exhalation, while
- Thoracic flexion is enhanced by inhalation.

The influences of breathing on the tone of extensor and flexor muscles would therefore seem to be somewhat more complex than Goodheart's suggestions indicate, with an increase in tone being evident in the extensors of the thoracic spine during exhalation, while, at the same time, the flexors of the cervical and lumbar spine are also toned. Similarly, inhalation increases tone in the flexors of the thoracic spine and the extensors of the cervical and lumbar regions.

Goodheart's proposed pattern of breathing during application of SCS would therefore increase tone in some of the tissues being treated, while inhibiting their antagonists.

Since the 'finger spread', which he also advocates during SCS, increases strength/tone in the tissues being treated, the use of a held breath would seem to require more discrimination than the simple injunction to hold the breath in inhalation when treating flexor muscles and in exhalation when treating extensors.

Why spread the fingers?

Strain/counterstrain methods act upon the muscle spindles which lie throughout the muscle, with greatest concentration in the centre, around the belly (Gowitzke & Milner 1980). There are many more spindles found in muscles with an active (phasic) function than are found in those with a stabilising, postural (tonic) function.

The role of spindles (based on the complex interplay between intra- and extrafusal fibres) is as a length comparator, as well as a means for supplying the central nervous system with information as to the rate of change (Figs 5.1 and 5.2). Spindles also exert an effect on the strength displayed by the muscle, a phenomenon which is used in applied kinesiology (AK) and which Goodheart has incorporated into his version of SCS methodology.

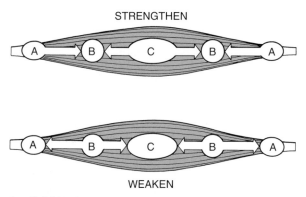

STRENGTHEN

WEAKEN

A = Golgi tendon organs
B = belly of muscle
C = muscle spindle

Figure 5.1 Proprioceptive manipulation of muscles. Pressure directed away from the belly of a muscle (B) towards the Golgi tendon organs (A) produces relaxation of the muscle, while pressure towards the belly of a muscle (B) from the region of the Golgi tendon organs (A) tones 'strengthens' it. Pressure near the belly of the muscle (B) towards the muscle spindle (C) weakens it, while pressure away from the spindle (C), near the belly (B), tones/'strengthens' it.

Spindle density is not uniform, for example muscles in the cervical region contain a high density of muscle spindles, especially the deep suboccipital muscles. Peck et al (1984) report that rectus capitis posterior minor muscles are rich in proprioceptors, containing an average of 36 spindles/g muscle. Rectus capitis posterior major muscles average 30.5 spindles/g muscle. In contrast, the splenius capitis contains 7.6 spindles/g muscle, while gluteus maximus contains only 0.8 spindles/g muscle.

If the operator's thumbs are placed about 5 cm apart over the belly of the muscle, where spindles are most densely sited, and heavy pressure is exerted by means of the thumbs pushing towards each other – parallel with the fibres of the muscle in question – a weakening effect will be noted if the muscle has been previously tested and is now tested again (see Fig. 5.1).

The explanation lies in the neurology, as Walther explains:

The digital manoeuvre appears to take pressure off the intrafusal muscle fibres, causing a decrease in the afferent nerve impulse and, in turn, causing temporary [minutes at most] inhibition of the extrafusal fibres.

If this experiment fails at first it may be because the precise location of spindles has not been influenced and repetition is called for (and this is especially likely in muscles with sparse spindle presence, see above regarding spindle density).

This effect of 'weakening' a muscle can be reversed by means of the precisely opposite manipulation of the spindles, in which the thumbs which are pressing into the tissues are 'pulled' apart. This will only 'strengthen' a hypotonic or inhibited, weak muscle and will not enhance the strength of an already strong one.

Recall that Goodheart suggests applying SCS techniques to muscles only when they initially test as being of 'normal' strength, and which test as becoming weak following a short – 3-second – isometric contraction, which he maintains indicates a neuromuscular imbalance, possibly involving neuromuscular spindle cell function.

The introduction of a spread of the fingers over the spindle cells, during the time in which the tissues in which the spindles lie are being held in a

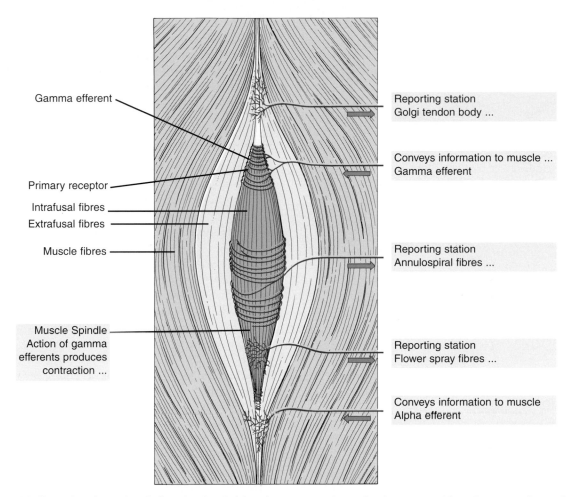

Figure 5.2 Illustration of muscle spindles, showing Golgi tendon organs and neural pathways to and from these reporting stations.

position of ease, strengthens the muscle and inhibits the antagonist to that muscle; a combination of influences which apparently enhances the process of balancing of neuromuscular function and reduces the time required for the spindle to 'reset'.

Testing the muscle by means of a short, strong isometric contraction after such SCS treatment should now fail to result in its weakening, according to Goodheart's approach.

Psoas treatment using Goodheart's protocol

The supine patient is asked to contract the muscle maximally against the operator's resist-ance, by means of hip flexion, adduction and external rotation, for 3 seconds (Fig. 5.3A).

If the muscle tests as being weaker than previously, it is considered suitable for Goodheart's SCS approach.

The tender point for psoas usually lies in the belly of the muscle where it crosses the pubic bone. This is palpated by a finger and thumb, or two fingers, while the hip is taken into flexion in order to shorten psoas. Fine-tuning is introduced to remove sensitivity from the palpated point (Fig. 5.3B).

Goodheart's refinements are now added, as the patient is asked to inhale deeply and to hold the breath, while at the same time the operator

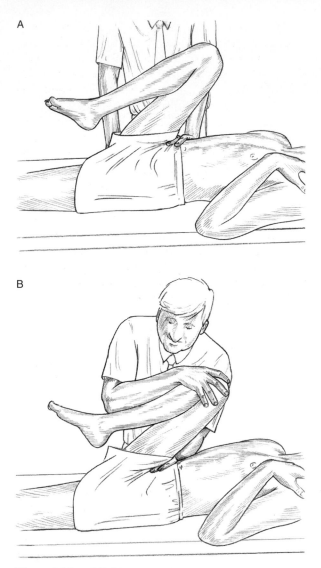

Figure 5.3A and B Treatment of psoas dysfunction using Goodheart's protocol to achieve ease. (**A**) hand position, (**B**) final position of ease.

strongly spreads the fingers[1] which are in contact with the tender point. This is held for 30 seconds, with the patient being told to let the breath go when they feel any sign of strain in holding it.

---

[1] Walthers (1988) advises that in areas where a two-finger stretch is not possible, a stretch applied by one finger will be found to effectively influence the amount of time needed to hold the position of ease.

After 30 seconds, the patient's leg is very slowly and passively returned to a neutral position. A retest of the effects of a short, strong isometric contraction should no longer produce a weakening effect and symptoms of psoas imbalance should be reduced or normalised.

Goodheart's coccygeal lift technique

Different uses of what appear to be SCS mechanisms have been evolved by clinicians such as George Goodheart and Marsh Morrison (see induration technique described in Ch. 1, p. 9, and the inguinal lift method later in this chapter, p. 92).

Goodheart has described a method which seems to rely on the crowding, or slackening, of spinal dural tissues, with the coccyx being used as the means of achieving this. Startling results in terms of improved function and release of hypertonicity in areas some distance from the point of application are claimed (Goodheart 1985). Goodheart's term for this is a 'filum terminale cephalad lift': it is proposed that this be shortened to 'coccygeal lift', at least in this text.

This method focuses on normalising flexion/extension dysfunction between the spinal column and the spinal cord, despite the spiral nature of the manner in which the spine copes with forced flexion (Illi 1951).

Goodheart and Walther report that there is frequently a dramatic lengthening of the spinal column after application of the coccygeal lift procedure with Goodheart mentioning specifically that, in good health, there should be no difference greater than about half an inch in the measured length of the spinal column sitting, standing and lying, using a tapeless measure which is rolled along the length of the spine.

Goodheart quotes from the work of Upledger and of Breig in order to substantiate physiological and pathological observations which he makes relating to the dura, its normal freedom of movement, and some of its potential for problem-causing when restricted (Breig 1978, Upledger 1984).

Breig states that, using radiography, microscopic examination and mechano-elastic models, it has been shown that there are deforming forces, which relate to normal movements of the spine, impinging on the spinal cord and meninges, from the brain stem to the conus medullaris and the spinal nerves.

Upledger, in discussion of the physiological motion of the central nervous system recalls that, when assisting in neurosurgery in 1971, in which extradural calcification was being removed from the posterior aspect of the dural tube in the mid-cervical region, his task was to hold the dura with two pairs forceps during the procedure. However, he states:

The membrane would not hold still, the fully anaesthetised patient was in a sitting position … and it became apparent the movement of the dural membrane was rhythmical, independent of the patient's cardiac or respiratory rhythms.

Goodheart states:

Tension can be exerted where the foramen magnum is attached to the dura, and also at the 1st, 2nd and 3rd cervicals, which if they are in a state of fixation can limit motion. The dural tube is completely free of any dural attachment all the way down to the 2nd anterior sacral segment where finally the filum terminale attaches to the posterior portion of the 1st coccygeal segment. The release which comes from the coccygeal lift cannot be just a linear longitudinal tension problem. The body is intricately simple and simply intricate and once we understand the closed kinematic chain and the concept of the finite length of the dura, we can see how spinal adjustments can sometimes allow compensations to take place.

What is happening?

The anatomy of what is happening and the process of utilising this procedure is briefly explained as follows (Sutherland 1939, Williams & Warwick 1980):

- The dura mater attaches firmly to the foramen magnum, axis and 3rd cervical vertebrae, and possibly to the atlas, with a direct effect on the meninges.
- Its caudad attachments are to the dorsum of the 1st coccygeal segment by means of a long filament, the filum terminale.
- Flexion of the spine alters the length of the intervertebral canal, while the cord and the

dura have a finite length (the dura being approximately 2.5 inches longer than the cord, allowing some degree of slack when the individual sits), which Goodheart reasons requires some form of 'arrangement' between the caudal and the cephalad attachments of the dura, a 'take-up' mechanism to allow for maintenance of proper tension on the cord.
- Measurement of the distance between the external occipital protuberance to the tip of the coccyx shows very little variation from the standing to the sitting and lying positions. However, if all the contours between these points are measured in the different positions, a wide variation is found: the greater the degree of difference the more likely there is to be spinal dysfunction and, Goodheart postulates, dural restriction and possible meningeal tension.
- Tender areas of the neck flexors or extensors are used as the means of monitoring the lift of the coccyx which is to follow: as the palpated pain and/or hypertonicity eases, so is the ideal degree of lift being approached.

Method

- With the patient prone, the operator stands at waist level. After palpation and identification of the area of greatest discomfort and/or hypertonicity in the cervical spinal musculature with the operator's cephalad hand, the index finger of the caudad hand is placed so that the tip of the index or middle finger is on the very tip of the coccyx, while the hand and fingers follow precisely the contours of the coccyx and sacrum (Figs 5.4A and 5.4B).
- This contact slowly and gently takes out the available slack as it lifts the coccyx, along its entire length including the tip, directly towards the painful contact on the neck, using anything up to 15 lb (7.5 kg) of force.
- If the painful monitoring point does not ease dramatically, the direction of lift is altered (by a few degrees only) slightly towards one shoulder or the other.
- Once the pain has been removed from the neck point, and without inducing additional pain in

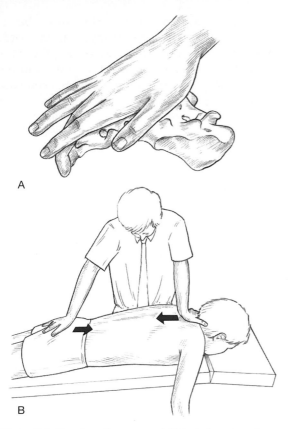

A

B

Figure 5.4 Goodheart's coccygeal lift technique for release of dural restrictions (see text). Operator's left hand is monitoring sensitivity ('tender point') in the cervical region as the coccyx is eased towards the head.

the coccyx, this position is maintained for up to 1 minute.

- Additional ease to the restricted or torsioned dural sleeve can be achieved by using the hand which is palpating the cervical structures to impart a gentle caudal traction by means of holding the occipital area in such a way as to lightly compress it while easing it towards the sacrum (so moving the upper three cervical segments inferiorly) as the patient exhales. This hold is maintained for 4 or 5 cycles of breathing.

Goodheart and others report dramatic changes in function, lengthening of the spine so that it measures equally in all positions, reduction in cervical dysfunction, removal of chronic headaches and release of tension in psoas and piriformis.

Variations The author has commonly found the following variations to make application of the coccygeal lift less difficult to achieve:

- Once identified, the patient can apply the compression force to the tender area which is being used as a monitor until ease is achieved. This frees the operator so that positioning and application of the coccygeal lift is less stressful. The position described above, as advised by Goodheart and Walther, can be awkward if the operator is slight and the patient tall.
- A side-lying position of the patient can allow for an even less uncomfortable (for the operator) application of the procedure. In this instance, the patient monitors the pain in the cervical area once the operator has identified it. The operator stands at upper thigh level, behind the side-lying patient and, using the fifth finger aspect of the cephalad hand to achieve contact along the whole length of the coccyx, with the elbow braced against the hip/abdomen area, the force required to achieve the lift is applied by means of the operator leaning into the hand contact while the caudad hand stabilises the anterior pelvis of the patient.

As in Jones' SCS methods, the patient reports on the changes in palpated pain levels until a 70% reduction is achieved.

MORRISON'S 'INGUINAL LIFT'

American chiropractor Marsh Morrison was responsible for popularising a number of methods which bear a close resemblance to strain/counterstrain and certainly fall into the context of positional release methods.

His 'induration' technique was described in Chapter 1 (p. 9), and in this section a method which has a passing similarity to Goodheart's coccygeal lift method is presented.

Morrison maintained that most women who periodically wear high heels present with a degree of what he termed 'pelvic slippage' (Morrison 1969). The use of the approach described below is meant to enable low back adjustments to 'hold'. He recommended its application when low back problems failed to respond to more usual methods, since he maintained that the pelvic imbalance could act to prevent the normalisation of spinal dysfunction.

Method

- The patient lies supine with legs apart.
- The superior margin of the pubis should be palpated, close to the inguinal area. Pain will be found on the side of 'slippage'. This painful site is palpated by the patient and the same reporting of a numerical value for the pain as was described in detail in Chapter 3 (p. 50) should be used, with the objective of reducing pain during the procedure, from a starting level of 10, by at least 70%.
- The patient (if male) should be asked to hold the genitals towards the non-treated side. Whether the patient is male or female a second person should be in the room, since the operator is in a vulnerable position when engaging the inguinal area.
- The operator stands to the side of the patient just below waist level on the side to be treated, and places the flat table-side hand on the inner thigh so that the web between finger and thumb comes into contact with the tendon of gracilis, at the ischiopubic junction.
- It is important to have the contact hand on the gracilis tendon relaxed, not rigid, with the 'lift' effort being introduced via a whole-body effort, rather than by means of pushing with that hand, in order to minimise the potential sensitivity of the region.
- Light pressure, superiorly directed, is then made to assess for discomfort. If the pressure is tolerable, the hemipelvis on the affected side is 'lifted' towards the shoulder on that side until pain reduces adequately in the palpated point, and this position is held for 30 seconds.

- The author has found that introduction of a degree of lift towards the ceiling via the contact hand (sometimes involving support from the other hand) often allows for a greater degree of pain reduction in the palpated point.

Morrison described 'multiple releases' of tension in supporting soft tissues, as well as a more balanced pelvic mechanism.

The author confirms that this is an extremely valuable method which can be applied to lower abdominal 'tension' as well as to pelvic imbalances.

By removing the tension from highly stressed ligamentous and other soft tissues in the pelvis, some degree of rebalancing normalisation occurs. Whether this involves the same mechanisms as are thought to occur when SCS is applied, or whether it relates directly to Goodheart's coccygeal lift method, remains for further evaluation. It is an example of positional release, involving a palpated pain point which is used as a monitor, and so fits well with Jones' methodology.

Summary

Goodheart has brought some unique insights into the application of positional release techniques, most notably the ability to rapidly identify where tender points are likely to be situated – in tissues shortened at the time of stress or strain; the use of strength testing prior to and after treatment to evaluate the need and the success of the procedure; the use of respiratory assistance as well as neuromuscular stretch to facilitate the resetting of the spindles; and the use of coccygeal lift as a potential means of achieving whole-spine and dural release.

REFERENCES

Breig A 1978 Adverse Mechanical Tension in the CNS. John Wiley, New York

Cummings J, Howell J 1990 The role of respiration in the tension production of myofascial tissues. J American Osteopathic Association 90(9): 842

Goodheart G 1984 Applied Kinesiology – 1982 workshop procedure manual, 20th edn. Privately published, Detroit

Goodheart G 1985 Applied Kinesiology – 1985 workshop procedure manual, 21st edn. Privately published, Detroit

Gowitzke B, Milner M 1980 Understanding the Scientific Bases of Human Movement. Williams & Wilkins, Baltimore

Illi F 1951 The Vertebral Column. National College of Chiropractic, Chicago

Kisselkova, Georgiev J 1976 Applied Physiology 46: 1093–1095

Korr I 1975 Proprioceptors and somatic dysfunction. J American Osteopathic Association 74: 638–650

Lewit K 1991 Manipulative Therapy in Rehabilitation of the Locomotor System. Butterworths, London

Morrison M 1969 Lecture notes. Seminar, September 1969 at Charing Cross Hotel, London

Peck D, Buxton D F, Nitz A A 1984 Comparison of spindle concentrations in large and small muscles acting in parallel combinations. J Morphology 180: 243–252

Sutherland W 1939 The cranial bowl. Privately published, Mankato, Minnesota

Upledger J 1984 Cranial Sacral Therapy. Eastland Press, Seattle

Walther P 1988 Applied Kinesiology Synopsis. Systems DC, Pueblo, Colorado

Williams P, Warwick R 1980 Gray's Anatomy. W B Saunders, Philadelphia

6

SCS for muscle pain (plus INIT and self-treatment)

MUSCLE PAIN

Pain is the most frequent presenting symptom in medical practice in the industrialised world. Muscle pain forms a major element of that category of symptoms and according to the leading researchers into the topic, Melzack and Wall (1988), myofascial trigger points are a key element in all chronic pain, and are often the main factor maintaining it.

It is clearly of major importance that practitioners and therapists have available in their repertoire safe and effective methods for handling myofascial pain syndromes, such as the current epidemic of muscle pain associated with chronic fatigue, now defined as fibromyalgia, or 'fibromyalgia syndrome' (FMS).

Travell and Simons (1986) have demonstrated the distinct connection between myofascial trigger point activity and a wide range of pain problems and sympathetic nervous system aberrations. Trigger (and other non-referring pain) points commonly lie in muscles which have been stressed in a variety of ways, often as a result of postural imbalances (Barlow 1959, Goldthwaite 1949), congenital factors – warping of fascia via cranial distortions (Upledger 1983), short leg problems or small hemipelvis – occupational or leisure overuse patterns (Rolf 1977), emotional states reflecting into the soft tissues (Latey 1986), referred/reflex involvement of the viscera producing facilitated (neurologically hyper-reactive) segments paraspinally (Beal 1983, Korr 1976) and trauma (see Chapter 2 for discussion of the evolution of dysfunction).

What causes the trigger point to develop?

Janet Travell and David Simons are the two physicians who, above all others, have helped our understanding of trigger points. Simons (Lewit & Simons 1984) has described the evolution of trigger points as follows:

In the core of the trigger lies a muscle spindle which is in trouble for some reason. Visualise a spindle like a strand of yarn in a knitted sweater ... a metabolic crisis takes place which increases the temperature locally in the trigger point, shortens a minute part of the muscle (sarcomere) – like a snag in a sweater – and reduces the supply of oxygen and nutrients into the trigger point. During this disturbed episode an influx of calcium occurs and the muscle spindle does not have enough energy to pump the calcium outside the cell where it belongs. Thus a vicious cycle is maintained and the muscle spindle can't seem to loosen up and the affected muscle can't relax.

Simons has tested his concept and found that at the core of a trigger point there is an oxygen deficit compared with the muscle tissue which surrounds it.

Travell (Travell & Simons 1992) has confirmed that the following factors can all help to maintain and enhance trigger point activity:

- Nutritional deficiency, especially vitamin C, B-complex and iron
- Hormonal imbalances (low thyroid, menopausal or premenstrual situations, for example)
- Infections (bacteria, viruses or yeast)
- Allergies (wheat and dairy in particular)
- Low oxygenation of tissues (aggravated by tension, stress, inactivity, poor respiration).

The repercussions of trigger point activity go beyond simple musculoskeletal pain – take for example their involvement in hyperventilation, chronic fatigue and apparent pelvic inflammatory disease.

Muscle pain and breathing dysfunction

Trigger point activity is particularly prevalent in the muscles of the neck/shoulder region which also act as accessory breathing muscles, particularly the scalenes. In situations of increased anxiety and chronic fatigue the incidence of borderline or frank hyperventilation is frequent and may be associated with a wide range of secondary symptoms including headaches, neck, shoulder and arm pain, dizziness, palpitations, fainting, spinal and abdominal discomfort, digestive symptoms relating to diaphragmatic weakness and stress, as well as the anxiety-related phenomena of panic attacks and phobic behaviour (Bass & Gardner 1985).

Clinically, where upper chest breathing is a feature, the upper fixators of the shoulders and the intercostal, pectoral and paraspinal muscles of the thoracic region are likely to palpate as tense, often fibrotic, with active trigger points being common (Roll et al 1987). Successful breathing retraining and normalisation of energy levels seems in such cases to be accelerated and enhanced following initial normalisation of the functional integrity of the muscles involved in respiration, directly or indirectly (latissimus dorsi, psoas, quadratus lumborum).

Pelvic pain and myofascial trigger points

Slocumb (1984) has shown that in a large proportion of chronic pelvic pain problems in women, often destined for surgical intervention, the prime cause involves trigger point activity in muscles of the lower abdomen, perineum, inner thigh and even on the walls of the vagina.

THE EVOLUTION OF MUSCLE DYSFUNCTION

Progressive adaptation

Selye has described the progression of changes in tissues which are being locally stressed (local adaptation syndrome), such as is occurring in many of the examples given by Liebenson (1996). Stress in this context is seen as anything at all which requires the muscle to adapt to it. In soft tissue settings this often involves trauma or microtrauma, allowing what Liebenson called 'post-trauma adhesion formation' to occur.

Selye described an initial alarm (acute inflammatory) stage followed by a stage of adaptation or resistance, when stress factors are continuous or repetitive, at which time muscular tissue may become progressively fibrotic. If such a change is taking place in muscle which has a postural rather than a phasic function, the entire muscle structure will shorten, rather than just the fibres being influenced, and parts of the muscle may become fibrotic (Janda 1985, Selye 1984).

Clearly such fibrotic tissue, lying in altered (shortened) muscle, cannot simply 'release' itself in order to allow the muscle to achieve its normal resting length (a prerequisite for the normalisation of trigger point activity). Along with various forms of stretch (passive, active, muscle energy techniques, propriceptive neuromuscular facilitation, etc.), it has been noted in Chapter 2 that inhibitory pressure is commonly employed in treatment of trigger points.

Such pressure technique methods (analogous to acupressure or shiatsu methodology) are often successful in achieving at least short-term reduction in trigger point activity and are variously dubbed 'neuromuscular techniques' (NMT) (Chaitow 1991a). Application of inhibitory pressure may involve elbow, thumb, finger or mechanical pressure (a wooden, rubber-tipped T-bar is commonly employed in the USA) or cross-fibre friction.

In addition, various positional release methods, including SCS, have been used to successfully release hypertonicity, improve function and reduce perceived pain.

A combination of inhibitory pressure and SCS, followed by stretching, can be employed in a sequential manner – known as integrated neuromuscular inhibition technique, or INIT (see below, p. 110) – in order to deliver the benefits of all these methods in a single coordinated manner.

Gutstein's model

Gutstein (1955) called localised functional sensory and/or motor abnormalities of musculoskeletal tissue (comprising muscle, fascia, tendon, bone and joint) 'myodysneuria' (now known as fibromyalgia, formerly 'fibrositis' and 'muscular rheumatism'). He sees the causes of such changes as multiple. Among them are:

- Acute and chronic infections which, it is postulated, stimulate sympathetic nerve activity via the toxic debris which results from their activities
- Excessive heat or cold, changes in atmospheric pressure and draughts
- Mechanical injuries, both major and repeated minor microtraumas
- Postural strain and unaccustomed exercises which may predispose towards soft tissue changes by lowering the threshold for future stimuli, involving the process of sensitisation or facilitation.
- Allergic and endocrine factors which can cause imbalance in the autonomic nervous system
- Inherited factors which make adaptation and adjustment to environmental factors inefficient
- Arthritic changes: since muscles are the active components of the musculoskeletal system, it is logical to assume that their overall structural and functional state influences joints. Chronic spasm, contraction and shortening of muscles may contribute towards osteoarthritic changes, which themselves produce further neuromuscular modification and new symptoms
- Visceral diseases which intensify and precipitate somatic symptoms in the distribution of their spinal and adjacent segments. Paraspinal muscles become hypertonic as a result of organ dysfunction which 'feeds back' into the tissues alongside the segment which innervates them.

Diagnosis of myodysneuria was made according to some of the following criteria, according to Gutstein (1955):

- A varying degree of muscular tension and contraction was found to be present, although sometimes adjacent, non-indurated tissue was more painful than the contracted soft tissues.
- Sensitivity to pressure or palpation of affected muscles and their adjuncts was the main method of assessment.

- When contraction was marked, the application of deep pressure to demonstrate tenderness was needed.

An epidemic of muscle pain problems seems currently to affect most industrialised societies. A detailed evaluation of aspects of this topic is appropriate in the context of the describing of positional release techniques in general and strain/counterstrain in particular, since they have shown themselves to be extremely useful in treating both myofascial pain problems (trigger points), as well as the far less responsive problems associated with fibromyalgia syndrome (FMS) – described below.

Pathophysiology of fibromyalgia/fibrositis/myodysneuria

The changes which occur in tissue involved in the onset of myodysneuria/fibromyalgia, according to Gutstein, are thought to be initiated by localised sympathetic predominance, associated with changes in the hydrogen ion concentration and the calcium and sodium balance in the tissue fluids. These changes are associated with vasoconstriction and hypoxia/ischaemia (Petersen 1934).

Pain results, it is thought, as these alterations affect the pain sensors and proprioceptors. Muscle spasm and hard, nodular, localised tetanic contractions of muscle bundles, together with vasomotor and musculomotor stimulation, intensify each other, creating a vicious cycle of self-perpetuating impulses (Bayer 1950).

There are varied and complex patterns of referred symptoms which may result from such 'trigger' areas, as well as local pain and minor disturbances. Such sensations as aching, soreness, tenderness, heaviness and tiredness may all be manifest, as may modification of muscular activity due to contraction resulting in tightness, stiffness, swelling, etc.

Since the period in which Gutstein was researching this area (mainly the 1940s and 1950s), a great deal of research has been carried out, which has resulted in the production of strict guidelines for a diagnosis of fibromyalgia by the

---

Box 6.1   American College of Rheumatology criteria for the diagnosis of fibromyalgia

1. History of widespread pain

Pain is considered widespread when *all* of the following are present:
- pain in the left side of the body
- pain in the right side of the body
- pain above the waist
- pain below the waist.

In addition, the patient should complain of pain in the spine or the neck or front of the chest, or thoracic spine or low back

2. Pain in 11 of 18 palpated sites

There should be pain on pressure (around 4 kg of pressure maximum) on not less than 11 of the following sites:
- Either side of the base of the skull where the suboccipital muscles insert
- Either side of the side of the neck between the 5th and 7th cervical vertebrae (technically described as between the 'anterior aspects of intertransverse spaces')
- Either side of the body on the midpoint of the muscle which runs from the neck to the shoulder (upper trapezius)
- Either side of the body on the origin of the supraspinatus muscle which runs along the upper border of the shoulder blade
- Either side, on the upper surface of the rib, where the second rib meets the breast bone, in the pectoral muscle
- On the outer aspect of either elbow just below the prominence (epicondyle)
- In the large buttock muscles, either side, on the upper outer aspect in the fold in front of the muscle (gluteus medius)
- Just behind the large prominence of either hip joint in the muscular insertion of piriformis muscle
- On either knee in the fatty pad just above the inner aspect of the joint.

American College of Rheumatology (Wolfe et al 1990). These are given in Box 6.1.[1] Associated conditions which predispose towards, and accompany fibromyalgia, are given in Box 6.2.

Do trigger points cause fibromyalgia?

Myofascial pain syndrome (MPS) is a disorder in which pain of a persistent aching type is referred to a target area (usually localised rather than

---

[1] There are criteria from other experts in the study of fibromyalgia which are at variance with those listed in Box 6.1.

Box 6.2 Main associated conditions which predispose towards and accompany fibromyalgia

These include the following (Block 1993, Duna & Wilke 1993, Fishbain 1989, Goldenberg 1993a, Jacobsen 1992, Kalik 1989, Rothschild 1991):

- 100% of people with FMS have muscular pain, aching and/or stiffness (especially in the morning)
- Almost all suffer fatigue and badly disturbed sleep with consequent reduction in production of growth hormone
- Symptoms are almost always worse in cold or humid weather
- The majority of people with FMS have a history of injury – sometimes serious but often only minor – within the year before the symptoms started
- 70% to 100% (different studies show variable numbers) are found to have depression (though this is more likely to be a result of the muscular pain rather than part of the cause)
- 73% to 34% have irritable bowel syndrome
- 56% to 44% have severe headaches
- 50% to 30% have Raynaud's phenomenon
- 24% suffer from anxiety
- 18% have dry eyes and/or mouth (sicca syndrome)
- 12% have osteoarthritis
- 7% have rheumatoid arthritis
- An as yet unidentified number of people with FMS have had silicone breast implants and a newly identified silicone breast implant syndrome (SBIS) is now being defined
- Between 3 and 6% are found to have substance (drugs/alcohol) abuse problems

---

Box 6.3 Similarities and differences between FMS and MPS

FMS and MPS are *similar* (or identical) in that both:

- Are affected by cold weather
- May involve increased sympathetic nerve activity and may involve conditions such as Raynaud's phenomenon
- Have tension headaches and paraesthesia as a major associated symptom
- Are unaffected by anti-inflammatory, pain-killing medication whether of the cortisone type or standard formulations.

FMS and MPS are *different* in that:

- MPS affects males and females equally, fibromyalgia mainly females
- MPS is usually local to an area such as the neck and shoulders, or low back and legs, although it can affect a number of parts of the body at the same time while fibromyalgia is a generalised problem, often involving all four 'corners' of the body at the same time.
- Muscles which contain areas which feel 'like a tight rubber band' are found in the muscles of around 30% of people with MPS and more than 60% of people with FMS
- People with FMS have poorer muscular endurance than do people with MPS
- MPS can sometimes be severe enough to cause disturbed sleep; in fibromyalgia the sleep disturbance has a more causative role, and is a pronounced feature of the condition
- Patients with MPS usually do not suffer from morning stiffness whereas those with fibromyalgia do
- Fatigue is not usually associated with MPS while it is common in fibromyalgia
- MPS can sometimes lead to depression (reactive) and anxiety whereas in a small percentage of fibromyalgia cases (some leading researchers believe) these conditions can be causative
- Conditions such as irritable bowel syndrome, dysmenorrhoea and a subjective feeling of 'swollen joints' are noted in fibromyalgia, but seldom in MPS
- Low-dosage tricyclic antidepressant drugs are helpful in dealing with the sleep problems associated with FMS, and many of the symptoms of fibromyalgia – but not those of MPS
- Exercise programmes (cardiovascular fitness) can help some fibromyalgia patients; according to experts, but this is not a useful approach in MPS.

---

general such as in FMS) by trigger points lying some distance away from the site of reported pain (see Fig. 6.1). This phenomenon has long been recognised as a cause of severe and chronic pain in many people. Since some experts insist that the 'tender' points which are palpated when diagnosing fibromyalgia need to refer pain elsewhere if they are to be taken seriously in the diagnosis (thus making them trigger points by definition) the question needs to be asked whether MPS is not the self-same condition as FMS?

The answer is – not quite.

Scandinavian researchers showed in 1986 that around 65% of people with fibromyalgia had identifiable trigger points, and it is clear therefore that there is an overlap between FMS and MPS (Henriksson 1993).

Baldry (1993), a leading British physician/acupuncturist, has summarised the similarities and differences between these two conditions and these are given in Box 6.3.

What is happening in the FMS patient's muscles?
(Goldenberg 1989, 1994, Henriksson 1994, Moldofsky 1993)

Many of the adaptations and changes described above are likely to be taking place in the muscles

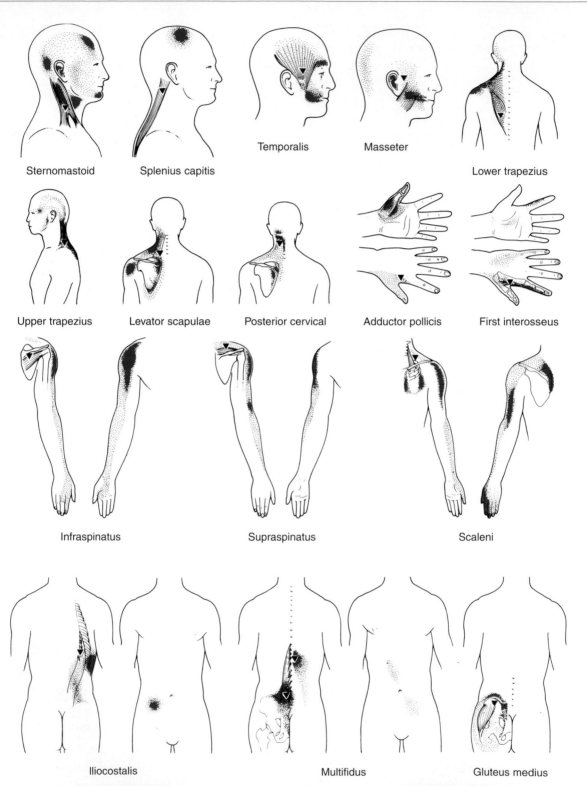

Sternomastoid

Splenius capitis

Temporalis

Masseter

Lower trapezius

Upper trapezius

Levator scapulae

Posterior cervical

Adductor pollicis

First interosseus

Infraspinatus

Supraspinatus

Scaleni

Iliocostalis

Multifidus

Gluteus medius

Figure 6.1 A selection of the most commonly found examples of representations of trigger sites and their reference (or target) areas. Trigger points found in the same sites in different people will usually refer to the same target areas.

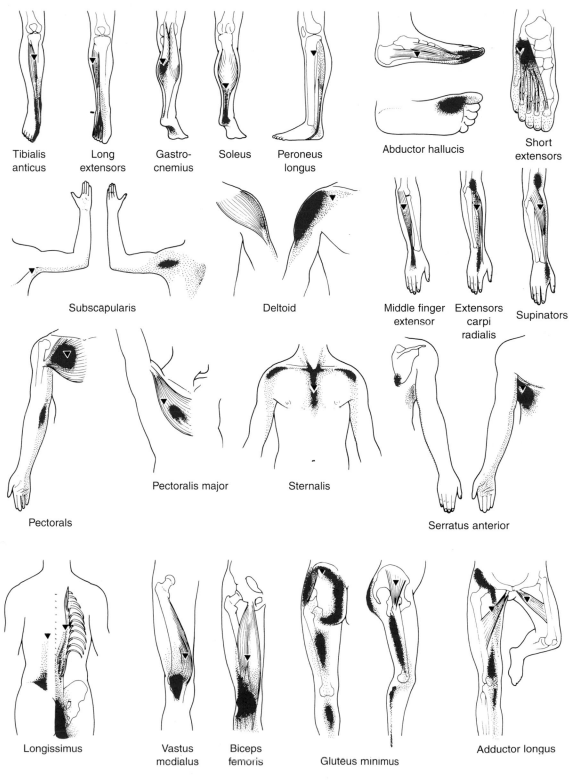

Tibialis anticus

Long extensors

Gastro-cnemius

Soleus

Peroneus longus

Abductor hallucis

Short extensors

Subscapularis

Deltoid

Middle finger extensor

Extensors carpi radialis

Supinators

Pectorals

Pectoralis major

Sternalis

Serratus anterior

Longissimus

Vastus medialus

Biceps femoris

Gluteus minimus

Adductor longus

of anyone with fibromyalgia – plus a number of additional factors:

- A biochemical imbalance seems to be present which may be the direct result of the negative effect of disturbed sleep – this leads to inadequate growth hormone production and therefore poor repair of minor muscle damage.
- There are also commonly lower than normal levels of serotonin in the blood and tissues, resulting in lowered pain thresholds, because of the reduced effectiveness of the pain-killing influence of endorphins and also due to the increased presence of substance P.
- The sympathetic nervous system – controlling as it does the degree of muscle tone – can become disturbed leading to muscle ischaemia, resulting in additional presence of substance P and increased pain sensitivity.
- Some researchers (Duna & Wilke 1993) propose that all these elements combine in fibromyalgia including:
  - disordered sleep, which leads to reduced growth hormone production
  - low levels of serotonin, leading to reduced natural pain-killing effects of endorphins
  - disturbed sympathetic nervous system, which has resulted in muscle ischaemia and increased pain sensitivity.

All these disturbances involve substance P being released, leading to low pain thresholds and activation of latent trigger points, with fibromyalgia as the end result.

Other researchers propose that a great deal of 'microtrauma' of muscles occurs in FMS patients (for reasons not yet clear, but genetic predisposition is a possibility) leading to calcium leakage in the tissues, which increases muscle contraction, further reducing oxygen supply. This microtrauma seems also to be associated with a reduction in the muscle's ability to produce energy, so causing it to fatigue more easily and to be unable to pump the excess calcium out of the cells.

A similar mechanism is said by Travell and Simons to be involved in myofascial trigger point activity (Simons 1986)

James Daley has tested just what happens in the muscles of people with chronic fatigue syndrome (CFS) (ME) when they exercise. Tests involving people with FMS (Bennett 1990) gave similar results, which were that these people's muscles produced excessive lactic acid which added to their discomfort. Some of the patients showed a dramatic rise in blood pressure during exercise; about a third had erratic breathing when exercising and many also had low carbon dioxide levels when resting – an indication of a hyperventilation tendency (see Ch. 2 for the implications of this).

There are clearly numerous interacting causative elements operating in both FMS and MPS and many treatment methods have shown benefit; manual therapy (see below, p. 108), nutritional and herbal treatment, stress reduction, breathing and postural re-education, exercise (in some cases), electro-acupuncture, hypnotherapy, homeopathy, cardiovascular training, biofeedback and cognitive-behavioural modification – among others – have all been shown to be useful in encouraging recovery (Abraham et al 1992, Deale & Wessley 1994, DeLuze et al 1992, Ferraccioli 1989, Fisher et al 1989, Gemmell et al 1991, Goldenberg et al 1991, Haanen et al 1991, Kacera 1993, Kleijnen et al 1992, McGain et al 1988, Sandford Kiser et al 1983, Warot et al 1991).

There is some evidence that progressive cardiovascular training (graduated training through exercise) improves muscle function and reduces pain in FMS, but this is not thought desirable (and is often quite impossible anyway because of the degree of fatigue) in CFS (ME) (Goldenberg 1993b).

Outlook for FMS and MPS?

The outlook for people with myofascial pain syndrome (MPS) is excellent, since the trigger points usually respond quickly to appropriate techniques, where the outlook for fibromyalgia is less positive, with a lengthy treatment and recovery phase being the norm. Research indicates that a number of approaches can minimise the suffering, including application of SCS and other osteopathic manipulative techniques (see later in this chapter for details).

Trigger points are certainly part – in some cases the major part – of the pain suffered by people with fibromyalgia (and they certainly are if pressure on the 'tender point' produces pain in a target area). Trigger points can be eliminated in various ways, one of which involves an integrated use of different soft tissue approaches, INIT, a method which is discussed later in this chapter (p. 110).

Terminology

Dr Craig Liebenson, a Los Angeles chiropractor and researcher, explains some of the difficulties we experience when describing soft tissue changes (Chaitow, 2001). He explains that muscles are often said to be 'short', 'tight', 'tense', or 'in spasm'; however, these terms are often used very loosely (Liebenson 2001):

In order to provide proper indications for the use of appropriate soft tissue techniques we should define our treatment objectives. Muscles suffer either neuromuscular, viscoelastic, or connective tissue alterations. A tight muscle could have either increased neuromuscular tension or connective tissue fibrosis.

Liebenson (2001) continues:

Muscle spasm is a neuromuscular phenomenon relating either to upper motor neuron disease or an acute reaction to pain or tissue injury. Electromyographic (EMG) activity is increased in these cases. Examples include spinal cord injury, reflex spasm such as appendicitis or acute lumbar antalgia with loss of flexion relaxation response (Triano & Schultz 1987). Long lasting noxious stimulation has been shown to activate the flexion withdrawal reflex (Dahl et al 1992).

Tension without EMG elevation

Increased muscle tension can occur without a consistently elevated EMG. An example is in trigger points, in which case a muscle fails to relax properly. Muscles housing trigger points have been shown to have dramatically different levels of EMG activity within the same functional muscle unit. Hubbard and Berkoff (1993) showed EMG hyper-excitability in the nidus of the trigger point in a taut band which had a characteristic pattern of reproducible referred pain.

Increased stretch sensitivity

Other influences are described by Liebenson (2001): 'Increased sensitivity to stretch can also lead to increased muscle tension. This has been shown to occur under conditions of local ischaemia (Mense 1993). According to Janda neuromuscular tension can also be increased by central influences due to limbic dysfunction (Janda 1991).'

He continues his discussion of these muscle states:

Muscle stiffness is a viscoelastic phenomenon described by Walsh (1992). This has to do with fluid mechanics and viscosity of tissue. It is not a neuromuscular phenomenon. Fibrosis occurs in muscle or fascia gradually and is typically related to post-trauma adhesion formation. Lehto found that fibroblasts proliferate in injured tissue during the inflammatory phase (Lehto et al 1986). If the inflammatory phase is prolonged then a connective tissue scar will form as the fibrosis is not absorbed.

Trigger point influence

Some of the influences of trigger points are also touched on by Liebenson (2001):

Various studies have demonstrated that trigger points in one muscle are related to inhibition of another functionally related muscle (Headley 1993, Simons 1993). In particular, it was shown by Simons (1993) that the deltoid muscle can be inhibited when there are infraspinatus trigger points present. Headley (1993) has shown that lower trapezius inhibition is related to trigger points in the upper trapezius.

Facilitation/sensitisation

Facilitation, which was discussed in Chapter 2, describes how local areas become increasingly sensitised due to stress of any sort, and helps to explain some of the benefits achieved via 'spontaneous release by positioning', first described by Jones in 1964 after he had noted that a patient with a severe lesion, which was interfering with normal movement and function, gained considerable release when he was positioned in such a way that the discomfort was stopped.

It can be assumed that the factor of increased sensitisation, or facilitation, reduces during the period of pain cessation which occurs during the holding of the 'ease' position in positional release.

A corollary to the decrease in sensitisation would be that for a time following the treatment, the patient would be liable to recurrence of the problem as a result of residual sensitisation and the long-lasting effects of conditioning. This liability should be gradually reversed as calmer and more balanced neural inputs and responses become the norm.

Korr (1976) has proposed a mechanism involving the gamma motor system and muscle proprioceptors as one of the common causes of sustained muscle contraction associated with somatic dysfunction and the process of facilitation/sensitisation. He proposed that manipulative procedures involving high-velocity, short-amplitude forces, as well as muscle energy techniques, can act to force the central nervous system to correct abnormally high excitation of the muscle spindles, and to so allow the muscle to return to its normal length and the joint to its normal motion.

Similar reasoning, with regard to decreasing muscle spindle activity, can be applied to functional positional release techniques, which, instead of forcing a contracted muscle towards its restriction barrier, allow it to continue to shorten until it relaxes normally. In both direct (forcing through a barrier of restriction) and indirect (moving away from the barrier) procedures, afferent input to the cord may be reduced for a sufficient time, and to a sufficient degree, to allow the sensitisation to decrease below a critical level. That is, afferent input would be reduced either directly, or via central brain influences, to a level below that required to sustain sensitisation and therefore dysfunctional patterns of behaviour, in this instance sustained inappropriate degrees of contraction and hypertonicity.

Local facilitation

According to Korr (1976), a trigger point is a localised area of somatic dysfunction which behaves in a facilitated manner, i.e. it will amplify and be affected by any form of stress imposed on the individual whether this is of a physical, chemical or emotional nature.

A trigger point is palpable as an indurated, localised, painful entity with a reference (target) area, to which pain or other symptoms are referred (Chaitow 1991b).

Muscles housing trigger points can frequently be identified as being unable to achieve their normal resting length using standard muscle evaluation procedures (Janda 1983). The trigger point itself commonly lies in fibrotic tissue, which has evolved as the result of exposure of the tissues to diverse forms of stress, and always lies in hypertonic bands of myofascial tissue.

Trigger point characteristics summarised

- The leading researcher into trigger points, Janet Travell, defines trigger points as: hyper-irritable foci, lying within taut bands of muscle, which are painful on compression and which refer pain or other symptoms at a distant site'.
- Embryonic trigger points will develop as 'satellites' of existing triggers in the target area, and in time these will produce their own satellites.
- According to Melzack, nearly 80% of trigger points are in exactly the same positions as known acupuncture points as used in traditional Chinese medicine (Melzack & Wall 1988).
- Painful points ('tender points') which do not refer symptoms to a distant site are often latent triggers, which need only to have imposed additional degrees of stress in order to create greater facilitation, and to so be transformed into active triggers.
- The taut band in which triggers lie will twitch if a finger is run across it, and is tight but not usually fibrosed, since it will commonly soften and relax if the appropriate treatment is applied – something fibrotic tissue cannot do.
- Muscles which contain trigger points will often hurt when they are contracted (i.e. when they are working) and they will almost always be painful if stretched forcefully.
- Trigger points are areas of increased energy consumption and lowered oxygen supply due

to inadequate local circulation. They will therefore add to the drain on energy and the fatigue being frequently experienced.

- The muscle in which trigger points lie cannot reach its normal resting length – it is being held almost constantly in a shortened position (making it an ideal target for the methods of SCS, since such muscles will happily be shortened further but will resist being lengthened).

- Until the muscle housing a trigger point can reach its normal resting length without pain or effort, treatment of a trigger point will only achieve temporary relief as it will reactivate after treatment.

- Stretching of the muscles housing a trigger point, using either active or passive methods, is a useful way of treating the shortness as well as the trigger point, since this can reduce the contraction (taut band) as well as increasing circulation to the area – something which SCS can also achieve.

- There are many variably successful ways of treating trigger points (see below, p. 106) including acupuncture, procaine injections, direct manual pressure (with the thumb, etc.), stretching the muscle, ice therapy, etc. Whatever is done though, unless the muscle can be induced to reach its normal resting length, any such treatment will be of limited value.

- Some of these methods (pressure, acupuncture) cause the release in the body and the brain of natural pain-killing substances – endorphins – which explains one of the ways in which pain is reduced. Pain is also relieved when one sensation (finger pressure, needle) is substituted for another (the original pain). In this way pain messages are partially or totally blocked, or partially prevented from reaching or being registered by the brain.

- Methods which improve the circulatory imbalance will affect trigger points, which contain areas of ischaemic tissue, and in this way appear to deactivate them.

- The target area to which a trigger refers pain will be the same in everyone if the trigger point is in the same position – but this pattern of pain distribution does not relate to known nerve pathways or to acupuncture meridian pathways.

- The way in which a trigger point relays pain to a distant site is thought to involve one of a variety of neurological mechanisms which probably involve the brain 'mislocating' pain messages which it receives via several different pathways. (The truth is that, as yet, we do not know how trigger points produce their symptoms.)

- Trigger points lie in parts of muscles most prone to mechanical stress, often close to origins and insertions as discussed earlier in this chapter (see central and attachment point discussion below).

- Trigger points involve a self-perpetuating cycle (pain leading to increased tone leading to more pain) and will almost never deactivate unless adequately treated.

Different types of trigger points
(Simons & Travell 1998)

Central triggers

- Central trigger points form in the centre of the muscle's fibres, close to the motor endplate (neuromuscular junction).

- Excess acetylcholine (ACh) is released at the synapse, usually associated with overuse or strain, leading to release of calcium.

- Resulting ischaemia creates an O_2 deficit and energy crisis.

- Without available ATP, calcium ions, which are keeping the gates open for ACh to keep flowing, cannot be removed.

- A chemically sustained contracture (without motor potentials) is different from a contraction (voluntary with motor potentials) and a spasm (involuntary with motor potentials).

- Actin–myosin filaments shorten in the area of the motor endplate.

- A contracture 'knot' forms the characteristic trigger point nodule.

- The remainder of the sarcomeres of that fibre are stretched, creating the palpable taut band.

- Massage, stretch applications and other modalities such as positional release techniques disturb the sarcomeres, alter the chemistry, and/or possibly damage the endplate, disrupting the cycle so that the tissues relax, often in seconds, often permanently.

Attachment triggers

- Attachment trigger points form at junctures of myofascial and tendinous or periosteal tissues.
- Awareness of a muscle's fibre arrangement (fusiform, pennate, bipennate, multipennate, etc.) and attachment sites, will help to locate trigger points rapidly, since their sites are predictable.
- Tension from taut bands on periosteal or connective tissues can lead to enthesopathy or enthesitis, as recurring concentrations of muscular stress provoke inflammation, with a strong tendency towards fibrosis and calcific deposition.
- Periosteal pain points may be palpated at the attachments.

Choice of trigger point treatment

- Central trigger points should be addressed with their contracted central sarcomeres and local ischaemia in mind.
- Since the end of the taut band housing the trigger point is likely to create enthesopathy, stretching the muscle before releasing its central trigger point might further irritate or inflame the attachments.
- Techniques should first be applied to relax the taut fibres before manual elongations are attempted (e.g. positional release, gliding strokes and/or myofascial release).
- Stretches, particularly active range of motion, should be applied gently until reaction is noted, to avoid tissue insult.
- Attachment trigger points seem to respond to ice applications rather than to heat.
- Gliding techniques should be applied from the centre of the fibres out towards the attachments, unless contraindicated (as in some extremity tissues).
- By elongating the tissue towards the attachment, sarcomeres which are shortened at the

centre of the fibre will be lengthened and those which are over-stretched near the attachment sites will have their tension released.
- When passive stretching is applied, care should be taken to assess for tendinous or periosteal inflammation, in order to avoid placing more tension on already distressed connective tissue attachments (e.g. better to use methods to reduce hypertonicity rather than initiating stretching, and positional release achieves this effectively).
- As will be explained later in this chapter a sequential combination of methods, including positional release, can effectively achieve trigger point deactivation and enhanced function.

Correct choice of treatment is vital. Unless soft tissue and other changes as described above (and their causes) are accurately identified, no therapeutic method will do more than produce short-term relief.

In order for restrictions, imbalances and malcoordination in the musculoskeletal system to be satisfactorily addressed, and where possible reversed, the individual needs to be appropriately treated as well as taught improved patterns of use. In order for appropriate treatment to be offered, assessment methods are needed which lead to identification of:

- Patterns of misuse
- Postural imbalances
- Shortened postural muscles
- Weakened muscles
- Patterns of functional malcoordination and imbalance
- Local changes within muscles (such as trigger points) and other soft tissues
- Joint restrictions
- Functional imbalances in gait, respiration, etc.

Of equal importance is the need for the availability of a repertoire of therapeutic modalities and methods, which can be tailored to the particular needs of the individual and the tissues being addressed.

For example, functional or positional release methods such as SCS, or acute-phase muscle energy technique (MET) methods, can produce a neurological release of hypertonicity or spasm, and are therefore most appropriate in circumstances of acute dysfunction, or where hypertonicity is a key feature of a problem. While it is not possible to modify fibrotic changes by means of positional release, the enhanced circulation which results from such methods (see Ch. 1) offers benefits to tissues which have been relatively oxygen-starved.

Similarly, it would be perfectly appropriate to attempt to use stronger MET methods (described below) in treatment of chronic fibrotic tissues, in which circumstances gentler (SCS, for example) methods might only be useful in reducing hypertonicity and enhancing circulation prior to more vigorous approaches being used. Neuromuscular techniques could be usefully applied in both settings (indirect positional release or direct MET methodology) and in both acute or chronic settings (Chaitow 1991a).

GENERAL TREATMENT METHODS

A wide variety of treatment methods has been advocated in treating trigger points, including inhibitory (ischaemic compression) pressure methods (Chaitow 1982, 1989, Nimmo 1966), acupuncture and/or ultrasound (Kleyhans & Aarons 1974), chilling and stretching of the muscle in which the trigger lies (Travell & Simons 1986), procaine or xylocain injections (Slocumb 1984), active or passive stretching (Lewit 1992), and even surgical excision (Dittrich 1954).

Clinical experience, confirmed by the diligent research of Travell and Simons, has shown that while all or any of these methods can successfully inhibit trigger point activity in the short term, in order to completely eliminate the noxious activity of such a disruptive structure, more needs to be done, therapeutically speaking, to the local tissues, in order to stretch the muscle to a more normal length.

Travell and Simons have shown that whatever initial treatment is offered to inhibit the neurological hyper-reactivity of the trigger point, the muscle in which it lies has to be made capable of

reaching its normal resting length following such treatment, or else the trigger point will rapidly reactivate.

In treating trigger points, the method of chilling the offending muscle (housing the trigger), while holding it at stretch in order to achieve this end, was advocated by Travell and Simons, while Lewit espoused the muscle energy method of a physiologically induced postisometric relaxation (or reciprocal inhibition) response, prior to passive stretching. In recent publications, Travell and Simons have moved towards Lewit's viewpoint, using postisometric relaxation (MET) as a starting point before stretching offending muscles (Travell & Simons 1992).

Both methods are commonly successful, although a sufficient degree of failure occurs (trigger rapidly reactivates or fails to completely 'switch off') to require investigation of more successful approaches.

One reason for failure of muscle-stretching methods may relate to the possibility of the tissues which are being stretched not being the precise ones housing the trigger point, and this was the factor which initiated the evolution of INIT as described below (p. 110).

Re-education and elimination of causes

Common sense, as well as clinical experience, also dictates that the next stage of correction of such problems should involve re-education (postural, breathing, relaxation, etc.), as well as the elimination of factors which contributed to the problem's evolution. This might well involve ergonomic evaluation of home and workplace, as well as the introduction and dedicated application of re-education methods.

Muscle energy technique

A popular method for achieving tonus release in a muscle prior to stretching involves introduction of an isometric contraction to the affected muscle (producing postisometric relaxation through the influence of the golgi tendon organs) or to its antagonist (producing reciprocal inhibition) (Chaitow 1991a).

The original use of isometric contractions prior to stretching was in proprioceptive neuromuscular facilitation techniques (PNF), which emerged from physical medicine in the early part of the 20th century. PNF advocated a full-strength contraction against operator-imposed resistance, whereas in most forms of muscle energy technique (MET) methodology, derived from osteopathic research and clinical experience, a partial (not full-strength) isometric contraction is performed prior to the stretch, in order to preclude tissue damage or stress to the patient and/or therapist, which PNF not infrequently produces (Greenman 1989, Hartman 1985).

Strain/counterstrain and muscle problems

As described in Chapter 3, Jones (1981) has shown that particular painful tender points – relating to joint or muscular strain, chronic or acute – can be used as monitors, pressure being applied to them as the body or body part is carefully positioned in such a way as to remove or reduce the pain felt in the palpated point.[2]

When the position of ease is attained in which pain vanishes or markedly eases from the palpated tender point, the stressed tissues are felt to be at their most relaxed – and clinical experience indicates that this is so, since they palpate as 'easy' rather than having a sense of being 'bound', or tense.

Strain/counterstrain and trigger points

Simons and Travell (1998) discuss strain/counterstrain in relation to the treatment of trigger points, and suggest that most of the tender points listed in Jones' original book (Jones 1981), and many of those described in subsequent PRT texts

(D'Ambrogio & Roth 1997), are close to attachment trigger point sites. This is, however, not universally true: 'Of the 65 tender points [in Jones' original book], nine were identified at the attachment region of a named muscle. Forty-four points were located either at the region of a muscular attachment where one might find an attachment trigger point, or, occasionally, at the belly of a muscle where a central trigger point might be located'. (see discussion earlier in this chapter relating to attachment and central trigger points).

D'Ambrogio and Roth (1997) state, 'There appears to be a close association between the tender points used in positional release therapy and [those used] by Jones'. If at least some, and possibly the majority, of Jones' tender points, are demonstrably the same entities as Simons and Travell's trigger points, logic suggests that a therapeutic approach which effectively deactivates one (the tender point) should beneficially influence the other (trigger point). The lead author of this text suggests that clinical evidence supports this supposition, especially when the positional release method is combined with other approaches such as ischaemic compression and muscle energy technique (MET), which have a good track record in trigger point deactivation.

Is SCS of value in fibromyalgia?

Osteopathic physicians utilising SCS and muscle energy techniques as well as other osteopathic methods, have conducted numerous studies involving patients with a firm diagnosis of FMS. Among the studies in which SCS was a major form of treatment of FMS are the following:

1. Doctors at the Chicago College of Osteopathic Medicine (led by Drs A Stoltz and R Kappler) measured the effects of osteopathic manipulative therapy (OMT – which included both SCS and MET) on the intensity of pain from tender points in 18 patients who met all the criteria for FMS. Each had six visits/treatments and it was found, over a 1-year period, that 12 of the patients responded well, in that their tender points became less sensitive (14% reduction against a 34% increase in the six patients who did

---

[2] Tender points, as described by Jones, are found in tissues which were short rather than being stretched at the time of injury (acute or chronic) and are usually areas in which the patient was unaware of pain previous to their being palpated. They seem to equate in most particulars with 'Ah Shi' points in traditional Chinese medicine.

not respond well). Most of the patients – the responders and the non-responders who had received SCS and MET – showed (using thermographic imaging) that their tender points were more symmetrically spread after the course than before. Activities of daily living were significantly improved and general pain symptoms decreased (Stoltz 1993).

2. Osteopathic physicians at Kirksville College of Osteopathic Medicine treated 19 patients classified as having fibromyalgia syndrome, using SCS and MET approaches, for 4 weeks, one treatment each week. 84.2% of the patients showed improved sleep patterns and 94.7% reported a significant reduction in pain after this short course of treatment (Lo et al 1992).

3. Doctors at Texas College of Osteopathic Medicine selected three groups of FMS patients, one of which received OMT, another had OMT plus self-teaching (study of the condition and self-help measures) and a third group received only moist-heat treatment. The group with the lowest level of reported pain after 6 months of care was that receiving OMT, although benefits were also noted in the self-teaching group (Jiminez et al 1993).

4. Another group of doctors from Texas, in a study involving 37 patients with FMS (Rubin et al 1990), tested the differences resulting from using:
– drugs only (ibuprofen, alprazolam)
– osteopathic treatment (including SCS) plus medication
– osteopathic treatment plus a dummy medication (placebo)
– a placebo only.
The results showed that:
– Drug therapy alone resulted in significantly less tenderness being reported than did drugs and osteopathy, or the use of placebo and osteopathic treatment, or placebo alone.
– Patients receiving placebo plus osteopathic manipulation reported significantly less fatigue than the other groups.
– The group receiving medication and (mainly) osteopathic soft tissue manipulation showed the greatest improvement in their quality of life.

Hypothesis

The author hypothesises that partial contraction (using no more than 20–30% of patient strength, as is the norm in MET procedures) may sometimes fail to achieve recruitment and activation of the fibres housing the trigger point being treated, since light contractions of this sort fail to recruit more than a small percentage of the muscle's potential.

Subsequent stretching of the muscle may, therefore, only marginally involve the critical tissues surrounding and enveloping the myofascial trigger point. Failure to actively stretch the muscle fibres in which the trigger is housed might account for recurrence of trigger point activity in the same site, a short time following treatment. Repetition of the same stress factors which produced it in the first place could undoubtedly also be a factor in such recurrence – which emphasises the need for re-education in rehabilitation.

A method (integrated neuromuscular inhibition technique – INIT) which achieves precise targeting of these tissues (in terms of tonus release and subsequent stretching) would therefore seem to offer advantages because of a more precise targeting of the contraction and stretch, employing SCS as part of its methodology. This approach is described below.

Before treating a tender or trigger point, with whatever method, it is necessary to find it. How accurate are palpation methods?

Palpation tests for tender and trigger points

In 1992 a study was conducted by two leading figures in the study of myofascial pain, in order to see how accurate palpation for tender points and trigger points in myofascial tissues were, when used by experts who would be making the all-important diagnosis of FMS or MPS (Wolfe et al 1992). Volunteers from three groups were tested – some with FMS, some with MPS and some with no pain or any other symptoms.

The FMS patients were easily identified – 38% of the FMS patients were found to have trigger points.

Of the MPS patients, only 23.4% were identified as having trigger points and of the normal volunteers less than 2% had any.

Most of the MPS patients had tender points in sites usually tested in FMS and would have qualified for this diagnosis as well.

Recommended trigger point palpation method

There are a variety of palpation methods by means of which trigger (or tender) points can rapidly be identified, among which the simplest and possibly the most effective is use of what is termed 'drag' palpation, as discussed in Chapter 4 (Chaitow 1991b). A light passage of a single digit, finger or thumb, across the skin ('feather-light touch') elicits a sense of hesitation, or 'drag', when the skin has an increased water content compared with surrounding skin. This increased hydrosis, sweat, seems to correlate with increased sympathetic activity, which accompanies local tissue dysfunction in general and trigger point activity in particular (Lewit 1992).

Lewit (1992) additionally suggests that the skin overlying a trigger point will exhibit reduced elasticity when lightly stretched apart, as compared with surrounding skin. He terms such areas as 'hyperalgesic skin zones' and identifies a further characteristic: a reduced degree of movement of the skin over the underlying fascia, palpable when attempting to slide or 'roll' the skin.

These three features of skin change (reduced movement of skin on fascia, reduced local elasticity and increased hydrosis) offer simple and effective clues as to underlying dysfunction.

Systematic approaches to the charting of trigger point locations (and their deactivation) are offered by systems such as neuromuscular technique (NMT), in which a methodical sequence of palpatory searches are carried out, based on the trigger point 'maps' as described by Simons and Travell (1998, Chaitow & DeLany 2000). When attempting to palpate for trigger points at depth, not simply using skin signs, a particularly useful phrase to keep in mind is that used by Stanley Lief DC, co-developer of NMT: 'To discover local changes [such as trigger points] it is necessary to constantly vary palpation pres-

sure, to "meet and match" tissue tensions' (Chaitow 1996). D'Ambrogio and Roth (1997), put it differently: 'Tissue must be entered gently, and only necessary pressure must be used to palpate through the layers of tissue'.

INIT hypothesis
(Chaitow 1994)

Clinical experience indicates that by combining the methods of direct inhibition (pressure mildly applied, continuously or in a make-and-break pattern) with the concept of SCS and MET, a specific targeting of dysfunctional soft tissues should be achieved.

 INIT method 1

It is reasonable to assume, and palpation confirms, that when a trigger point is being palpated by direct finger or thumb pressure, and when the very tissues in which the trigger point lies are positioned in such a way as to take away the pain (entirely or at least to a great extent), the most (dis)stressed fibres in which the trigger point is housed are in a position of relative ease (Fig. 6.2).

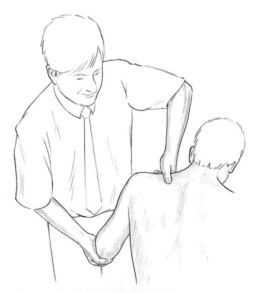

Figure 6.2A   First stage of INIT in which a tender/pain/trigger point in supraspinatus is located and ischaemically compressed, either intermittently or persistently.

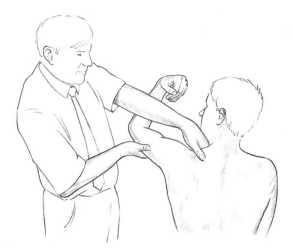

Figure 6.2B   The pain is removed from the tender/pain/trigger point by finding a position of ease which is held for at least 20 seconds, following which an isometric contraction is achieved involving the tissues which house the point.

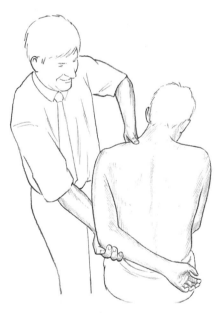

Figure 6.2C   Following the holding of the isometric contraction for an appropriate period, the muscle housing the point of local soft tissue dysfunction is stretched. This completes the INIT sequence.

At this time the trigger point would be under direct inhibitory pressure (mild or perhaps intermittent) and would have been positioned so that the tissues housing it are relaxed (relatively or completely).

Following a period of 20–30 seconds of this position of ease and inhibitory pressure, the patient could be asked to introduce an isometric contraction into the tissues and to hold this for 7–10 seconds – involving the precise fibres which had been repositioned to obtain the strain/counterstrain release. The effect of this isometric contraction would be to produce (following the contraction) a degree of reduction in tone in these tissues (as a result of postisometric relaxation). The hypertonic or fibrotic tissues could then be gently stretched, as in any muscle energy procedure, with the strong likelihood that the specifically targeted fibres would be stretched.

INIT method 2

Instead of an isometric contraction followed by stretch (following on from the holding of a position of ease as described above), an isolytic approach could be used.

The muscle receiving attention would be actively contracted by the patient at the same time that a stretch was being introduced – resulting in mild trauma to the muscle and the breakdown of fibrous adhesions between it and its interface and within its structures (Mitchell et al 1979).

To introduce this method into trigger point treatment, following the application of inhibitory pressure and SCS release, the patient is asked to contract the muscles around the palpating thumb or finger (lying on the now-inhibited pain point, in tissues which are 'at ease') with the request that the contraction should not be a full-strength effort since the operator intends to gently stretch the tissues while the contraction is taking place.

This isotonic-eccentric effort – designed to reduce contractions and break down fibrotic tissue – should target precisely the tissues in which the trigger point being treated lies buried. Following the isolytic stretch, the tissues could benefit from effleurage and/or hot and cold applications, to ease local congestion. An instruction should be given to avoid active use of the area for a day or so.

Treating muscle pains using SCS

When muscles hurt, SCS can be applied using Jones' or Goodheart's guidelines, as explained in Chapters 1 and 3. Jones has provided a formula which can be applied to any pain points, whether of muscle or joint origin, as to the position of ease which is most likely to assist in resolution of the pain, albeit sometimes only temporarily. He has shown that tender or pain points on the anterior surface require flexion, while those on the posterior surface require extension. The further the tender points are from the midline, the more side-bending and/or rotation will be needed to achieve ease. Apart from these general guidelines, all the protocol for successful use of SCS requires is that as the procedure is performed, the reported degree of pain in the palpated point should be reduced by at least 70% and the position held for at least 1 minute, and ideally 90 seconds, before a slow return to neutral is carried out.

As long as these criteria are met, and no additional pain is introduced, or increased elsewhere during the procedure, a successful outcome can be anticipated.

Goodheart has simplified the way in which we can target tender point location, by noting that the point needed to monitor any given dysfunction will be found in the tissues which are antagonists to the muscles active when painful movements are performed, or which result in restriction.

An additional possibility is to simply treat anything which palpates, or which is reported, as tender, using the methods as outlined.

In regard to myofascial trigger points, the integrated use of inhibitory pressure, strain/counterstrain and a form of muscle energy technique – applied to a trigger point or other area of soft tissue dysfunction involving pain or restricted range of motion (of soft tissue origin) – is an efficient approach, allowing as it does a precise targeting of the culprit tissues. The use of an isolytic approach as part of this sequence will be more easily achieved in some regions rather than others – upper trapezius posing less of a problem in terms of positioning and application than might, for example, quadratus lumborum.

SCS used alone, without the initial ischaemic compression and subsequent MET, remains the most gentle of approaches.

When confronted by soft tissue changes of a sensitive and painful nature in a person for whom vigorous or painful treatment (or anticipated reactions to treatment based on their degree of arousal and general health status) would be undesirable, SCS and other functional approaches (see Chapters 1 and 7) offer useful therapeutic options. SCS is also, as has been demonstrated, ideal for self-treatment, and guidelines for self-treatment using SCS for some of the 'fibromyalgia tender points' are provided below.

SPECIFIC MUSCLE DYSFUNCTION – SCS APPLICATIONS

The description of SCS treatment methods for those muscles included in this summary should be seen as representative, rather than comprehensive. It is assumed that once the basic principles of SCS application have been understood, and the methods as developed by Jones and Goodheart and described in earlier chapters (particularly Chapter 4) have been practiced, the following selection of muscles should suffice as exemplars.

In all descriptions it is assumed that one of the practitioner's digits will be monitoring the tender point. In some instances it is suggested that the practitioner should encourage the (intelligent and cooperative) patient to apply the monitoring pressure on the tender point, if two hands are needed by the practitioner to efficiently and safely position the patient into 'ease'. The tender points described are those identified either by Jones (1981), or by D'Ambrogio and Roth (1997), and may be used to treat the named muscles if these are hypertonic, painful or are in some way contributing to a joint dysfunction. It is worth re-emphasising that where chronic changes have evolved in muscles (e.g. fibrosis) positional release may be able to ease hypertonicity, and reduce pain, but cannot of itself modify tissues, which have altered structurally.

- In all instances of treatment of muscle pain using SCS, the position of ease should be held for not less than 90 seconds, after which a very slow return is made to neutral.

- No 'new' or additional pain should be caused by the positioning of the tender point tissues into ease.

 Upper trapezius

Tender points are located approximately centrally in the posterior or anterior fibres (Fig. 6.3).

Method The supine patient's head is side-flexed towards the treated side while the practitioner uses the positioning of the ipsilateral arm to reduce reported tender point pain by at least 70% (Fig. 6.4). The position of ease usually involves shoulder flexion, abduction and external rotation.

 Subclavius

Tender point lies inferior to central portion of clavicle, on its undersurface (Fig. 6.5).

Method Patient is side-lying, with ipsilateral shoulder in slight extension, forearm behind

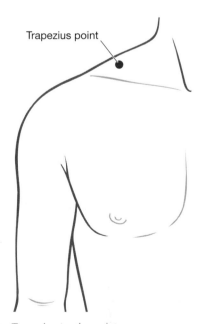

Figure 6.3   Trapezius tender point.

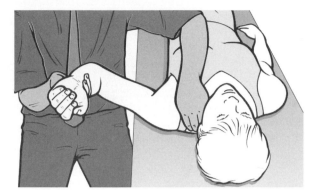

Figure 6.4   Treatment of trapezius tender point.

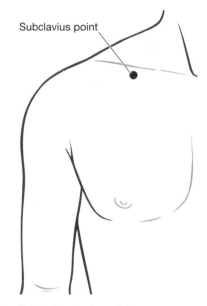

Figure 6.5   Subclavius tender point.

patient's back. The practitioner applies slight compression to the ipsilateral shoulder in a medial direction, with fine-tuning possibly involving protraction until reported sensitivity in the palpated point drops by at least 70% (Fig. 6.6).

 Subscapularis

Tender point lies close to the lateral border of the scapula, on its anterior surface (Fig. 6.7).

Method The patient lies close to the edge of the table with the arm held slightly ($\pm 30°$) in

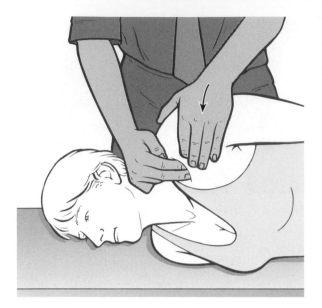

Figure 6.6   Treatment of subclavius tender point.

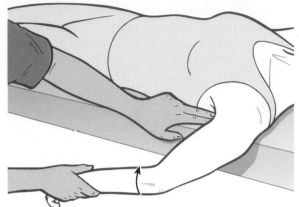

Figure 6.8   Treatment of subscapularis tender point.

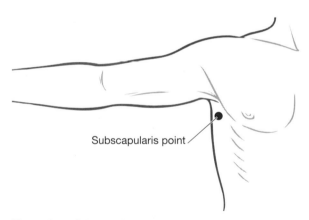

Figure 6.7   Subscapularis tender point.

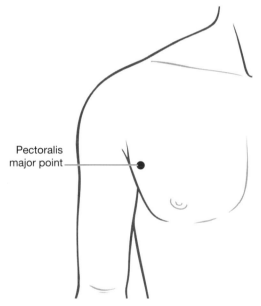

Figure 6.9   Pectoralis major tender point.

abduction, extension and internal rotation at the shoulder (Fig. 6.8). Slight traction on the arm may be used for fine-tuning, if this significantly reduces reported sensitivity.

Pectoralis major

Tender point lies on the muscle's lateral border close to the anterior axillary line (Fig. 6.9).

Method The patient lies supine as the ipsilateral arm is flexed and adducted at the shoulder,

taking the arm across the chest (Fig. 6.10). Fine-tuning involves varying the degree of flexion and adduction, which can at times usefully be amplified by applied traction to the arm (but only if this reduces the reported sensitivity in the tender point).

Pectoralis minor

Tender point is just inferior and slightly medial to the coracoid process (and also on the anterior

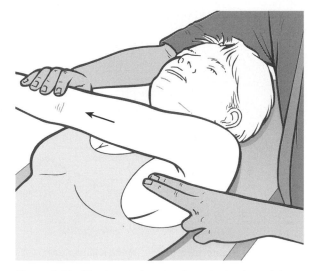

Figure 6.10   Treatment of pectoralis major tender point.

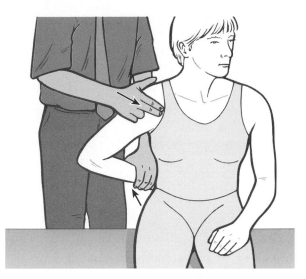

Figure 6.12   Treatment of pectoralis minor tender point.

surfaces of ribs 2, 3 and 4 close to the mid-clavicular line) (Fig. 6.11).

Method The patient is seated and the practitioner stands behind. The patient's arm is taken into extension and internal rotation, bringing the flexed forearm behind the back (Fig. 6.12). The hand which is palpating the tender point is used to introduce protraction to the shoulder while at the same time compressing it anteromedially to

fine-tune the area and reduce reported sensitivity by at least 70%.

Pubococcygeus dysfunction

Tender point lies on the superior aspect of the lateral ramus of the pubis, approximately a thumb width from the symphysis (Fig. 6.13).

Method The patient is supine as the ipsilateral leg is flexed (Fig. 6.14) until sensitivity in the palpated point drops by at least 70%. Long-axis

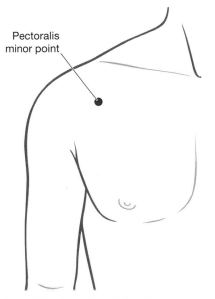

Pectoralis
minor point

Figure 6.11   Pectoralis minor tender point.

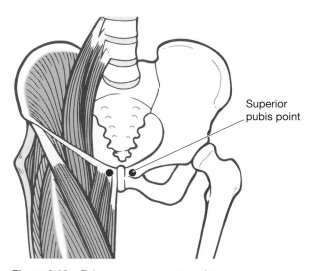

Superior
pubis point

Figure 6.13   Pubococcygeus tender point.

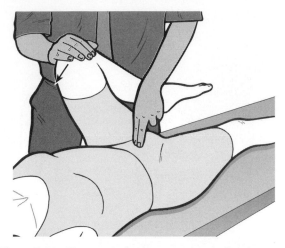

Figure 6.14 Treatment of pubococcygeus dysfunction.

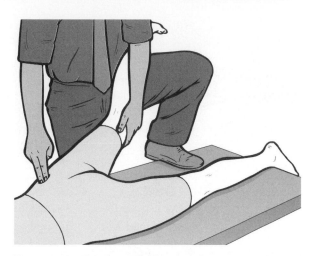

Figure 6.16 Treatment of gluteus medius tender point.

compression through the femur towards the pelvis may be useful for fine-tuning.

Gluteus medius

Tender point lies laterally, on the posterior superior iliac spine (Fig. 6.15).

Method The prone patient's ipsilateral leg is extended at the hip and abducted (Fig. 6.16) until reported pain reduces by at least 70%.

Medial hamstring

Tender point is found on the tibia's posteromedial surface on the tendinous attachment of semimembranosis (Fig. 6.17).

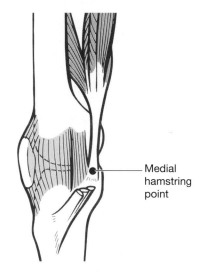

Figure 6.17 Medial hamstring tender point.

Method The patient is supine, affected leg off the edge of the table so that thigh is extended and slightly abducted, and knee is flexed (Fig. 6.18). Internal rotation of the tibia is applied for fine-tuning to reduce reported sensitivity in the tender point by at least 70%.

Lateral hamstring

Tender point is found on the tendinous attachment of biceps femoris on the postero-lateral surface of the head of the fibula (Fig. 6.19).

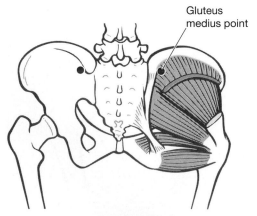

Figure 6.15 Gluteus medius tender point.

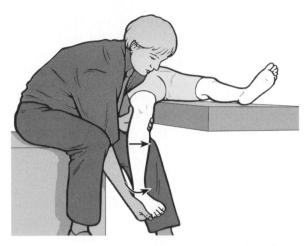

Figure 6.18   Treatment of medial hamstring tender point.

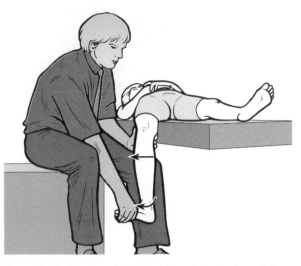

Figure 6.20   Treatment of lateral hamstring tender point.

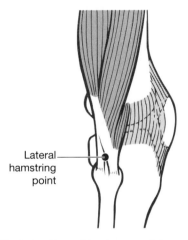

Lateral hamstring point

Figure 6.19   Lateral hamstring tender point.

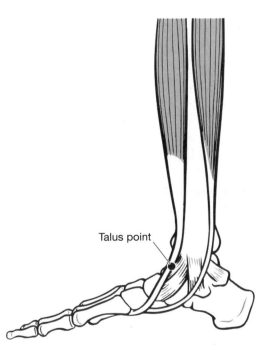

Talus point

Figure 6.21   Tibialis anterior tender point.

Method The patient is supine, affected leg off the edge of the table so that thigh is extended and slightly abducted, and knee is flexed (Fig. 6.20). Adduction or abduction, as well as external or internal rotation of the tibia, is introduced for fine-tuning, to reduce reported sensitivity in the tender point by at least 70%.

Tibialis anterior

Tender point is found in a depression on the talus, just medial to the tibialis anterior tendon, anterior to the medial malleolus (Fig. 6.21).

Method The prone patient's ipsilateral knee is flexed as the foot is inverted and the ankle internally rotated to fine-tune (Fig. 6.22), until reported sensitivity in the palpated tender point reduces by at least 70%.

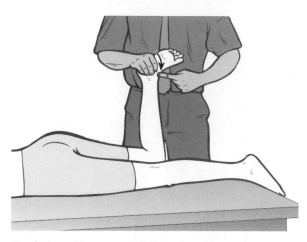

Figure 6.22 Treatment of tibialis anterior tender point.

Self-treatment SCS methods for fibromyalgia patients

The following are self-treatment methods, useful for people with fibromyalgia symptoms, which utilise SCS in relieving pain and tension from key 'tender point' sites which are used in the diagnosis of the condition (see Box 6.1, p. 98).

What should emerge, if the patient follows the guidelines as described below, is a sense of their being able to treat their own pain by this simple, non-invasive method.

Using the tender points

As described earlier in this chapter (p. 98), the diagnosis of FMS depends on there being at least 11 tender points present out of 18 tested, using a set amount of pressure (not more than 4 kg).

It should be explained to the patient that:

1. As they palpate the point they should do so just hard enough to produce a discomfort which they can use to guide them to a position of ease, using a method such as: '10 = the pain on pressure; find the position which equals 3 or less'.
2. They should be told that any movements they carry out should create no new pain as they perform the procedure and should not make any existing pain worse.

3. They should remain in the position of ease, once found, for not less than 1 minute and should then slowly return to a neutral position.
4. They should understand clearly that a position of ease for a tender point on the front of the body probably involves bending forwards slightly and vice versa, and that the guidelines given below for individual 'points' or muscles will be a guide only, not an absolute prescription, since they may well find other positions which provide greater ease.

These are the instructions, given in lay terms, which can be spelled out and demonstrated to the patient for self-treatment of the most accessible of the tender points (any of which can of course be treated by the clinician using the guidelines as described in the self-treatment notes).

Patient's instructions for self-treatment

Guidelines for the basic rules to be followed during self-treatment are summarised in Box 6.4.

1. Suboccipital muscles

To use SCS on these muscles you should be lying on your side with your head on a low pillow. These points lie at the base of your skull in a hollow just to the side of the centre of the back of the neck. Palpate the tender point on the side which is lying on the pillow with the hand on that same side, and press just hard enough to register the pain and score this in your mind as a '10'. The muscles at the base of the skull, when tender, need the head to be taken backwards and

---

Box 6.4 Patient's self-treatment guidelines

Remember the basic rules:

- Find a pain point
- Press on it hard enough to score '10'
- Move the body or part of the body around slowly until the pain is reduced to a 3, causing no additional pain or new pain anywhere else
- Stay in that position of ease for 1 minute
- Slowly return to neutral.

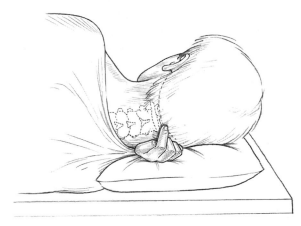

Figure 6.23 Strain/counterstrain self-treatment for suboccipital tender point.

usually leaned and perhaps turned towards the side of pain to ease the tenderness you are causing by your pressure (Fig. 6.23).

First, just take the head slightly backwards very slowly as though you are looking upwards. If the palpated pain changes give it a score. If it is now below '10' you are on the right lines. Play around with slightly more backward bending of the neck, done very slowly, and then allow the head to turn and perhaps lean a little towards the pain side. Keep 'fine-tuning' the position as you slowly reduce the pain score. You should eventually find a position in which it is reduced to 3 or less.

If the directions described above do not achieve this score reduction, the particular dynamics of your muscular pain might need you to turn the head away from the side of pain, or to find some other slight variation of position to achieve ease.

Once you have found the position of maximum ease, just relax in that position.

You do not need to maintain pressure on the tender point all the time; just test it from time to time by pressing.

Remember also that the position which eases the tenderness should not produce any other pain – you should be relatively at ease when resting with the pain point at ease. Stay like this for at least 1 minute and then SLOWLY return to a neutral position, turn over, and treat the other side in the same way.

2. Lateral neck tender points

These points lie near the side of the base of the neck between the transverse processes of the 5th and 7th cervical vertebrae. You can find the tenderness by running a finger very lightly – skin on skin, no pressure – down the side of your neck starting just below the ear lobe. As you run down you should be able to feel the slight 'bump' as you pass over the tips of the transverse processes – the part of the vertebrae which sticks out sideways.

When you get to the level of your neck which is about level with your chin, start to press in lightly after each 'bump'. Try to find an area of tenderness on one side (Fig. 6.24).

Once you have found this, sit or lie and allow the head to bend forwards (use a cushion to support it if you are lying on your back). As with the first point treated you will find that tenderness will be reduced as you take the head forwards. Find the most 'easy' position by experimenting with different amounts of forward-bending. The tenderness will be reduced even more as you fine-tune the position of your head and neck by slightly side-bending and turning the head either towards or away from the pain side – whichever gives the best results in terms of your 'pain score'. When you get the score down to a 3 or less stay in that position for at least 1 minute and then

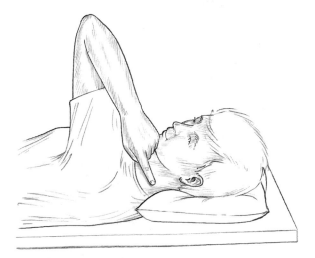

Figure 6.24 Strain/counterstrain self-treatment for lateral cervical tender point.

SLOWLY return to neutral and seek out a tender point on the other side of the neck, and treat it also.

3. Midpoint of upper trapezius muscle

The trapezius muscle runs from the neck to the shoulder and you can get an easy access to tender points in it by using a slight 'pinching' grip on the muscle using your thumb and index finger of (say) the right hand to gently squeeze the muscle fibres on the left until something very tender is found. If pressure is maintained on this tender point for 3 or 4 seconds it might well start to produce a radiating pain in a distant site, probably the head, in which case the tender point is also a trigger point (the same could be true of any of the tender points you are going to palpate but this one is one of the likeliest and commonest to refer pain elsewhere) (Fig. 6.25).

To treat the tenderness you should lie down on the side opposite that which you are treating (i.e. treated side is uppermost).

Lightly pinch/squeeze the point to produce a score of 10 and try altering the position of the arm, perhaps taking it up and over your head to 'slacken' the muscle you are palpating, or altering the neck position by having it side-bent towards the painful side on a thick cushion. Fine-tune the arm and head positions until you reduce the score in your pain point (don't pinch it all the time, just intermittently to test whether a new position is allowing it to ease).

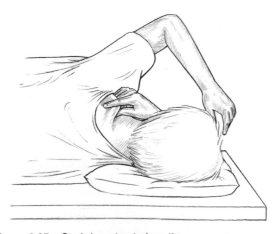

Figure 6.25 Strain/counterstrain self-treatment for tender point in middle fibres of upper trapezius muscle.

Once you find your position of ease (score down to 3 or less) stay in that position for not less than 1 minute, then SLOWLY return to a neutral position, sit up and seek out a tender point in much the same position on the other side.

4. Origin of the supraspinatus muscle above the shoulder blade

Lie on your back, head flat on the floor/bed/surface, and resting your elbow on your chest, ease your hand over your opposite shoulder area to feel with the tips of your fingers for the upper surface (nearest your neck) of your other shoulder blade.

Run your fingers along this upper surface towards the spine until you come to the end of the shoulder blade and there press into the muscles a little, looking for an area of great tenderness (most people are tender here).

You may need to press a little downwards, or back towards the shoulder or in some other direction until your find what you are looking for and can score the sensitivity as a '10'.

With your affected side (the side being treated) arm resting at your side and while your finger remains in contact with the tender point, bend the arm on the affected side so that your fingertips rest close to your shoulder. Now bring the elbow on the affected side towards the ceiling, VERY SLOWLY, and let it fall slightly away from the shoulder about half way to the surface on which you are lying (Fig. 6.26).

This should reduce the score. Now start to use 'fine-tuning' of the arm position in which you rotate the bent arm gently at the shoulder, twisting so that the elbow comes towards the chest and the hand moves away from the shoulder, very slightly, until the pain is down to a score of about 3. Hold this position for at least 1 minute, and then SLOWLY return to neutral and do the same on the other arm.

5. 2nd rib tender points

Sitting in a chair, rest a middle finger on the upper border of your breast bone, and move it

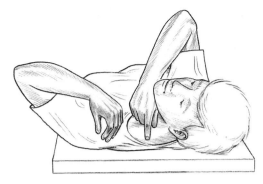

Figure 6.26   Strain/counterstrain self-treatment for supraspinatus tender point.

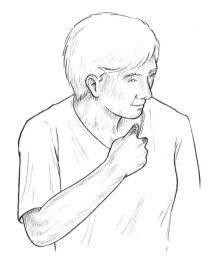

Figure 6.27   Strain/counterstrain self-treatment for second rib tender point.

slowly sideways until you touch the end of your collar bone where it joins your breast bone. Now run the finger towards your shoulder for not more than an inch along the collar bone and then down towards the chest half an inch or so. You should feel first a slight 'valley' before you come to the 2nd rib (you cannot touch the 1st rib because it is hidden behind the collar bone). Press the upper surface of the 2nd rib firmly and it should be tender, perhaps very tender (Fig. 6.27).

Maintain the pressure and score '10' and then begin to take that score down by firstly bending the head and your upper back forwards, slightly (very slightly) towards the side of the pain point, until you feel the pain reduce. Find the most 'easy' position of forward and slightly side-bending and then see whether slightly tilting the head one way or the other helps to reduce the score even more. Try also to take a full deep breath in and then slowly let the breath go, and see which part of the breathing cycle eases the tenderness most. Once you have the score down to a 3 or less, add in that most 'easy' phase of the breath (hold the breath at that phase which eases the pain most) for 10–15 seconds. Then breathe normally, but retain the position of ease for at least 1 minute before SLOWLY returning to neutral and seeking out the tender point on the other side for similar attention.

REFERENCES

Abraham G et al 1992 Management of FMS – use of magnesium and malic acid. J Nutritional Medicine 3: 49–59

Baldry D 1993 Acupuncture, Trigger Points and Musculoskeletal Pain. Churchill Livingstone, Edinburgh

Barlow W 1959 Anxiety and muscle tension pain. British J Clinical Practice 13: 5

Bass C, Gardner W 1985 Respiratory abnormalities in chronic symptomatic hyperventilation. Br Medical J 290(6479): 1387–1390

Bayer H 1950 Pathophysiology of muscular rheumatism. Zeitschrift fur Rheumatologie 9: 210

Beal M 1983 Palpatory testing of somatic dysfunction of patients with cardiovascular disease. J American Osteopathic Association, July

Bennett R 1990 Presentation on muscle microtrauma. First National Seminar for Patients, Columbus, Ohio, April 1990. Report in Fibromyalgia Network, May 1993

Block S 1993 Fibromyalgia and the rheumatisms. Controversies in Rheumatology 19(1): 61–78

Chaitow L 1982 Described in: Neuro-Muscular Technique. Thorsons, Wellingborough

Chaitow L 1989 Described in: Soft Tissue Manipulation. Thorsons, Wellingborough

Chaitow L 1991a Soft Tissue Manipulation. Thorsons, Wellingborough

Chaitow L 1991b Palpatory Literacy. HarperCollins, London

Chaitow L 1994 INIT in treatment of pain and trigger points. Br J Osteopathy XIII: 17–21

Chaitow L 1996 Modern Neuromuscular Techniques. Churchill Livingstone, Edinburgh

Chaitow L 2001 Muscle Energy Techniques. Churchill Livingstone, Edinburgh

Chaitow L, DeLany J 2000 Clinical Application of Neuro-muscular Techniques. Vol. 1 .The Upper Body. Churchill Livingstone, Edinburgh

Dahl J B, Erichsen C J, Fuglsang-Frederiksen A, Kehlet H 1992 Pain sensation and nociceptive reflex excitability in surgical patients and human volunteers. Br J Anaesthesia 69: 117 121

D'Ambrogio K, Roth G 1997 Positional Release Therapy. Mosby, St. Louis, Missouri

Deale A, Wessley S 1994 A cognitive–behavioural approach to CFS. The Therapist 2(1): 11–14

DeLuze C et al 1992 Electroacupuncture in fibromyalgia. Br Medical J November: 1249–1252

Dittrich R 1954 Somatic pain and autonomic concomitants. American J Surgery

Duna G, Wilke W 1993 Diagnosis, etiology and therapy of fibromyalgia. Comprehensive Therapy 19(2): 60–63

Ferraccioli G et al 1989 EMG-biofeedback in fibromyalgia syndrome. J Rheumatology 16: 1013–1014

Fishbain D 1989 Diagnosis of patients with myofascial pain syndrome. Archives of Physical & Medical Rehabilitation 70: 433–438

Fisher P et al 1989 Effect of homoeopathic treatment of fibrositis (primary fibromyalgia). Br Medical J 32: 365–366

Gemmell H et al 1991 Homoeopathic Rhus toxicodendron in treatment of fibromyalgia. Chiropractic J Australia 21(1): 2–6

Goldenberg D 1989 Fibromyalgia and its relationship to chronic fatigue syndrome, viral illness and immune abnormalities. J Rheumatology 16(19): 92

Goldenberg D 1993a Fibromyalgia, chronic fatigue syndrome and myofascial pain syndrome. Current Opinion in Rheumatology 5: 199–208

Goldenberg D 1993b Fibromyalgia: treatment programs. J Musculoskeletal Pain 1(3/4): 71–81

Goldenberg D 1994 Presentation to the 1994 American College of Rheumatology Conference

Goldenberg D et al 1991 Impact of cognitive–behavioural therapy on fibromyalgia. Arthritis and Rheumatism 34(19): 190

Goldthwaite J 1949 Essentials of Body Mechanics. J B Lippincott, Philadelphia

Greenman P 1989 Manual Medicine. Williams and Wilkins, Baltimore

Gutstein R 1955 A Review of myodysneuria (fibrositis). American Practitioner and Digest of Treatments 6(4)

Haanen H et al 1991 Controlled trial of hypnotherapy in treatment of refractory fibromyalgia. J Rheumatology 18: 72–75

Hartman L 1985 Handbook of osteopathic technique. Hutchinson, London

Headley B J 1993 Muscle inhibition. Physical Therapy Forum 24

Henriksson K 1993 Proceedings from Second World Congress on Myofascial Pain and Fibromyalgia. J Musculoskeletal Pain 1: 3–4

Henriksson K 1994 Reported in: Fibromyalgia Network Compendium May/July 1993. Fibromyalgia Network, Tucson, Arizona

Hubbard D R, Berkoff G M 1993 Myofascial trigger points show spontaneous needle EMG activity. Spine 18: 1803–1807

Jacobsen S 1992 Dynamic muscular endurance in primary fibromyalgia compared with chronic myofascial pain syndrome. Archives of Physical & Medical Rehabilitation 73: 170–173

Janda V 1983 Muscle function testing. Butterworths, London

Janda V 1985 In: Glasgow E (ed) Aspects of Manipulative Therapy. Churchill Livingstone, Edinburgh

Janda V1991 Muscle spasm – a proposed procedure for differential diagnosis. Manual Medicine 1001: 6136–6139

Jiminez C et al 1993 Treatment of FMS with OMT and self-learned techniques. J American Osteopathic Association 93(8): 870

Jones L 1981 Strain/counterstrain. Academy of Applied Osteopathy, Colorado Springs

Kacera W 1993 Fibromyalgia and chronic fatigue – a different strain of the same disease? Canadian J Herbalism XIV(IV): 20–29

Kalik J 1989 Fibromyalgia: diagnosis and treatment of an important rheumatologic condition. J Osteopathic Medicine 90: 10–19

Kleijnen J et al 1992 Ginkgo biloba. The Lancet 340

Kleyhans A, Aarons 1974 Digest of Chiropractic Economics, September

Korr I 1976 Spinal cord as organiser of the disease process. Academy of Applied Osteopathy Yearbook, Colorado Springs

Latey P 1986 Muscular manifesto. Privately published, London

Lehto M, Jarvinen M, Nelimarkka O 1986 Scar formation after skeletal muscle injury. Archives of Orthopedic Trauma Surgery 104: 366–370

Lewit K 1992 Manipulation in Rehabilitation of the Locomotor System. Butterworths, London

Lewit K, Simons D 1984 Myofascial pain – relief by postisometric relaxation. Archives of Physical & Medical Rehabilitation 65: 462–464

Liebenson C 1996 Rehabilitation of the Spine – a practitioners manual. Williams and Wilkins, Baltimore

Liebenson C 2001 In: Chaitow L (ed) Muscle Energy Techniques. Churchill Livingstone, in press

Lo K et al 1992 Osteopathic manipulative treatment in fibromyalgia syndrome. J American Osteopathic Association 92(9): 1177

McCain G et al 1988 Controlled study of supervised cardiovascular fitness training program. Arthritis and Rheumatism 31: 1135–1141

Melzack R, Wall P 1988 The Challenge of Pain. Penguin, London

Mense S 1993 Nociception from skeletal muscle in relation to clinical muscle pain. Pain 54: 241–290

Mitchell F, Moran P, Pruzzo N 1979 Evaluation of Osteopathic Muscle Energy Procedure. Valley Park

Moldofsky H 1993 Fibromyalgia, sleep disorder and chronic fatigue syndrome. Ciba Foundation Symposium. Chronic Fatigue Syndrome 173: 262–270

Nimmo R 1966 Receptor tonus technique. Lecture notes, London

Petersen W 1934 The Patient and the Weather: autonomic disintegration. Edward Bros, Ann Arbor

Rolf I 1977 The Integration of Human Structures. Harper and Row, New York

Roll M et al 1987 Acute chest pain without obvious cause before age 40. J Psychosomatic Research 31(2): 215–221

Rothschild B 1991 Fibromyalgia: an explanation for the aches and pains of the nineties. Comprehensive Therapy 17(6): 9–14

Rubin B et al 1990 Treatment options in fibromyalgia syndrome. J American Osteopathic Association 90(9): 844–845

Sandford Kiser R et al 1983 Acupuncture relief of chronic pain syndrome correlates with increased plasma metenkephalin concentrations. Lancet (ii): 1394–1396

Selye H 1984 The Stress of Life. McGraw Hill, New York

Simons D G 1993 Referred phenomena of myofascial trigger points. In: Vecchiet L, Albe-Fessard D, Lindlom U (eds) New trends in referred pain and hyperalgesia. Elsevier, Amsterdam

Simons D & Travell J 1998 Myofascial pain and dysfunction Vol. 1 (2nd edn). Williams and Wilkins, Baltimore

Simons D 1986 Fibrositis/fibromyalgia – a form of myofascial trigger point? American Medicine 81(3A): 93–98

Slocumb J 1984 Neurological factors in chronic pelvic pain trigger points and abdominal pelvic pain. American J Obstetrics and Gynecology 49: 536

Stoltz A 1993 Effects of OMT on the tender points of FMS. J American Osteopathic Association 93(8): 866

Travell J, Simons D 1986 Trigger Point Manual. Williams and Wilkins, Baltimore

Travell J, Simons D 1992 Myofascial Pain and Dysfunction – the trigger point manual. Williams and Wilkins, Baltimore

Triano J, Schultz A B 1987 Correlation of objective measure of trunk motion and muscle function with low-back disability ratings. Spine 12: 561

Upledger J 1983 Craniosacral Therapy. Eastland Press, Seattle

Walsh E G 1992 Muscles, Masses and Motion – the physiology of normality, hypotonicity, spasticity, and rigidity. MacKeith Press, Blackwell Scientific Publications, Oxford

Warot D et al 1991 Comparative effects of Ginkgo biloba extracts on psychomotor performance and memory in healthy subjects. Therapie 46(1): 33–36.

Wolfe F, Smythe H, Yunus M et al 1990 American College of Rheumatology 1990 Criteria for classification of fibromyalgia. Arthritis and Rheumatism 33: 160–172

Wolfe F, Simons D et al 1992 The fibromyalgia and myofascial pain syndromes. J Rheumatology 19(6): 944–951

7

SCS (and SCS variations) in hospital settings

SPECIAL PROBLEMS

Acutely ill patients have very special problems and needs when being considered for manual treatment. These relate to their inability to be moved more than a little, their difficulty in cooperating in a manual treatment because of 'multiple intravenous and subclavian taps, monitors or various types of catheters', as well as their current particular state of vulnerability, either due to illness or to their being pre- or post-surgical (Schwartz 1986).

Edward Stiles, then director of osteopathic medicine at Waterville Osteopathic Hospital in Maine, evaluated the usefulness of osteopathic attention to patients in hospital settings (Stiles 1976). He found that general osteopathic attention is of value in treating pre- and post-operative patients, especially with regard to excursion of the rib cage in order to establish a maximum ventilating ability:

This is particularly important for patients undergoing upper gastrointestinal or thoracic surgery, since a decrease in excursion of the rib cage can increase the patient's susceptibility to splinting of the thoracic cage and impede ventilating ability.

Few methods achieve this end more effectively than the application of variants of positional release methods, which are particularly relevant in the context of pain, restriction and limitation of the ability to manipulate the patient's position, as described in Chapter 3.

Positional release in pregnancy

Stiles (1976) discusses the value of positional release methods in treating a wide range of

125

problems arising in hospitalised patients, including those who are pregnant:

Pregnant patients commonly complain of pain in the back and/or legs. This usually can be relieved by osteopathic care, particularly functional techniques [see Chapter 8, p. 144 for correcting any somatic dysfunction in the lumbar area, sacrum, pelvis, and lower extremities. Functional techniques also allow for continued manipulative care right up to the time of delivery.

The potential value and importance of methods which are non-invasive and easily adapted to bed-ridden patients or those in considerable pain or distress, speaks for itself. The methods themselves are outlined by osteopathic physician Harold Schwartz, who has applied SCS methods to a severely ill, bed-bound population in a hospital setting. This involved patients in medical and surgical, obstetric and paediatric wards, including pre- and post-surgical patients, some of whom had undergone cystotomy, gastrotomy and other major surgery at the James A Taylor Hospital, Columbus, Ohio, which at the time of the report had 50 acute and 38 intermediate care beds.

Schwartz (1986) confirms Jones' assertion that all counterstrain positions are capable of being modified and applied to bed-bound patients, saying that, 'without exception, this observation has been found to be valid'.

SCS for respiratory distress

Schwartz (1986) also notes that SCS, which is the primary manipulative method routinely used in the hospital, is of particular value in mobilisation of the mechanical aspects of respiration, including, 'clavicle, ribs, sternum and anterior and posterior vertebral segments, as well as the diaphragm'. Patients due for surgery are routinely treated in order to normalise respiratory function, as well as being treated for post-operative ileus.

POST-OPERATIVE USES OF POSITIONAL RELEASE

Jerry Dickey (1989) has focused attention on the particular needs of the many thousands of people undergoing surgery each year via median sternotomy, in which the rib cage is opened anteriorly to allow access to the heart and other thoracic structures:

More than 250 000 patients undergo coronary bypass graft surgery (in the US alone) accomplished via the median sternotomy incision, an approach that has been gaining widespread acceptance. This surgical approach has been associated with a growing number of patients with structural complaints.

In this form of surgery an incision is made from the suprasternal notch to below the xiphoid process. The soft tissues below the skin are treated with diathermy to stem bleeding and the sternum is divided by an electric bone saw, the exposed edges being covered with bone wax. The sternum is then retracted with the upper level being placed at the level of the 2nd rib. Following whatever surgical intervention is involved, the sternal margins are brought together and held by stainless steel sutures. There are often drainage tubes exiting from below the xyphoid following surgery.

The degree of stress and injury endured by all the tissues of the region are clearly major, especially considering that the open-chest situation may have been maintained for many hours. The sequels to this trauma are many and varied, as Dickey explains, and include, 'dihescence, substernal and pericardial infection, nonunion of the sternum, pericardial constriction, phrenic nerve injuries, rib fractures and brachial plexus injuries'. The last two possible after-effects are probably related, according to Dickey (1989). Fully 23.5% of patients undergoing these procedures develop brachial plexus injuries, and he reports on this surgical procedure being carried out experimentally on ten cadavers, of which seven sustained first rib fractures with the fractured ends often impaling the lower trunks of the brachial plexus.

While such negative effects are usually noted immediately post-operatively many problems do not emerge until later, and these might include the structural and functional changes in chest mechanics that do not become evident for weeks or months, particularly restrictions affecting thoracic vertebrae and the rib cage, as well as fascial and diaphragmatic changes.

Dickey (1989) outlines a number of appropriate manual methods for helping in recovery, including positional release methods. He stresses the importance of structural evaluation and treatment both before and after surgery, with the manual therapeutic methods being of various types, but it is specifically the positional release approach which is discussed in the context of this book.

Because of the wide retraction involved, the upper ribs (because of their firmer attachments) sustain the greatest degree of strain. Interosseous contraction, fascial strain and diaphragmatic dysfunction may all be palpable and to an extent remediable.

It is as well to be reminded that patients undergoing this form of surgery are likely to be past middle-age, commonly with a range of existing musculoskeletal restrictions and dysfunctions, and therefore with a limited prospect of normal function being completely restored.

Testing and treating fascial patterns

Commencing around 4 weeks post-surgery, the first step suggested in aiding recovery from this trauma involves a fascial release method.

The patient should be supine. The operator places one hand between the scapulae with the other hand resting on the surface of the midline of the sternum (Fig. 7.1). Each hand should be turned independently in a clockwise and then an anticlockwise direction, allowing assessment of the 'tissue preference pattern', as the skin and fascia are taken in their respective directions of motion towards whichever restriction barriers they currently exhibit.

In other words, the motion of the hands on the tissues is asking, 'in which direction do the tissues most easily move?', as the anterior and posterior assessment is made.

Normal, unstressed, tissues exhibit an equal excursion in both directions of rotation, although this is seldom found in adults, even if surgical trauma has not been a factor (Zink et al 1979).

Whichever direction of rotation is most 'easy' should be held – simultaneously front and back, each in their preferred direction – until tension

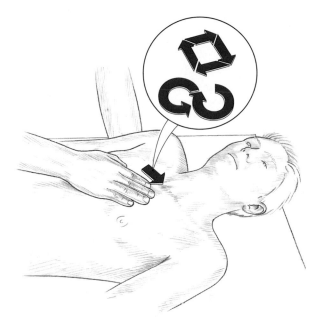

Figure 7.1 Release of traumatised fascial structures. In this figure, the operator's left hand lies between the patient's scapulae while the right hand lies on the sternum. The hands independently assess the 'tissue preference patterns' (Dickey 1989). These positions of ease are held in order to allow distorted fascial patterns to modify or normalise.

eases. This will commonly release recently acquired stress patterns in the fascia, possibly revealing older patterns which can then be addressed.

This approach should be applied at least weekly until distorted fascial patterns are resolved or cease to alter, possibly indicating an intractably fixed state.

Indirect rib treatment

Dickey suggests that following the non-specific fascial release method described above, standard rib function tests should be performed in order to identify ribs which are not symmetrical in their range of movement during the respiratory cycle, so that treatment can be introduced in order to assist in normalising what has become restricted.

In the early post-operative phase, a classical osteopathic positional release approach is suggested (Kimberly 1980).

Method The patient sits on one side of a treatment table and the operator sits facing the opposite way on the other side. In this way, by half-turning towards the patient, there is easy operator access to the lateral chest wall.

Having previously identified ribs which are restricted in their range of motion using standard assessment procedures, the operator places his hands so that the index and middle fingers of one hand contact the restricted rib to be treated, facing forwards along the anterior aspect of the rib, while the other index and middle finger contact the same rib, facing backwards along the posterior aspect (Figs 7.2A and 7.2B). The thumbs rest touching each other, tip-to-tip, at the mid-axillary line.

The patient is asked to sit erect and to gently lean towards the operator, so that the ribs and the fingers make good contact. In this way no force is exerted by the operator towards the ribs and the patient controls the degree of pressure being applied, which should be just enough to maintain firm contact.

At this point, the patient is asked to slightly rotate their trunk towards the side opposite that being treated, which effectively eases the rib away from its demifacets. When the operator senses that this has been achieved, the patient is instructed to partially inhale and then exhale in order for an evaluation to be made as to which phase of the cycle induces the greatest sense of palpable ease, freedom from tension. This evaluation is communicated to the patient, who is asked to hold the breath in the phase that induces maximum ease for as long as is comfortable.

As this process is continuing, the operator should be maintaining the contact on the rib in order to achieve its maximal degree of ease. Any sense that 'bind' is returning calls for a slight modification in the direction in which the rib is being held.

The patient may need to repeat the breathing phase several times in order to achieve freedom of motion for a restricted rib at any treatment

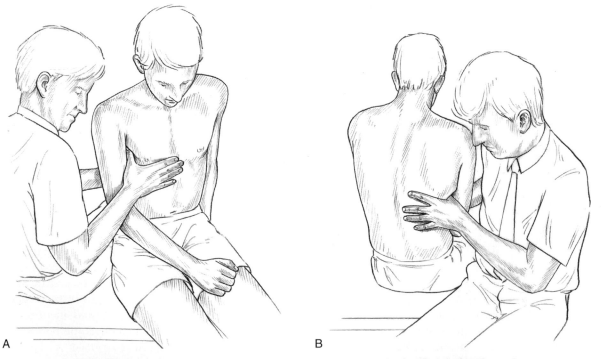

A   B

Figure 7.2A and B The operator achieves firm but gentle contact of a previously identified dysfunctional rib (elevated, depressed, restricted). The patient controls the degree of hand pressure by leaning towards the operator and then slightly turning towards the side opposite that being treated, which releases the demifacets. The patient then inhales and exhales as the operator assesses the phase at which the rib is most at ease. The patient holds this phase for as long as is comfortable, one or more times, until improved function is noted (Kimberly 1980, Dickey 1989).

session, which should be repeated not less than weekly until the ribs have all been released to the degree that is possible.

The SCS techniques for rib dysfunction correction outlined in Chapter 3 (p. 56) should also be employed in order to support the method described above.

Improving lymphatic drainage

In patients who have undergone surgery as described, there may well be lymphatic stasis, as evidenced by swelling/oedema in the region of the posterior axillary fold. Dickey suggests that the operator should, 'assess the tissue preference patterns of the upper arm and the forearm, independently'.

Once established, both sites should be taken towards the direction of the tissue preference, 'with slight compression through the elbow and the shoulder until he or she perceives the tension relaxing'. This approach is repeated at each visit until tissue drainage is normal.

It is not difficult to see the similarities between the post-operative methods suggested by Dickey and the concepts of SCS and functional technique as described elsewhere. The commonality is the sensing of directions of ease in tissues, along with a supportive, non-invasive holding of the tissues in that state until resolution occurs, whether the structures being treated are osseous (ribs) or soft (fascia, muscle).

Unlike SCS, these methods do not involve the use of pain-monitoring points, with the position of maximal ease being achieved entirely by means of palpation assessment.

FURTHER HOSPITAL APPLICATIONS OF SCS

SCS is also used in hospital settings as an adjunctive treatment of patients with congestive heart failure, respiratory failure, pneumonia, bronchitis and asthma.

Other conditions which call for SCS in hospital settings include acquired positional pain, especially after spinal anaesthesia, or after the return to a normal position following a lithotomy position, after perineal surgery.

Schwartz suggests that SCS can be used in differential diagnosis in acute pain situations. He gives examples of an apparent acute abdominal pain below and to the right of the umbilicus. This is where pain would be palpated were there a flexion strain of the 11th thoracic vertebrae, as well as if there were acute appendicitis. If pain returns rapidly after an SCS application to the point, appendicitis is strongly indicated.

A second example is given of the diagnostic potential of SCS in the case of a differential assessment between myocardial infarction and acute costochondritis. The latter is often rapidly amenable to SCS treatment using a tender point in one of the left costal interspaces, while the myocardial infarction would not respond to such treatment.

Schwartz (1986) suggests that:

Literally thousands of hospital days could be saved by judicious osteopathic examination for interspace dysfunction and appropriate counterstrain treatment.

Schwartz's description of the tender point

Schwartz's description of tender points is based directly on Jones' work. The points are used as monitors in SCS application, and are described as being, 'pea-sized bundles or swellings of fascia, muscle tendrils, connective tissue and nerve fibres as well as some vascular elements'.

Interestingly, unlike many other authors, he notes that, 'generally, but not always, pressure on the tender point will cause pain at a site distant to the point itself', which of course defines such a point as a trigger point, as well as a tender point (see Chapter 6, p. 109). He acknowledges that 'tender points' resemble both Chapman's neurolymphatic reflexes and Travell's myofascial trigger points (Owens 1982, Travell 1949).

Schwartz highlights the difference between SCS and other methods which use such points in treatment by saying, 'other methods invade the point itself, for example by needle in acupuncture, injection of Lidocaine into the point, or the use of pressure or ultrasound to destroy the tender point'.

When using SCS, if a position of ease is achieved and tenderness vanishes from the palpated point, one of a number of sensations may become apparent to the operator, a 'sudden release', or a 'wobble', or a 'give', or a 'melting away', all of which indicate a change in the tissues in response to the positional change which has been brought about by the operator.

The two phases of the positioning process are emphasised, the first being 'gross' movement which takes the area or the patient to the approximate position of ease, and 'fine-tuning' which takes the remainder of the pain from the tender point.

Special positions for bed-bound patients

The majority of spinal structure tender points were described in detail in Chapter 3 (p. 47 onward). In this summary of Schwartz's suggestions for bed-bound patients, only the particular modifications necessary in such a setting are emphasised.

Anterior cervical

The anterior cervical points located around the tips of the transverse processes are easily accessible in a bed-bound patient, as are the positions of ease (Fig. 7.3), which almost all require a degree of flexion and side-bending rotation, usually away from the side of pain.[1] The upper cervical anterior points tend to require more rotation in order to ease their discomfort than those in the lower cervical region.

Posterior cervical

The posterior cervical points lie on or around the tips of the spinous processes and require extension of the head on the neck, and/or the neck as a whole (Fig. 7.4), which is more easily achieved in bed-bound patients if they are side-lying, with – it is suggested – the painful side uppermost,

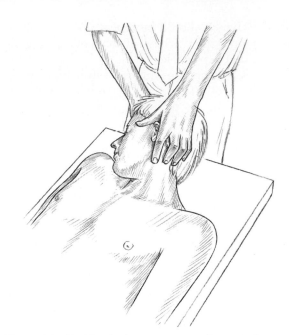

Figure 7.3 Positional release treatment of an anterior cervical strain (flexion) utilising a tender point as a monitor. Points in this area require more rotation than those in the lower cervical spine.

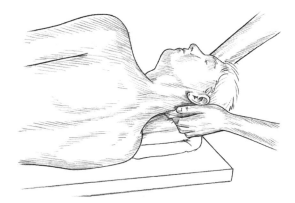

Figure 7.4 Patient side-lying: Positional release treatment of a posterior cervical strain (extension) utilising a tender point as a monitor. Points in this region require extension and some rotation and side-bending for 'fine-tuning' the position of ease.

since according to Schwartz's guidelines (based on Jones) the main side-bending and rotation needs to be towards the pain side, which would be difficult were the patient lying on that side.

The C3 posterior point may require extension or flexion to create ease and both directions should be gently attempted until the greatest reduction in sensitivity is achieved.

---

[1] According to Schwartz; the author, however, frequently finds rotation towards the pain more useful and suggests that readers experiment in order to confirm for themselves that rotation might indeed be in either direction, and that the patient's report of less pain and the feeling of greater ease in the palpated tissues is the most accurate guide to the final position.

Posterior thoracic and lumbar spinal

Posterior thoracic and lumbar spinal points lie close to the spinous processes in the upper thoracic and become increasingly lateral, lying on or around the transverse processes in the lower thoracic and lumbar vertebrae, in the lower thoracic spine.

The upper four thoracic segments are best treated with the patient side-lying with the arms resting, if possible, at the level of the shoulders (Fig. 7.5) and with the upper arm supported by a pillow in order to avoid the introduction of rotation. The patient should bend backwards to the level of the tender point in order to remove the palpated pain.

For the middle thoracic vertebrae, posterior points are also treated with the patient side-lying, but this time the arms are held above the head as the patient moves into extension.

The lower four thoracic vertebrae are treated for posterior tender points with the patient supine and the operator standing on the lesioned side, with one hand under the patient to palpate the point. The hand of the side opposite the pain is held and the arm drawn across the chest towards the operator, so that the shoulder on that side lifts 30–45° from the bed, at which time fine-tuning should remove residual pain.

If the patient's condition means that they cannot be turned onto their side, then the method suggested for the lower thoracic vertebrae can be substituted for the side-lying posture outlined above.

Posterior lumbar tender points

Posterior lumbar tender points which are described and illustrated in Chapter 3 (p. 48), and which are usually treated with the patient prone, can be dealt with efficiently in the side-lying posture.

L1, L2, L3 and L4 involve the side-lying patient, lesion side uppermost. L1 and L2 (Fig. 7.6) require the upper leg being taken into straight extension and then either abduction or adduction, and/or rotation (of the leg) one way or the other, whichever combination provides the greater ease. In treatment of L3 and L4, as well as upper-pole L5 (lying between the 5th lumbar spinous process and the 1st sacral spinous process) and the lower-pole L5 point (located midway on the body of the sacrum), abduction and extension of the leg is introduced and fine-tuning is achieved by variations in the degree of extension, as well as by the introduction of rotation internally or externally of the foot.

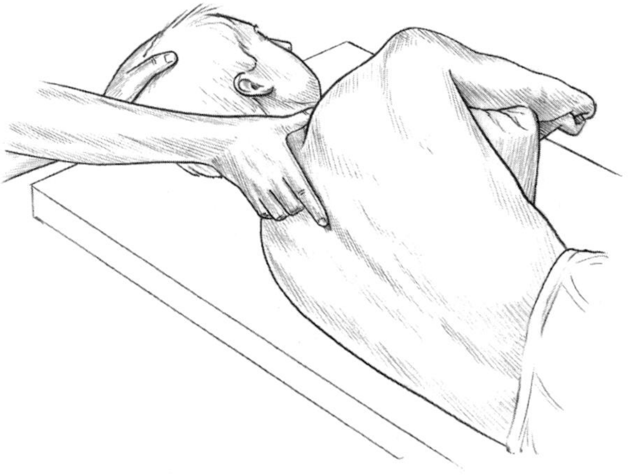

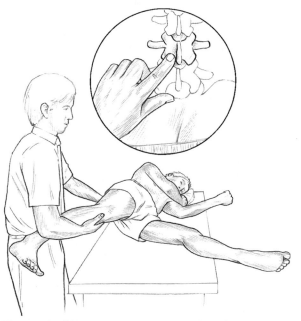

Figure 7.5 Side-lying position for treatment of extension strains in the thoracic or lumbar region. The patient is eased into extension until pain or palpated tension modifies appropriately.

Figure 7.6 Side-lying position for treatment of lower lumbar strains using the lower limb as a lever to achieve a position of ease. Fine-tuning may involve variations in rotation and/or flexion of the knee.

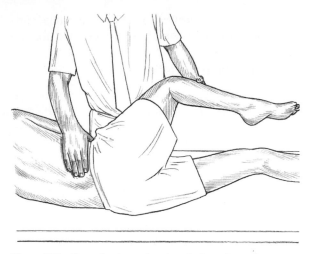

Figure 7.7 Some lumbar extension strains, where, for example, the tender point lies in the superior sacral sulcus, may ease if the hip is flexed in the side-lying position, as illustrated.

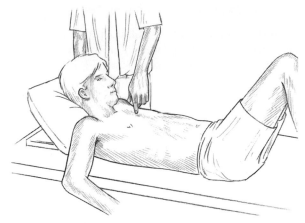

Figure 7.8 Thoracic spinal flexion strains – acute or chronic – are associated with tender points on the anterior thorax. Ease is achieved by introduction of flexion while the arms are held away from the trunk. Fine-tuning may involve head/neck rotation to one side or the other.

For treatment of what is known as the middle-pole L5 tender point (in the superior sulcus of the sacrum), the side-lying patient's upper leg (lesion side) is flexed at hip and knee and this rests on the operator's thigh. It is fine-tuned by movement of the leg into greater or lesser degrees of hip flexion (Fig. 7.7) and by the degree of abduction or abduction needed to produce ease. The patient's ipsilateral arm may then be used in fine-tuning by having it hang forward and down over the edge of the bed.

Anterior thoracic

Anterior thoracic tender points lie on the anterior or surface of the thorax, the first six on the midline and the lower ones slightly lateral to it, bilaterally at approximately 1–2 cm intervals (see Chapter 3, p. 47), so that from T8 onwards the tender points lie in abdominal musculature.

These points relate directly to respiratory dysfunction and respond dramatically quickly to SCS methodology. The improvement in breathing function is commonly immediately apparent to the patient. In bed-bound patients, the patient is supine and there is usually a need for pillows or bolsters to assist in supporting them as flexion is introduced (Fig. 7.8).

For the first six anterior thoracic tender points (lying on the sternum) the patient's arms are allowed to rest slightly away from the body, and the knees and hips are flexed, feet resting on the bed. The only movement usually needed to ease tenderness is flexion of the head and neck towards the chest (the lower the point the greater the degree of flexion). Fine-tuning involves movement of the head slightly towards or away from the palpated pain site.

For tender point treatment from T7 onwards, the patient's buttocks are rested on a pillow so that the segment involved is unsupported, allowing it to fall into flexion. Alternatively, the operator can support the flexed knees and bring them towards the head, so flexing the lumbar and thoracic spine (Fig. 7.9).

Fine-tuning may involve crossing the patient's ankles or side-bending to or away from the side of palpated tenderness, whichever combination reduces sensitivity more.

Anterior lumbar

Anterior lumbar (see Chapter 3, p. 47) tender points require a similar positioning to that called for by the thoracic points.

Rib dysfunction and interspace dysfunction

The appropriate treatment for rib dysfunction and interspace dysfunction is described in

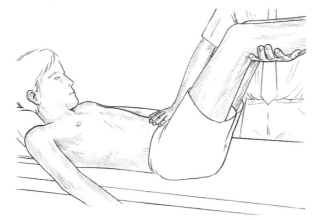

Figure 7.9 Positional release treatment of flexion strains of the lower thoracic and lumbar spine involve introduction of flexion via elevation of the flexed lower limb, with fine-tuning achieved by variations in limb positioning and/or side-bending.

Chapter 3 (pp. 56–60) and can be applied to bed-bound patients without any modification.

Schwartz reports that:

Interspace dysfunctions are implicated in costochondritis, the persistent chest pain of the patient who has suffered acute myocardial infarction, 'atypical' angina and anterior chest wall syndrome. They are strongly implicated along with depressed and elevated ribs in restricted motion of ribs … and thus contribute to the aetiology and morbidity of many respiratory illnesses.

Side-effects (McPartland 1996)

It is reported that between a quarter and a third of patients treated by SCS have some reaction, despite the gentleness of the approach. Very occasionally there are extensive 'muscle release' reactions. These are usually transitory and seldom last more than a few hours. However,

patients should be forewarned of the possibility to allay anxiety. No treatment is needed for the reaction if it occurs, as it is itself merely evidence of an adaptation process and passes rapidly.

'Stoic' patients

Since the process of finding a position of ease requires feedback from the patient, it is unlikely to be useful in patients who say that there is little or no pain (despite evidence to the contrary) and who would therefore have difficulty in reporting any change as positioning and fine-tuning were carried out. Such patients can be better treated using functional approaches, as described in Chapter 8, in which the operator relies on palpated tissue release or ease rather than on subjective information reported by the patient.

ADVANTAGES OF SCS IN THE HOSPITAL SETTING

SCS treatment is non-invasive and is anything but traumatic and can be applied to a patient in almost any degree of ill-health and distress.

Schwartz concludes:

It may be used on patients with fractures, as well as on post-surgical patients who have pain at the site of incision. It may also be used on patients who have osseous metastatic disease. If the part of the body that is to be treated can be moved by the patient it can safely be treated with SCS.

Results are claimed to be lasting and repetitive treatment is needed (in hospital settings) only if there is ongoing neurosensory reflex activity, or if the condition which produced the dysfunction in the first place is repeated or ongoing.

REFERENCES

Dickey J 1989 Postoperative osteopathic manipulative management of median sternotomy patients. J American Osteopathic Association 89(10): 1309–1322

Kimberly P (ed) 1980 Outline of osteopathic manipulative procedures. Kirksville College of Osteopathic Medicine, Kirksville

McPartland J M 1996 Personal communication

Owens C 1982 An endocrine interpretation of Chapman's reflexes. American Academy of Osteopathy, Newark, Ohio

Schwartz H 1986 The use of counterstrain in an acutely ill

in-hospital population. J American Osteopathic Association 86(7): 433–442

Stiles E 1976 Osteopathic manipulation in a hospital environment. J American Osteopathic Association 76: 243–258

Travell J 1949 Basis for multiple use of local block of somatic areas. Mississippi Valley Medical J 71: 13–21

Zink G et al 1979 An osteopathic structural examination and functional interpretation of the soma. Osteopathic Annals 7: 12–19

8

Functional technique

ORIGINS OF FUNCTIONAL TECHNIQUE

There is a long tradition in manipulative medicine in general, and osteopathy in particular, of positional release methods, often applied in an almost intuitive manner.

Hoover (1969a) quotes the words used by two osteopaths of his acquaintance who had been students of the founder of osteopathy, Andrew Taylor Still. They individually responded to a question as to what it was that they were doing while treating a patient, with the words, 'I am doing what the body tells me to do . .'.

All the words in the world cannot substitute for actually feeling what happens when these methods are applied and, for this reason, exercises later in this chapter will be included in order to help bring to life the meaning and feeling of the explanations for what is in essence the most simple, and yet one of the most potent, of manipulative methods; one which creates a situation in which dynamic homeostatic balance of the affected tissues is created; one in which self-repair can most easily occur.

The term 'functional technique' grew out of a series of study sessions held in the New England Academy of Applied Osteopathy in the 1950s under the general heading of, 'A functional approach to specific osteopathic manipulative problems' (Bowles 1955, 1956, 1957).

The methods involved were derived from traditional methods which dated back to the origins of osteopathy in the nineteenth century, but which had never been formalised or scientifically evaluated.

It was only in the 1950s and 1960s that research, most notably by Irvin Korr (1947), coincided with a resurgence of interest in this approach, largely as a result of the clinical and teaching work of HV Hoover, with the result that, 'functional technique has become quite comfortable in today's scientific climate, as well as streamlined and highly effective in practice' (Bowles 1981).

When considering the methodology of functionally orientated techniques, one distinctive difference stands out as compared with most other positional release methods, and with strain/counterstrain in particular.

In functional work, palpation for a 'position of ease' involves a subjective appreciation of tissue, as it is brought through positioning towards ease, to a state of 'dynamic neutral' (see Chapter 1), rather than relying on a report by the patient as to reduction in pain as positioning is pursued.

Theoretically (and usually in practice) the palpated position of maximum ease (reduced tone) in the distressed tissues should approximate the position which would have been found were pain being used as a guide as it would were either Jones' or Goodheart's approach being employed. Similarly, were the concept of 'exaggeration of distortion' or 'replication of position of strain' employed, the same end-position should be achieved, a position of dynamic neutral (see Chapter 1, Box 1.1, for summary of positional release variations).

Bowles (1956) gives an example:

A patient has an acute low back and walks with a list. A structural diagnosis is made and the fingertips palpate the most distressed tissues, within the area of most distress. The operator begins tentative positioning of the patient, preferably sitting. The fingertips pick up a slight change toward a dynamic neutral response, a little is gained, not much, but a little. A little, but enough so the original segment is no longer the most distressed area within the area of general distress. The fingers then move to what is now the most acute segment. As much feeling of dynamic neutral is obtained here as possible. Being temporarily satisfied with slight improvements here and there, this procedure continues until no more improvement is detectable. That is the time to stop.

Using tissue response to guide the treatment the operator has step-by-step eased the lesioning and corrected the structural imbalance to the extent that the patient is on the way to recovery.

FUNCTIONAL OBJECTIVES

Hoover (1957) has summarised the key elements of functional technique in diagnosis and treatment:

- Diagnosis of function involves passive evaluation as the part being palpated responds to physiological demands for activity made by the operator or the patient.
- Functional diagnosis determines the presence or absence of normal activity of a part which is required to respond as a part of the body's activities (say respiration, or the introduction of passive or active flexion or extension). If the participating part has free and 'easy' motion, it is normal. However, if it has restricted or 'binding' motion, it is dysfunctional.
- The degree of ease and/or bind present in a dysfunctional site when motion is demanded is a fair guide to the severity of the dysfunction.
- The most severe areas of observed or perceived dysfunction are the ones to treat initially.
- The directions of motion which induce ease in the dysfunctional sites indicate precisely the most desirable pathways of movement.
- Use of these guidelines automatically precludes undesirable manipulative methods, since an increase in resistance, tension or 'bind' would result from any movement towards directions of increased tissue stress.
- Treatment using these methods is seldom, if ever, painful and is well received by patients.
- The application requires focused concentration on the part of the operator and may be mentally fatiguing.
- Functional methods are suitable for application to the very ill, the extremely acute and the most chronic situations.

FUNCTIONAL EXERCISES

The exercises which are described in the text of this chapter are variously derived from the work of Johnston (1964), Stiles and colleagues (Johnston et al 1969, Johnston 1988), Greenman (1989), Hoover (1969b) and Bowles (1955, 1964, 1981).

Bowles is definite in his instructions to those attempting to learn to use their palpating contacts in ways which will allow the application of functional methods:

- The palpating contact ('listening hand') must not move.
- It must not initiate any movement.
- Its presence in contact with the area under assessment/treatment is simply to derive information from the tissue beneath the skin.
- It needs to be tuned into whatever action is taking place beneath the contact and must temporarily ignore all other sensations such as, 'superficial tissue texture, skin temperature, skin tension, thickening or doughiness of deep tissues, muscle and fascial tensions, relative positions of bones and range of motion'.
- All these signs should be assessed and evaluated and recorded separately from the functional evaluation, which should be focused single-mindedly on tissue response to motion:

It is the deep segmental tissues, the ones that support and position the bones of a segment, and their reaction to normal motion demands, that are at the heart of functional technique specificity.

Terminology

Bowles (1964) explains the shorthand use of these common descriptive words:

Normal somatic function is a well-organised complexity and is accompanied by an easy action under the functionally-orientated fingers. The message from within the palpated skin is dubbed a sense of 'ease' for convenience of description. Somatic dysfunction could then be viewed as an organised dysfunction and recognised under the quietly palpating fingers as an action under stress, an action with complaints, an action dubbed as having a sense of 'bind'.

In addition to the 'listening hand' and the sensations it is seeking, of ease and bind, Bowles suggests we develop a 'linguistic armament' which will allow us to pursue the subject of functional technique without 'linguistic embarrassment' and without the need to impose quotation marks around the terms each time they are used.

He therefore asks us to become familiar with the additional terms, 'motive hand', which indicates the contact hand which directs motion (or fingers, or thumb or even verbal commands for motion – active or assisted), and also 'normal motion demand' which indicates what it is that the motive hand is asking of the body part. The motion could be any normal movement such as flexion, extension, side-bending, rotation or combination of movements – the response to which will be somewhere in the spectrum of ease and bind, which will be picked up by the listening hand for evaluation.

At its simplest, functional technique sets up a 'demand–response' situation, which allows for the identification of dysfunction – as bind is noted – and which also allows for therapeutic intervention as the tissues are guided into ease.

Bowles' summary of functional methods

In summary, whatever region, joint or muscle is being evaluated by the listening hand the following results might occur:

- The motive hand makes a series (any order) of motion demands (within normal range) which includes all possible variations. If the response noted in the tissues by the listening hand is ease in all directions, then the tissues are functioning normally.
- The motive hand makes a series of motion demands which includes all possible variations. However, some of the directions of movement produce bind when the demand is within normal physiological ranges. The tissues are responding dysfunctionally.
- For therapy to be introduced in response to an assessment of bind relating to particular motion demands, the listening hand's feedback is required so that, as the motions which produced bind are reintroduced, movement is modified so that the maximum degree of ease possible is achieved:

Therapy is monitored by the listening hand and fine-tuned information as to what to do next is then fed back to the motive hand. Motion demands are selected which give an increasing response of ease and compliance under the quietly palpating fingers.

The results can be startling, as Bowles explains:

Once the ease response is elicited it tends to be self-maintaining in response to all normal motion demands. In short, somatic dysfunctions are no longer dysfunctions. There has been a spontaneous release of the holding pattern.

1. Bowles' functional exercise

- Stand up and place your fingers on your own neck muscles paraspinally, so that the fingers lie – very lightly, without pressing, but constantly 'in touch' with the tissues – approximately over the transverse processes.
- Start to walk for a few steps and try to ignore the skin and the bones under your fingers.
- Concentrate all your attention on the deep supporting and active tissues as you walk.
- After a few steps stand still and then take a few steps walking backwards, all the while evaluating the subtle yet definite changes under your fingertips.
- Repeat the process several times, once while breathing normally and once while holding the breath in, and again holding it out.
- Standing still, take one leg at a time backwards, extending the hip and then returning it to neutral before doing the same with the other leg.
- What do you feel in all these different situations?

This exercise should help to emphasise the 'listening' role of the palpating fingers and of their selectivity as to what it is to which they wish to listen.

The listening hand contact should be 'quiet, non-intrusive, non-perturbing' in order to register the compliance of the tissues and evaluate whether there is a greater or lesser degree of 'ease' or 'bind' on alternating steps and under different circumstances as you walk.

2. Stiles and Johnston's sensitivity exercise

Exercise 2(a) The time suggested for this exercise is 3 minutes.

- In a classroom setting, pair up with another person and have them sit, as you stand behind

them resting your palms and fingers over their upper trapezius muscle, between the base of the neck and shoulder.
- The object is to evaluate what happens under your hands as your partner takes a deep inhalation.
- This is not a comparison of inhalation with exhalation, but is meant to help you assess how the areas being palpated respond to inhalation – do they stay easy, or do they bind?
- You should specifically **not** try to define the underlying structures or their status in terms of tone or fibrosity, simply assess the impact, if any, of inhalation on the tissues.
- Do the tissues resist, restrict, bind or do they stay relaxed?
- Compare what is happening under one hand with what is happening under the other during inhalation.
- Reverse the roles and have your partner assess you in the same manner to see which hand palpates the area of greatest bind on your inhalation.

Exercise 2(b) The time suggested for this exercise is 5–7 minutes.

- Go back to the starting position where you are palpating your original partner who is seated with you standing behind.
- The objective this time is to map the various areas of 'restriction' or bind in the thorax, anterior and posterior, as your partner inhales.
- In this exercise try not only to identify areas of bind but assign what you find into 'large' (several segments) and 'small' (single segment) categories.
- To commence, place a hand, mainly fingers, on (say) the upper left, upper thoracic area, over the scapula, and have your partner inhale deeply several times, firstly when seated comfortably, hands on lap, and then with the arms folded on the chest (exposing more the costovertebral articulation).
- After several breaths with your hand in one position resite the hand a little lower, or more medially or laterally as appropriate, until the entire back has been 'mapped' in this way.
- Remember that you are not comparing how the tissues feel on inhalation as compared with

exhalation, but how different regions compare (in terms of ease and bind) with each other in response to inhalation.

● Map the entire back and front of the thorax in this way – for location of bind and for 'size' of the restricted area.

● Go back to any 'large' areas of bind and see whether you can identify any 'small' areas within them, using the same simple contact and inhalation as the motion component.

● Individual spinal segments can also be mapped by sequentially assessing them one at a time as they respond to inhalations.

● Switch places, so that your partner now has the opportunity to assess you.

● As you sit having your thorax assessed, take the opportunity to ask yourself how you would normally handle the information you have uncovered in your 'patient':

– Would you try in some way to mobilise what appears to be restricted?

– If so, how?

– Would your therapeutic focus be on the large areas of restriction or the small ones?

– Would you work on areas distant from or adjacent to the restricted areas?

– Would you try to achieve a release of the perceived restriction by trying to move it mechanically towards and through its resistance barrier, or would you rather be inclined to try to achieve release by some indirect approach, moving away from the restriction barrier?

– Or, do you try a variety of approaches, mixing and matching until the region under attention is free or improved?

There are no correct or incorrect answers to these questions; however, the various exercises in this section (and elsewhere in the book) should open up possibilities for other ways being considered, ways which do not impose a solution but allow one to emerge.

Exercise 2(c) The time suggested for this exercise is 5–7 minutes.

● Go back to the original 'doctor/patient' setting, with your partner seated, arms folded on the chest, and you standing behind with your listening hand/fingertips placed on the upper left thorax, on or around the scapula area.

● Your motive hand is placed at the cervicodorsal junction, so that it can indicate to your partner your request that she move forward of the midline (dividing the body longitudinally in the coronal plane), not into flexion but in a manner which carries the head and upper torso anteriorly.

● The movement will be found to be more easily accomplished if your partner has arms folded, as suggested above.

● The repetitive movement forwards, into the position described, and back to neutral, is initiated by the motive hand, while the listening hand evaluates the changes created by this.

● The comparison which is being evaluated is of one palpated area with another, in response to this normal motion demand. As Johnston, Stiles and colleagues (1967) state it: 'It is not anterior direction of motion compared with posterior direction, but rather a testing of motion into the anterior compartment only, comparing one area with the ones below and the ones above, and so on'.

● Your listening hand is asking the tissues whether they respond easily or with resistance to the motion demanded of the trunk. In this way try to identify those areas, large and small, which bind as the movement forward is carried out.

● Compare these areas with those identified when the breathing assessment was used.

The patterns elicited in Exercise 2(c) involved movement initiated by yourself, whereas the information derived from 2(a) and 2(b) involved intrinsic motion, initiated by exaggerated respiration. Stiles and his colleagues have in these simple exercises taken us through the initial stages of palpatory literacy in relation to how tissues respond to motion self-initiated or externally-induced.

Implications Other ways of using the information gathered during Exercise 2(c) are further expanded:

In this particular testing what you have been doing is changing the positional relationship of the shoulders and the hips. Clues about this shoulder-to-hips relationship, elicited at the restricted area in this way, can become criteria for you in picking the technique you may want to use to effectively change the specific dysfunction being tested … We feel that a better chance of 'correction' may be established if you use a technique which will take the dysfunctional area and deal not only with the flexion–extension component, the side-bending and the rotation, but also see that the shoulders are properly positioned in relation to the hips.

Hoover poses a number of questions in the following exercises ('experiments' he calls them) the answers to which should always be 'yes'. If your answers are indeed positive at the completion of the exercise then you are probably sensitive enough in palpatory skills to be able to effectively utilise functional technique.

3. Hoover's clavicle exercise

Exercise 3(a) Suggested time for this exercise is 5 minutes. The question posed in this part of the exercise is, 'Does the clavicle move in a definite and predictable manner?'.

- Stand facing your seated partner and place the pads of the fingers of your right hand (listening hand) onto the skin above the right acromioclavicular joint.
- With your left hand, hold the right arm just below the elbow. Ensure that your partner is relaxed and that you have the full weight of the arm and that they do not assist or hinder in any way as the exercise is carried out (Fig. 8.1).
- Ensure that you have this cooperation by raising and lowering the arm several times.
- Slowly and deliberately take the arm back from the midline, just far enough to sense a change in the tissues under your palpating hand and then return it to neutral. Avoid quick movements so that the sensations being palpated are accurately noted. Repeat this movement several times so that this single movement's influence can be assessed. Recall the question posed by Hoover for consideration as you make this passive movement of the arm.
- Now take the arm forward of the midline, until you sense a tissue change under your listening hand's fingertips. Repeat this single movement several times; forward and back to neutral, repeat and repeat, assess all the while.

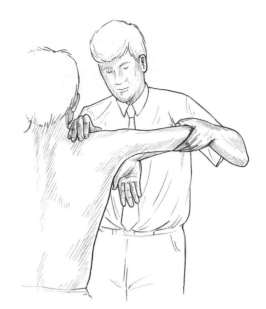

Figure 8.1 Assessing for positions which induce ease or bind in the acromioclavicular joint. The fully supported arm is passively moved in various directions (Exercises 3a, 3b and 3c, Hoover 1969b).

- Introduce abduction of the arm from its neutral position and then return it to neutral several times. Then introduce adduction – bringing the arm across the front of the trunk slightly – before returning it to neutral. Repeat this several times.
- In a similar manner, starting from and returning to neutral, assess the effect on ease and bind of a slowly introduced degree of internal and then external rotation, conducted individually. What was the response of individual physiological movements to the question, 'Does the clavicle move in a definite and predictable manner?'

The answer to the question posed should be that the clavicle does indeed move in a definite and predictable manner when demands for motion are made upon it.

Exercise 3(b) Suggested time for this exercise is 5 minutes. The question posed in this exercise is, 'Are there differences in ease of motion and feeling of tissues of the clavicle when it is caused to move in different physiological motions?'.

- Adopt the same starting position as in 3(a) and then move your partner's arm backwards into extension very slowly as you palpate tissue change at the lateral end of the clavicle.

● Compare the feelings of ease and bind as you then take the arm into flexion, bringing it forward of the body.

● Then compare the feelings of ease and bind as you abduct and adduct the arm sequentially, passing through neutral as you do so.

● Compare the ease and bind sensations as you internally and externally rotate the arm.

In this exercise, instead of individual motion demands assessed on their own, you have the chance to evaluate what happens in the tissues being palpated as opposite motions are introduced sequentially without a pause.

The question posed asks that you decide whether there were directions of motion which produced altered feelings of ease in the tissues.

The answer should be that there are indeed usually identifiable differences or aberrations of motion and tissue texture when the clavicle is caused to move in different physiological motions.

Exercise 3(c) Suggested time for this exercise is 5 minutes. The question posed in this exercise is, 'Can the differences of ease of motion and tissue texture be altered by moving the clavicle in certain ways?'.

● Repeat the introductory steps and commence by flexing the arm, and bringing it forwards of the midline until you note the clavicle beginning to move and the texture under palpation changing to bind. Then move the flexed arm backwards into extension until the clavicle starts to move and the sensation of bind is noted. Between these two extremes lies a position of maximum ease, a position of physiological balance, in this plane of motion (forward and backward of the midline). It is this state of balance which you need to establish.

● Starting from this balanced point of ease, use the same guidelines for assessing the point at which the clavicle starts moving and bind is noted, as you seek a point of balance between abduction and adduction of the arm.

● When you find the combined position of maximal ease, having explored flexion/extension and abduction/adduction, and starting from that position, you need to find the point of ease between the extremes where clavicle movement and bind are noted as you introduce internal and external rotation.

● Once this is established you have achieved a reciprocal balance between the arm and the clavicle.

You should have effectively answered question 3(c), since it should now become clear that aberrations of motion and tissue texture can be changed by motion of the clavicle.

The experiment continues

Starting from this position of reciprocal balance, reassess, as you did in the first part of the whole exercise (p. 140), all the individual directions of motion of the arm (flexion, abduction, etc.).

Unlike the first part of the exercise, however, you will not be starting from the position in which the arm hangs at the side, but rather from a point of dynamic balance in which the tissues are at their most relaxed.

What you are seeking now are single motions of the arm/clavicle which are free, which produce the least sense of bind and the greatest sense of ease, starting from this balanced position.

When such a motion is identified:

This one motion is continued slowly and gently as long as the sensory hand reports improving conditions, if a state is reached in which movement in that one direction increases bind and does not make movement more easy and tissue texture more normal, the sequence of physiological motions are again checked.

What Hoover is taking us towards in this exercise is the point at which we no longer impose action on the body, but follow it – where we allow the tissues to guide us towards their most desired directions of motion and positional ease.

In effect, what he has done, if we can follow his instructions up to this point, is to bring us to the start of treating using functional technique. The process described above, of finding physiological, dynamic balance and then seeking the pathways of greatest ease for the tissues, is functional technique in action. Still, using the clavicle as our example, the further evolution of the process described, in which the tissues guide the operator, requires a great deal of practice. Hoover explains:

The operator relaxes and becomes entirely passive as his sensory or listening hand detects any change in the clavicle and its surrounding tissues. A change in the clavicle and its surrounding tissues, if felt by the sensory hand, sends information to the reflex centres which relay an order to the motor hand to move the arm in a manner so as to maintain the reciprocal balance, or neutral. If this is the proper move there will be a feeling of increasing ease of motion and improved tissue texture. This process continues through one or more motions until the state of maximum ease or quiet is attained.

4. Hoover's thoracic exercise

Exercise 4(a) Suggested time for this part of the exercise is 4 minutes.

● You are standing behind your seated partner, whose arms are folded on their chest. Having previously assessed by palpation, observation and examination the thoracic or lumbar spine of your partner, lightly place your listening hand on those segments which are most restricted or in which the tissues are most hypertonic.

● Wait and do nothing as your hand 'tunes' in to the tissues. Make no assessments as to structural status. Wait for at least 15 seconds. Hoover says:

The longer you wait the less structure you feel. The longer you keep the receiving fingers still, the more ready you are to pick up the first signals of segment response when you proceed to induce a movement demand.

● With your other hand, and by voice, guide the patient into flexion and then extension. The motive hand should apply very light touch, just a suggestion of which direction you want movement to take place. The listening hand does nothing but wait to feel the functional response of ease and bind as the spinal segments move into flexion and then extension.

● A wave-like movement should be noted as the segment being palpated is involved in the gross motion demanded of the spine. A change in the tissue tension under palpation should be noted as the various phases of the movement are carried out.

● Practice the assessment at various segmental levels and try to feel the different status of the palpated tissues during the phases of the process, as bind starts, becomes more intense, eases somewhat and then becomes very easy before a hint of bind reappears and then becomes intense again.

Decide where the maximum bind is felt and where maximum ease occurs. These are the key pieces of information required for functional technique as you assiduously avoid bind and home in on ease.

● Try also to distinguish between the bind which is a normal physiological response to an area coming towards the end of its normal range of movement, and the bind which is a response to dysfunctional restriction.

● Switch places and allow your partner to evaluate you in the same way.

Exercise 4(b) Suggested time for this part of the exercise is 3 minutes.

● Return to the starting position as in 4(a) and, while palpating an area of restriction or hypertonicity, induce straight side-bending to one side and then the other while assessing for ease and bind in exactly the same way as in 4(a).

● Change places and allow your partner to do this to you.

Exercise 4(c) Suggested time for this part of the exercise is 3 minutes.

● Return to the starting position as in 4(a) and 4(b) and while palpating an area of restriction or hypertonicity, induce rotation to one side and then the other while assessing for ease and bind in exactly the same way as in 4(a) and 4(b).

Exercise 4(d)

● Return to the starting position as in 4(a) and, while palpating an area of restriction or hypertonicity, induce straight side-bending to one side and then the other while assessing for ease and bind in exactly the same way as in 4(a).

● Change over to allow your partner to do this to you.

Different responses

Hoover describes variations in what might be felt as the response of the tissues as palpated during these various positional demands:

1. Dynamic neutral This response to motion is an indication of normal physiological activity. There is minimal signalling during a wide range of motions in all directions. Hoover states it in the following way:

This is the pure and unadulterated unlesioned (i.e. not dysfunctional) segment, exhibiting a wide range of easy motion demand–response transactions.

2. Borderline response This is an area or segment which gives some signals of some bind fairly early in a few of the normal motion demands. The degree of bind will be minimal and much of the time ease, or dynamic neutral, will be noted. Hoover states that, 'most segments act a bit like this', they are neither fully 'well' nor 'sick'.

3. The lesion response[1] This is where bind is noted almost at the outset of almost all motion demands, with little indication of dynamic neutral. Hoover suggests that you should:

Try all directions of motion carefully. Try as hard as you can to find a motion demand that doesn't increase bind, but on the contrary, actually decreases bind and introduces a little ease. This is possible. This is an important characteristic of the lesion [dysfunction].

Indeed, he states that the more severe the restriction the easier it will be to find one or more slight motion demands which produce a sense of ease or dynamic neutral, because the contrast between ease and bind will be so marked.

Hoover's summary

Practice is suggested with dysfunctional joints and segments in order to become proficient. Three major ingredients are required for doing this successfully, according to Hoover:

1. A focused attention to the process of motion demand and motion response, while whatever is being noted is categorised, as 'normal', 'slightly dysfunctional', 'frankly or severely dysfunctional', and so on.

2. A constant evaluation of the changes in the palpated response to motion in terms of ease and bind, with awareness that this represents increased and decreased levels of signalling and tissue response.

3. An awareness that in order to thoroughly evaluate tissue responses, all possible variations in motion demand are required, which calls for a structured sequence of movement demands.

Hoover suggests that these be verbalised (silently):

Mentally, set up a goal of finding ease, induce tentative motion demands until the response of ease and increasing ease is felt, verbalise the motion-demand which gives the response of ease in terms of flexion, extension, side-bending and rotation. Practice this experiment until real skills are developed. You are learning to find the particular ease-response to which the dysfunction is limited.

In addition, depending upon the region being evaluated, the directions of abduction, adduction, translation forwards, translation backwards, translation laterally and medially, translation superiorly and inferiorly, etc., need to be factored into this approach.

Greenman's functional exercise, below (p. 144), introduces some of these elements.

Bowles describes the goal

Charles Bowles summarises succinctly what is being sought:

The activity used to test the segment (or joint) is largely endogenous, the observing instrument is highly non-perturbational, and the information gathered is about how well or how poorly our segment of structure is solving its problems. Should we find a sense of easy and non-distorted following of the structures, we diagnose the segment as normal. If we find a sense of binding, tenseness, tissue distortion, a feeling of lagging and complaining in any direction of the action, then we know the segment is having difficulty properly solving its problems.

The diagnosis would be of dysfunction.

---

[1] Note the use of the word 'lesion' predates the introduction of the term 'somatic dysfunction' to describe abnormally restricted segments or joints. To update this term we should call this a 'dysfunctional response'.

5. Greenman's functional literacy exercise

Exercise 5(a) The time suggested for this exercise is 3 minutes.

● Stand behind your seated partner, whose arms are folded so that their hands hold their opposite shoulders.

● Place a listening hand somewhere on the upper thoracic spine, where tissue tightness or restriction has previously been identified.

● Your other hand should be placed on your partner's head in order to initiate movement into flexion and back to neutral several times as you palpate for the position which induces maximal ease under the listening hand.

● Then introduce a slow repetitive extension and back to neutral sequence, again noting where the position of maximal ease is achieved.

Is ease greater in flexion or extension?

Exercise 5(b) The time suggested for this exercise is 3 minutes.

● Return to neutral and introduce side-bending to the right and rotation to the left of the head and neck on the trunk, as you palpate the upper thoracic segment you have chosen. Do this several times and then reverse the directions so that the head/neck is side-bending to the left and rotating to the right repetitively. In which variation and direction do the tissues become easiest?

● Try to find a point somewhere between extreme side-bending left with rotation right and side-bending right with rotation left, where the palpated tissues feel most relaxed.

Exercise 5(c) The time suggested for this exercise is 3 minutes.

● Go back to neutral and introduce, and try to combine, the following motions as you palpate for ease and bind:
- small degrees of neck flexion combined with right side-bending and right rotation
- small degrees of neck flexion combined with left side-bending and left rotation.

Did you feel the same or different degrees of ease and bind in the palpated tissues during these motions?

● Switch positions with your partner and have your tissues evaluated.

6. Greenman's spinal 'stacking' method

The recommended time for this exercise is 10 minutes.

In previous exercises individual directions and some simple combinations of movement have been used to assess the response of the palpated tissues in terms of ease and bind. In this exercise pairs of motion demands are made (e.g. flexion and extension). However, each of these assessments, after the first one, commences from the point of ease discovered in relation to the previous motion demand assessed.

In this way, the ultimate position of maximal ease, of dynamic neutral, is equal to the sum of all the previously achieved positions of ease so that one position of ease is literally 'stacked' onto another.

● Stand behind your seated partner, whose arms are crossed on their chest, hands on shoulders.

● Place your listening hand on an upper thoracic segment and take your other arm across and in front of your partner's folded arms to embrace their opposite shoulder or lateral chest wall.

● Motion demands are made by verbal instruction as well as by slight encouragement from the motive hand.

● A series of assessments is made for ease (see Fig. 8.2) in each of the following pairs of direction:
- flexion and extension
- side-bending in both directions
- rotation in both directions
- translation anteriorly and posteriorly
- lateral translation in both directions
- translation cephalad and caudad (traction and compression)
- full inhalation and full exhalation.

● The last investigation should be of the influence on ease of the different phases of breathing, full inhalation and full exhalation. However, apart from this, the sequence in which the other movements are performed is irrelevant, as long

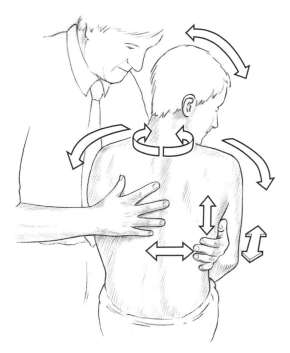

Figure 8.2 Functional palpation (or treatment) of a spinal region/segment during which all possible directions of motion are assessed for their influence on the sense of 'ease and bind' in the palpated tissues. After the first position of ease is identified (sequence is irrelevant) each subsequent assessment commences from the position of ease (or combined positions of ease) identified by the previous assessment(s) in a process known as 'stacking'.

as they are all introduced so that each subsequent motion demand commences from the position of ease previously discovered.

● The final respiratory demand indicates in which phase of breathing the most ease in the tissues is noted, and once this has been established that phase is 'stacked' onto the combined position of ease previously developed, and is held for anything from 90 seconds, after which the position of neutral is slowly readopted before the entire stacking sequence is performed again.

Functional treatment of the knee

Johnston (1964) describes the way in which an acute knee restriction might be handled using a functional approach. He stresses that the description given is unique to the particular pattern of dysfunction existing in the patient under consid-

eration and that quite different patterns of dysfunction and therapeutic input would be noted in each and every acute knee problem treated. We need to consider, in each case, 'this particular patient with this particular problem'.

A young male patient is described who had a painful left knee, of 3 months duration, which could not fully straighten following a period of extensive kneeling. On examination, the left leg remained slightly flexed at the knee, with tissues in the region somewhat warmer and more congested than in the normal right knee. Extension of the knee was painful and produced a rigid resistance as well as subjective pain.

Standing on the left of the patient the operator placed his right hand so that the palm was in contact with the patella, the thumb encircled the knee to contact the lateral aspect of the joint interspace while the second finger was in contact with the medial joint interspace. This listening hand maintained a contact light enough to appreciate subtle changes in tissue status (the sense of tension and rigidity in the tissues – described as bind) while also being able to assist in subsequent motion introduced by the other hand.

The left hand firmly held the patient's left ankle (Fig. 8.3A).

Initially the extreme sense of bind was assessed by slightly yet forcibly taking the joint into extension – straightening the leg a little. As the knee was then returned to its position of slight flexion the sense of ease was noted.

Exploration of various directions of motion were then evaluated for the response of ease and bind. This has the purpose of 'mapping out an enlarging pattern for the response of decreasing bind'. The knee was then moved into greater degrees of flexion, both elevated from the table and with the upper leg handing below the edge of the table (Figs 8.3B and 8.3C). Various motions were assessed, including abduction and adduction of the lower limb, internal and external rotation of the lower leg.

The greatest degree of ease was noted by the listening hand when the hip was flexed, the knee was markedly flexed and the lower leg was internally rotated and abducted.

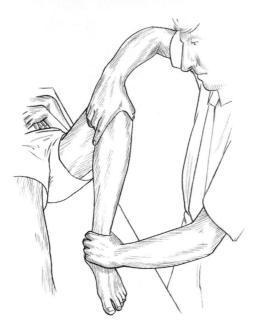

Figure 8.3A   Johnston's (1964) exercise for 'mapping out an enlarging pattern for the response of decreasing bind' in a knee joint.

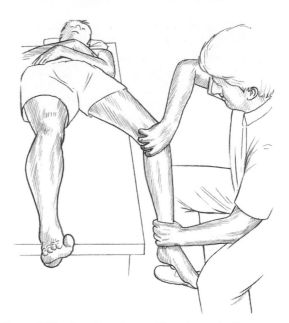

Figure 8.3C   An alternative position of ease for the strained knee may be found in which the hip is slightly extended and abducted while the lower limb is taken into flexion, abduction and/or internal rotation.

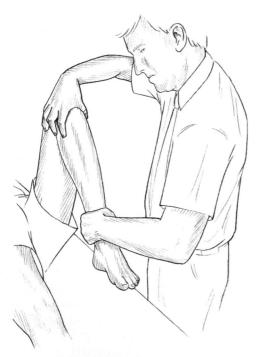

Figure 8.3B   Commonly a position of ease for the knee will be found in which introduction of hip and knee flexion is followed by the lower leg being internally rotated and abducted, while tissue status is monitored in the knee area.

Painless approach

Johnston highlights the value of such an approach in a painful condition:

Even when this testing involved the potentially painful ranges of motion, the increasing binding response at the fingertips is so immediate and is so dramatic a signal to the operator that the ranges need barely be entered.

Treatment was carried out, following this evaluation sequence, with the supine patient's leg supported as in the assessment process. The limb was raised to clear the table and taken into semi-flexion, as a torsion arc of internal rotation and abduction was introduced by the operator's left hand (holding the ankle), while the right hand monitored the response of the tissues around the knee, as well as supporting the knee in its flexed position.

Alternative ranges and motions were occasionally tested during the procedure in order to 're-clue' the operator's right hand to the sense of immediately increasing bind.

With the knee markedly flexed, the thigh slightly abducted, and the lower leg held in its 'ease' position of internal rotation and abduction, a 'sudden change' in tissue tension was noted, which allowed a sense of freedom as the leg was returned to its resting position. It remained slightly flexed but with objectively less rigidity, an assessed improvement of around 15% in terms of its degree of acuteness.

Repetition of the whole process

Precisely the same sequence of assessment and treatment was then repeated once more. This repetition is not a precise repositioning of the knee in the previous position of ease, but rather a further evaluation during which a new ideal position of 'balanced neutral' is determined by the process of palpation and motion. Having gone through this process once, the second sequence will usually reveal a slightly different pathway to a state of ease. In this instance, Johnston informs us that the subsequent evaluation of the position of maximal ease for the dysfunctional knee differed slightly from the previous one, as did the therapeutic holding position.

After these two functional treatments, the degree of dysfunction in terms of restriction and pain was reduced by approximately 40%.

At subsequent visits the process was carried further towards normalisation so that:

After five office visits during four weeks of continued improvement in use, the leg was able to be rested comfortably straight and the binding was no longer discernible at the knee.

It is the experience of those using functional technique that a less chronic, less 'organised' degree of dysfunction would respond more rapidly than one, such as the case described, in which soft tissue changes in response to the strained tissues had become established for several months.

This functional diagnostic and treatment process takes longer to describe than to accomplish, for, once the listening hand learns to evaluate ease and bind, and the operator learns to assess the variable positions open to motion, in any given setting, the whole process can take a matter of a very few minutes.

Functional treatment of the atlanto-occipital joint

This final 'exercise' is offered as a means of introducing functional technique methodology into clinical practice. It is almost universally applicable, has no contraindications, and builds on the basic exercises in functional methodology described in this chapter. The only situations in which it would be difficult or impossible to apply this method would be if the patient were unable to relax and allow the procedure to be completed, over a period of several minutes.

- Patient is supine.
- Practitioner sits at the head of the table, slightly to one side so that s/he is facing the corner.
- One hand (caudal hand) cradles the occiput with opposed index finger and thumb palpating the soft tissues adjacent to the atlas.
- The other hand is placed on patient's forehead or crown of head.
- The caudal hand searches for feelings of 'ease' or 'comfort' or 'release' in the tissues surrounding the atlas, as the hand on the head directs it into compound series of motions, one at a time.
- As each motion is 'tested' a position is identified where the tissues being palpated feel at their most relaxed or easy.
- This position of the head is used as the starting point for the next element in the sequence of assessment.
- In no particular order (apart from the first movements into flexion and extension), the following directions of motion are tested, seeking always the position of the head and neck which elicits the greatest degree of ease in the tissues around the atlas, to 'stack' onto the previously identified positions of ease.
  - flexion/extension (suggested as the first directions of the sequence)
  - side bending left and right
  - rotation left and right
  - antero-posterior translation (shunt, shift)
  - side-to-side translation
  - compression/traction.
- Once 'three dimensional equilibrium' has been ascertained (known as dynamic neutral), in

which a compound series of ease positions have been 'stacked', the patient is asked to inhale and exhale fully – to identify which stage of the breathing cycle enhances the sense of palpated 'ease' – and the patient is asked to hold the breath in that phase of the cycle for 10 seconds or so.

● The final combined position of ease is held for 90 seconds before SLOWLY returning to neutral.

● Note that the sequence in which directions of movements are assessed is not relevant – as long as as many variables as possible are employed in seeking the combined position of ease.

● The effect of this held position of ease is to allow neural resetting to occur, reducing muscular tension, and also to encourage improved circulation and drainage through previously tense and possibly ischaemic or congested tissues.

REFERENCES

Bowles C 1955 A functional orientation for technic, part 1. Academy of Applied Osteopathy Year Book, Colorado Springs

Bowles C 1956 A functional orientation for technic, part 2. Academy of Applied Osteopathy Year Book, Colorado Springs

Bowles C 1957 A functional orientation for technic, part 3. Academy of Applied Osteopathy Year Book, Colorado Springs

Bowles C 1964 The musculoskeletal segment as a problem-solving machine. Academy of Applied Osteopathy Yearbook, Colorado Springs

Bowles C 1981 Functional technique – a modern perspective. J American Osteopathic Association 80(5): 326–331

Greenman P 1989 Principles of manual medicine. Williams & Wilkins, Baltimore

Hoover H V 1957 Functional technique. Academy of Applied Osteopathy Yearbook, Colorado Springs

Hoover H 1969a Collected papers. Academy of Applied Osteopathy Yearbook, Colorado Springs

Hoover H V 1969b A method for teaching functional technic. Academy of Applied Osteopathy Yearbook, Colorado Springs

Johnston W 1964 Strategy of a functional approach in acute knee problems. Academy of Applied Osteopathy Yearbook, Colorado Springs

Johnston W 1988 Segmental definition (Part 1 January and Part 2 February). J American Osteopathic Association

Johnston W, Robertson A, Stiles E 1969 Finding a common denominator. Academy of Applied Osteopathy Yearbook, Colorado Springs

Korr I 1947 The neural basis for the osteopathic lesion. J American Osteopathic Association 47: 191

9

Facilitated positional release (FPR)

THE NATURE OF FPR
(Schiowitz 1990, 1991)

Stanley Schiowitz has described the method known as facilitated positional release (FPR), which uses elements of both SCS and functional technique, in what seems to produce an accelerated resolution of hypertonicity and dysfunction, to the extent that this is achievable via positional release mechanisms.

He explains that FPR is in line with other indirect methods, which adopt positional placement towards a direction of freedom of motion, and away from restriction barriers.

What is 'special' to this approach is that FPR adds to this absolute requirement (movement away from the barrier of restriction), the need for a prior modification of the sagittal posture – so that in a spinal area for example, a balance would first be achieved between flexion and extension. FPR then adds to this the 'facilitating' elements, which could involve either compression or torsion, or a combination of both, which induces an immediate tissue release in terms of hypertonicity or restriction of motion.

In spinal terms, the placing of regions into a neutral state, somewhere between extension and flexion, has the effect of releasing facet engagement.

The neurophysiology which Schiowitz describes in order to explain what happens during the application of FPR is based on the work of Korr (1975, 1976) and Bailey (1976) and correlates with the mechanisms suggested in Chapter 6 (p. 103), relating to the manner in which muscles respond to facilitation and sensitisation, as well as to the means whereby neural mechanisms can be induced to modify any increase in gamma motoneuron activity which may be affecting muscle spindle behaviour. 'This (reduction in gamma motoneuron activity) allows the extrafusal muscle fibres to lengthen to their normal relaxed state' (Carew 1985).

The placement of involved tissues or joints into a position of ease involves the operator fine-tuning the neurological feedback process, ensuring that the relaxation response is specific to the muscle fibres involved in the problem.

Do muscles cause joint problems or vice versa?

Janda (1988) states that it is not known whether dysfunction of muscles causes joint dysfunction or vice versa. However, he points to the undoubted fact that they massively influence each other, and that it is possible that a major element in the benefits noted following joint manipulation derives from the effects that such methods (high-velocity thrust, mobilisation, etc.) have on associated soft tissues.

Steiner (1994) has specifically discussed the role of muscles in disc and facet syndromes and describes a possible sequence of events as follows:

- A strain involving body torsion, rapid stretch, loss of balance, etc., produces a myotatic stretch reflex response in, for example, a part of the erector spinae.
- The muscles contract to protect excessive joint movement, and spasm may result if there is an exaggerated response and they fail to assume normal tone following the strain.
- This limits free movement of the attached vertebrae, approximates them and causes compression and, possibly, bulging of the intervertebral discs and/or a forcing together of the articular facets.
- Bulging discs might encroach on a nerve root, producing disc-syndrome symptoms.
- Articular facets, when forced together, produce pressure on the intra-articular fluid, pushing it against the confining facet capsule, which becomes stretched and irritated.

- The sinuvertebral capsular nerves may therefore become irritated, provoking muscular guarding, initiating a self-perpetuating process of pain–spasm–pain.

He continues:

From a physiological standpoint, correction or cure of the disc or facet syndromes should be the reversal of the process that produced them, eliminating muscle spasm and restoring normal motion.

He argues that before discectomy or facet rhizotomy is attempted, with the all-too-frequent 'failed disc-syndrome surgery' outcome, attention to the soft tissues and articular separation to reduce the spasm should be tried, to allow the bulging disc to recede and/or the facets to resume normal relationships.

Clearly, osseous manipulation often has a place in achieving this objective. However, the evidence of clinical experience indicates that a soft tissue approach may also be employed in order to allow restoration of functional integrity.

If, for example, joint restriction were the result of muscle hypertonicity, then complete or total release of this heightened tone would ensure a greater freedom of movement for the joint.

If, however, other intra-articular factors were causing the joint restriction then, although improvement of soft tissue status produced by a reduction in hypertonicity would ease the situation somewhat, the basic restriction would remain unresolved.

Focus on soft tissue or joint restriction using FPR

Schiowitz suggests that FPR can be directed towards either local palpable soft tissue changes, or as a means of modifying the deeper muscles which might be involved in joint restriction:

It is sometimes difficult … to make a clear diagnostic distinction as to which is the primary somatic dysfunction, changes in tissue texture or motion restriction. If in doubt, it is recommended that the palpable tissue changes be treated first. If motion restriction persists, then a technique designed to normalise deep muscles involved in the specific joint motion restriction should be applied.

In order to appreciate the way in which FPR is used examples of its application will be explained.

SOFT TISSUE CHANGES IN THE SPINAL REGION

Schiowitz follows Jones' guidelines, which state that soft tissue changes on the posterior aspect of the body are treated in part by taking them into a backward-bending direction, while those on the anterior aspect of the body require a degree of flexion to assist in their normalisation using FPR. However, he also reminds us that:

Some muscles have a contralateral side-bending function or a rotary component or both. Those muscles must be placed in their individual shortened positions. Careful localisation of the component motions of compression, forward- or backward-bending, and side-bending/rotation to the area of tissue texture change will allow a faster and more accurate result.

FPR for soft tissue changes affecting spinal joints

After placing the patient into a relaxed position, the first requirement is that the sagittal posture should be modified to create a flattening of the anteroposterior spinal curve in whichever spinal region needs treating, 'thus a mild reduction of the normal cervical and lumbar lordosis or the thoracic kyphosis is established', inducing a softening and shortening of the affected muscle(s).

Following this, additional elements of fine-tuning might involve compression and/or torsion (Fig. 9.1), in order that the dysfunctional tissue or articulation to be treated may be placed in such a manner that 'it moves freely or is pain-free, or both'.

The position of ease achieved by this fine-tuning is then held for 3–4 seconds, before being released so that the area can be re-evaluated.

The component elements which comprise the various facilitating forces, i.e. crowding or torsion, can be performed in any order.

Intervertebral application of FPR

When dealing with restrictions and dysfunctional states of the intervertebral (soft tissue) structures, Schiowitz suggests that the associated vertebrae be placed into 'planes of freedom' of motion. For this to be successful, the directions of

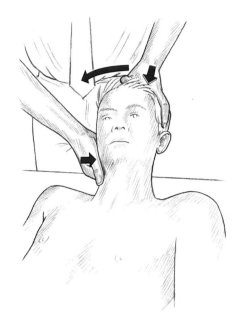

Figure 9.1   FPR treatment of anterior cervical dysfunction involves introduction of a reduced cervical curve followed by compression, side-bending and some slight torsion to achieve a sense of ease in palpated tissues.

'ease' and 'bind' of a given segment need first to be evaluated.

If, for example, there is a restriction of a cervical vertebra in which it is found that, in relation to the vertebrae below, it cannot easily extend, side-bend right and rotate right, it would be logical, in order to establish a position of ease, to take it into flexion, side-bending left and rotation left, in relation to the vertebrae below, as a first stage of application of FPR.

Cervical restriction – FPR treatment method

If, in such an example, there were obvious discomfort/pain or tissue changes palpable posterior to the articular facet of the third cervical vertebra, the following procedure (which needs to involve backward-bending because the tissues are on the posterior aspect of the body) might be suggested.

The patient would be supine on the table, the operator seated at the head of the table with a pillow on his lap. The patient would move to a position in which the head was clear of the end of the table and comfortably resting on the cushion. Contact would be made with the area of tissue texture alteration (right articular facet, third cervical vertebra) by the operator's left index-finger pad, while at the same time the head (occipital region) was being well supported by the right hand of the operator. It is via the activity of this right hand that further positioning would mainly be achieved.

As noted previously, the first priority in FPR is to reduce the sagittal curve and this would be achieved by means of a slight flexion movement, introduced by the left hand.

The second component, compression, would then be introduced by application of pressure through the long axis of the spine towards the feet. The changes in tissue tone thus induced should be easily palpable by the contact finger ('listening finger') as a reduction in the sense of 'bind'. No more than 0.5 kg (1 lb) of force should be involved in this compressive effort (Fig. 9.2A).

The next component of FPR in this instance would be the introduction of rotation/torsion and this could be achieved by slight extension and side-bending to the right over the operator's contact on the dysfunctional tissue, the right index finger. Cervical spinal mechanics dictate that side-bending is impossible without some degree of rotation taking place towards the same side. Therefore, rotation to the right would automatically occur as the neck was being side-bent over the finger, so further easing and softening the tissues being treated (Fig. 9.2B).

This final position would be held for 3–4 seconds, before slowly returning the neck and head to neutral for reassessment of the degree of tissue change/release achieved by the procedure.

Spinal joint – FPR treatment

The only difference between treating a soft tissue change which is affecting a spinal joint, and treating the spinal joint itself using FPR, is the degree of precision required in the positioning process.

Where the individual mechanics of restriction have been identified, the joint needs to be placed in 'all three planes of freedom of motion', into the directions of 'ease', using 'careful localisation of

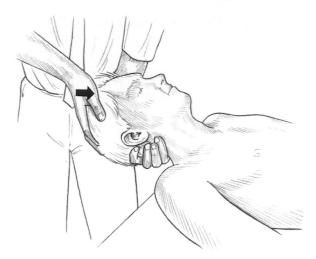

Figure 9.2A   FPR treatment of posterior cervical dysfunction involves introduction of a reduced cervical curve followed by compression, as palpating hand monitors tissues for a sense of ease.

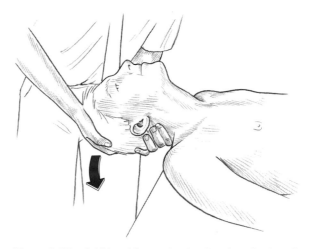

Figure 9.2B   Additional fine-tuning involves introduction of extension side-bending and some slight rotation until a sense of ease in palpated tissues is noted, and held for 4–5 seconds.

the component motions'. In other words, in flexion, side-bending and rotation, having taken care to commence from a position in which the normal sagittal curves have been somewhat reduced or neutralised.

Slight movement only for top cervical articulation

It is important to recall that in regard to the atlanto-occipital joint, flexion should require a slight degree of movement only, and that atlanto-occipital mechanics involves contralateral directions of motion, i.e. side-bending and rotation are in opposite directions, unlike the rest of the cervical spine where side-bending and rotation are towards the same side.

FPR treatment of thoracic region dysfunction

The patient should be seated for treatment of thoracic soft tissue dysfunction. The example relates to tissue tension in the area of the sixth thoracic vertebral transverse process, on the right.

The operator stands behind and to the right, having placed a contact, palpating or 'listening', (left index) finger on the area to be treated (Fig. 9.3).

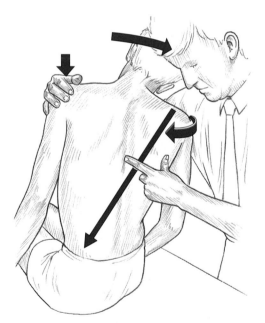

Figure 9.3 FPR treatment of thoracic region dysfunction (in this example 'tissue tension' to the right of the sixth thoracic vertebrae). One hand monitors tissue status as the patient is asked to 'sit straight' and to then slightly extend the spine. The operator then introduces compression from the right shoulder towards the left hip which automatically produces side-bending and rotation to the right. If ease is noted in the palpated tissues, the position is held for 4–5 seconds.

The operator places the right hand across the front of the patient's shoulders so that the operator's right hand rests on the patient's left shoulder and the operator's right axilla stabilises the patient's right shoulder.

In order to reduce the anteroposterior curves, the patient is then asked to sit up straight. In a controlled manner the patient is then told to 'lift the sternum towards the ceiling', so introducing a slight extension motion which is monitored by the contact (left index) finger in order to assess changes in tension/bind. This extension movement is slightly assisted, but not forced, by the operator's right hand/arm.

When some ease is noted, the operator uses compressive effort through the right shoulder (via his own right axilla). The suggestion given by Schiowitz is that, 'this compressive motion should be applied as close to the patient's neck as possible, and directed downwards towards the patient's left hip'.

Once again there is a monitoring, at the site of soft tissue tension, of the effects of this compressive effort.

In spinal structures other than the cervical spine, side-bending is normally always accompanied by rotation towards the opposite side, and the compressive effort through the right shoulder towards the left hip would therefore introduce both right side-bending and left rotation at the area being palpated. If this produces a significant palpable softening, or 'ease', of the previously tense tissues, the position would be held for 3–4 seconds before returning to a neutral position for reassessment.

Thoracic flexion restriction and FPR

Schiowitz gives the example of a sixth thoracic vertebra which is free in its motions on the seventh vertebra when it moves easily into extension, side-bending right and rotation to the right. The directions of restriction therefore, which would engage the barrier, would be into flexion, side-bending left and rotation left, and it is these directions of movement which would be utilised were a direct method being employed to overcome that barrier, possibly located in this instance at the right articular facet joint.

However, since FPR is an indirect method, it is towards the directions of ease that we need to travel in order to achieve release.

The starting positions (patient, operator, palpating digit at the right sixth articular facet, shoulder contacts) should be precisely as described above (p. 153) for tissue release. The compressive force would be applied straight downwards towards the monitoring finger. No increase in movement into extension is suggested, as this would reduce the chances of facet release.

When some ease was noted at this contact point from the compressive effort, a torsional side-bending and rotation movement to the right would be introduced until the freedom of motion was noted in the facet contact. This would be held for 3–4 seconds, then released. After repositioning into neutral, the range of motion which was previously restricted should be reassessed.

Prone treatment for thoracic flexion dysfunction

For the same restriction (difficulty in moving into flexion and side-bending rotation to the left) the patient could be lying prone with the operator standing beside the table on the side opposite the dysfunctional vertebral restriction.

The prone position would tend to introduce a mild degree of extension which can be enhanced by placement of a thin cushion under the patient's head/neck area.

In this example, standing on the left of the patient, the operator's left (monitoring) index finger would be placed on the right articular joint between the sixth and seventh thoracic vertebrae.

The operator's right hand would cup the area over the acromion process, pulling this towards the patient's feet, parallel to the table, until a desirable 'softening' of the tissues was noted by the palpating digit. This effort should be maintained as the operator leans backwards, in order to initiate a backward movement (towards the ceiling) of the patient's right shoulder, so introducing extension, together with side-bending and rotation of the thoracic spine towards the right, up to the palpating finger, all the while maintaining the compression effort (light but firm).

A sense of ease should be noted in the palpated region, at which time the various positions and directions of pull may be fine-tuned in order to enhance ease to an optimal degree. After holding the final position for 3–4 seconds, a return to neutral is allowed before reassessment of the dysfunctional area.

Thoracic extension restriction treatment

Were the initial intervertebral restrictions different from those described, in that the direction of ease was into flexion rather than extension, the same sequence would be used as in soft tissue release, reduction of anteroposterior curves, flexion into 'ease', followed by the other components of side-bending to the right and rotation to the right. All other elements remain the same.

What is being suggested, therefore, is that when there is ease in the direction of extension, this is not reinforced by backward-bending but that the modulating forces are restricted to compression, side-bending (Fig. 9.4) and rotation ('torsion'). However, when there is ease in the direction of flexion this is used as one of the modulating motions, along with compression and the 'torsion' elements.

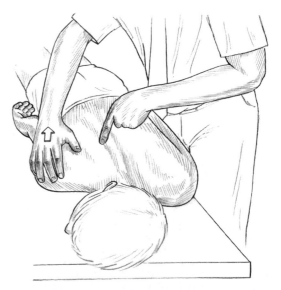

Figure 9.4 FPR treatment of thoracic flexion dysfunction.

FPR treatment for lumbar restrictions and tissue change

An example is given of an area of tissue tension located on the right transverse process of the fourth lumbar vertebra.

The patient lies prone with a pillow under the abdominal area, the purpose of which is to reduce the anterior lumbar curve. The operator stands to the right of the table, having marked the area of tissue tension with the right index finger. The operator's right knee is placed on the table at the level of the right hip joint, in order to offer a fulcrum over which the patient can be side-bent to the right (Fig. 9.5A).

The operator's left hand draws the patient's legs towards the right side of the table, which effectively side-bends the patient to the right. This motion is continued slowly until tissue

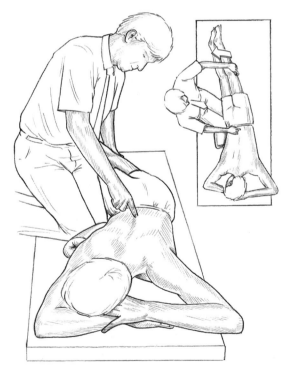

Figure 9.5 FPR treatment for lumbar restriction and tissue changes. Note that a pillow is used to reduce the anteroposterior curve of the lumbar spine while the operator introduces fine-tuning by positioning the legs to produce extension, side-bending and rotation until the palpating hand indicates that ease has been achieved. This is held for 3–4 seconds.

change (softening) is monitored by the index finger. At this time, the operator changes the position of the left hand so that it grasps the anterior surface, in order to be able to raise the thigh into extension, at the same time introducing external rotation until ease is noted at the palpated monitoring point.

This is held for 3 to 4 seconds before a return to neutral is allowed, followed by reassessment.

Variations

Depending upon the nature of specific spinal restrictions, the same general rules would be applied. The basic requirements involve a reduction in the anteroposterior curve, a degree of crowding, plus the spinal (or other) joint being taken to its combined positions of freedom of motion, away from the direction(s) of bind and into ease.

The examples given for thoracic and cervical normalisation using FPR should make the general principles clear.

MUSCULAR CORRECTIONS USING FPR

Schiowitz describes FPR application in treatment of piriformis and gluteal dysfunction.

The patient is prone with a cushion under the abdomen to neutralise the lumbar curve[1]. The operator is positioned seated on the side of dysfunction (right side in this example) facing cephalad. The operator's left hand monitors a key area of tissue dysfunction with the left hand (Fig. 9.6). The patient's flexed right knee and thigh are taken over the edge of the table and allowed to hang down supported at the knee by the operator's right hand. Flexion is introduced at the hip and knee by the operator, until an ease is sensed in the palpated tissues. The patient's thigh is then adducted towards the table until further ease is noted. The patient's knee is used as a lever to introduce internal or external rotation at the hip, whichever produces the greatest

---

[1] This is THE distinctive aspect of FPR, as compared with other indirect positional release methods.

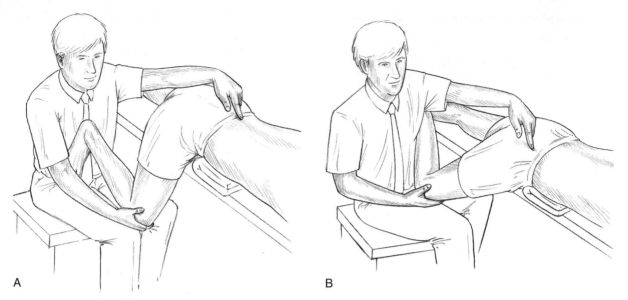

A   B

Figure 9.6A and B FPR for piriformis and gluteal dysfunction involves the patient lying prone with a cushion under the abdomen. For right-sided dysfunction the right leg is flexed at both hip and knee, and abducted over the edge of the table while internal rotation of the thigh is used to fine-tune a position of ease. Compression through the long axis of the femur is used to facilitate ease.

reduction in tension under the palpating hand/ finger (Fig. 9.6Λ).

Once this has been achieved, a degree of compression is introduced through the long axis of the thigh towards the monitoring hand, where a marked reduction in tissue tension should be noted. This is held for 3–4 seconds before release, return to neutral and reassessment (Fig. 9.6B).

The similarities and differences which exist when FPR and SCS, for example, are compared, should by now be clear (see the summary in Table 9.1).

The major advantage of FPR seems to lie in its reduced (hence 'facilitated') time for holding the position of ease.

Table 9.1 Similarities and differences between SCS and FPR

	SCS	FPR
Indirect approach	Yes	Yes
Monitoring contact	Pain point	Tissue tension
Find position of ease	Yes	Yes
Holding time	30–90 seconds	3–4 seconds
Uses facilitating crowding	No	Yes

Contraindications

There are no contraindications to FPR, except that its value lies most profoundly in acute and subacute problems, with its ability to modify chronic tissue changes being limited to the same degree as other positional release methods.

REFERENCES

Bailey H 1976 Some problems in making osteopathic spinal manipulative therapy appropriate and specific. J American Osteopathic Association 75: 486–499
Carew T 1985 The control of reflex action. In: Kandel E (ed) Principles of Neural Science, 2nd edn. Elsevier Science, New York

Janda V 1988 In: Grant R (ed) Physical Therapy of the Cervical and Thoracic Spine. Churchill Livingstone, New York
Korr I 1975 Proprioceptors and somatic dysfunction. J American Osteopathic Association 74: 638–650
Korr I 1976 Spinal cord as organiser of the disease process.

Academy of Applied Osteopathy Yearbook, Colorado Springs

Schiowitz S 1990 Facilitated positional release. J American Osteopathic Association 90(2): 145–156

Schiowitz S 1991 Facilitated positional release. In: DiGiovanna E (ed) An Osteopathic Approach to Diagnosis and Treatment. Lippincott, Philadelphia

Steiner C 1994 Osteopathic manipulative treatment – what does it really do? J American Osteopathic Association 94(1): 85–87

10

Cranial and TMJ positional release methods

CRANIAL STRUCTURES AND THEIR MOBILITY

There is little if any debate relating to the pliability, indeed the plasticity, of infant skulls. However, in order for cranial manipulation as currently taught and practiced to be taken seriously, it is necessary to establish whether or not there is evidence of verifiable motion between the cranial bones during and throughout adult life.

Sutherland (1939) observed mobile articulation between the cranial bones almost 100 years ago and researched the relevance of this for the rest of his life. He also described the influence of the intracranial ligaments and fascia on cranial motion, which he suggested acted (at least in part for they certainly have other functions) to balance motion within the skull. He further suggested that there existed what he termed a 'primary respiratory mechanism' which was the motive force for cranial motion.

This mechanism, he believed, was the result of the influence of a rhythmic action of the brain, which led to repetitive dilatation and contraction of cerebral ventricles and which was thereby instrumental in the pumping of cerebrospinal fluid.

The reciprocal tension membranes (mainly the tentorium cerebelli and the falx cerebri), which are themselves extensions of the meninges, along with other contiguous and continuous dural structures, received detailed attention from Sutherland.

He described these soft tissues as taking part in a movement sequence which, because of their direct link (via the dura and the cord) between the occiput and the sacrum, produced a total craniosacral movement sequence in which, as cranial motion took place, force was transmitted via the dura to the sacrum, producing in it an involuntary motion.

Five key elements of the cranial hypothesis, which Sutherland (1939) proposed, were:

- An inherent motility of the brain and spinal cord
- Fluctuating cerebrospinal fluid
- Motility of intracranial and spinal membranes
- Mobility of the bones of the skull
- Involuntary sacral motion between the ilia.

How do these propositions stand up to examination? The evidence is that inherent motility of the brain has been proven (Frymann 1971); however, the impact of this function on cranial bone mobility is possibly less than Sutherland imagined. Cranial motion probably contributes towards the composite of forces/pulses, which it has been suggested go towards producing what is known as the cranial rhythmic impulse – CRI (Greenman 1989, Magoun 1976, McPartland & Mein 1997).

The CSF fluctuates, but its role remains unclear in terms of cranial motion. Whether it helps drive the observed motion of the brain, or whether its motion is a byproduct of cranial (and brain) motion remains uncertain.

The intracranial membranous structures (falx, etc.) are clearly important, since they attach strongly to the internal skull and give shape to the venous sinuses. Dysfunction involving the cranial bones must therefore influence the status of these soft tissue structures, which strongly attach to them, and vice versa. To what degree they influence sacral motion is, however, questionable.

The bones of the skull can undoubtedly move at their sutures (Zanakis 1996). Whether this capacity is simply plasticity, which allows accommodation to intra- and extra-cranial forces, or whether the constant rhythmical motion, the CRI, drives a distinct cranial motion, is debatable. The clinical implications of restrictions of the cranial articulations seem to be proven, although dispute exists as to precise implications.

There seems to be involuntary motion of the sacrum between the ilia, but the means whereby this occurs remains unclear (or at least unproven), as does the significance of this motion in terms of cranial mechanics. Most cranial treatments, which attempt to normalise perceived restrictions, involve indirect, positional release-type techniques.

TREATMENT OF CRANIAL STRUCTURES

John Upledger, the internationally acknowledged craniosacral expert, suggests that in order for cranial structures to be satisfactorily and safely treated, 'indirect' approaches are best (Upledger & Vredevoogd 1983).

By following any restricted structure to its easy unforced limit, in the direction towards which it moves most easily ('the direction towards which it exhibits the greatest range of inherent motion') it may be noted that there is a sense in which the tissues wish to 'push back' from that extreme position, at which time the operator is advised to become 'immovable', not forcing the tissues against the resistance barrier, or trying to urge it towards greater 'ease', but simply refusing to allow movement. Upledger et al (1979) explains that, 'it is the inherent motion of the structure as it attempts to return to neutral, that pushes against you'.

It is not within the scope of this text to fully explore these concepts, some of which have been validated by animal and human research. However, a brief summary is needed in order for positional release applications to the cranial structures to be understood in the context of their clinical use (Chaitow 1999, Marmarou et al 1975, Moskalenko et al 1961, Upledger & Vredevoogd 1983).

Greenman (1989) summarises cranial flexibility as follows:

Craniosacral motion involves a combination of articular mobility and change in the tensions within the (intracranial) membranes. It is through the membranes attachment that the synchronous movement of the cranium and the sacrum occurs.

During cranial motion, he explains:

The sutures appear to be organised to permit and guide certain types of movement between the cranial bones. These are intimately attached to the dura, and the sutures contain vascular and nervous system elements. The fibres within the sutures appear to be present in directions, which permit and yield to certain motions.

In one model of cranial theory the movement of the cranial elements is said to be driven, at least in part, by a coiling and uncoiling process in which the cerebral hemispheres appear to swing upwards during what is known as cranial flexion, and then to descend again during the extension mode of the cranial cycle. As the flexion phase occurs, the paired and unpaired bones of the head are thought to respond in symmetrical fashion, which is both palpable and capable of being assessed for restriction. A variety of other theories exist to explain cranial motion (Heisey & Adams 1993), ranging from biomechanical explanations, in which respiration and muscular activity are the prime movers, to circulatory models, in which venomotion and cerebrospinal fluid fluctuations are responsible, and even compound 'entrainment' theories in which the body's multiple oscillations and pulsations combine to form harmonic influences (McPartland & Mein 1997). The truth is that while an undoubted, if minute (Lewandowski et al 1996) degree of motility (self-actuated movement) and mobility (movement induced by external features) can be demonstrated at the cranial sutures, many explanations for the mechanisms involved are as yet based on conjecture.

Motions noted at the sphenobasilar junction

During cranial flexion it is suggested by Upledger and Vredevoogd (1983) and others that the following movements take place simultaneously (it is important to realise that cranial motion is a plastic one rather than one involving gross movement):

- A reduction in the vertical diameter of the skull
- A reduction in the anteroposterior diameter, and

- An increase in the cranial transverse diameter.

These 'movements' are to be sure extremely small, in the region of 0.25 mm (250 microns) at the sagittal suture (Zanakis et al 1996).

Put simply, this means the skull gets 'flatter', narrower from front to back, and wider from side to side. This is all said to happen as the occiput is described as easing forwards at its base, causing the sphenoid to rise at its synchondrosis (Figs 10.1A and 10.1B). Because of its unique structure, this then causes the great wings of the sphenoid to rotate anteriorly, followed by the frontal and facial bones. The temporals and other cranial bones are then said to accommodate this motion by externally rotating.

Upledger's approach

The therapist attempting to ease the restricted cranial structure(s) in the direction of their greatest ease of motion commonly treats cranial restrictions, which have been identified by palpation methods. The practitioner then ensures that the cranial bones remain unmoving in that position of ease, until a sense is felt of an attempt by the structure to resume normal cranial

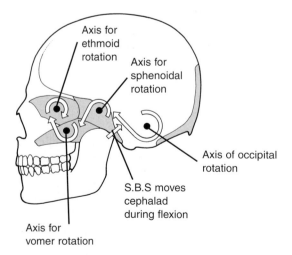
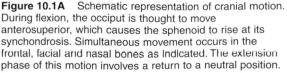

Figure 10.1A   Schematic representation of cranial motion. During flexion, the occiput is thought to move anterosuperior, which causes the sphenoid to rise at its synchondrosis. Simultaneous movement occurs in the frontal, facial and nasal bones as indicated. The extension phase of this motion involves a return to a neutral position.

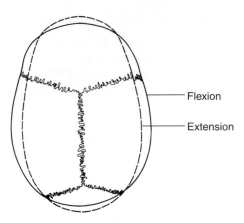

Figure 10.1B   The flexion phase of cranial motion ('inhalation phase') causes the skull as a whole to widen and flatten.

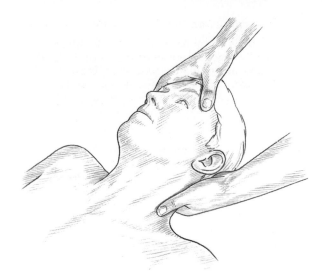

Figure 10.2   Sphenobasilar assessment: hand positions.

motion, as it 'pushes against' the operator's firm yet gentle resistance to motion.

Upledger explains what may happen next:

When the structure stops pushing against you it will travel farther in the direction of the ease of motion, often called 'the direction of ease'. As this movement away from you occurs, follow it, take up the slack, but without pushing. At the end of a cycle the motion will again move against you. [There are normally between 12 and 14 cycles of cranial respiratory motion per minute.] Once more you become immovable. Repeat this procedure through several more cycles of inherent craniosacral motion. Ultimately a tissue softening or release will occur. This is the therapeutic effect for which you have been waiting. The tissue has 'unlatched' itself. Follow a few cycles and re-evaluate for ease of motion and symmetry.

Caution

D'Ambrogio and Roth (1997) caution that:

With any cranial treatment it is recommended that certain precautions be taken. Symptoms and signs of space-occupying lesions and acute head trauma are clear contraindications. A history of seizures or previous cerebrovascular accident should be approached with caution.

Sphenobasilar assessment and treatment

In order to appreciate Upledger's directions, an exercise can be performed in which the patient is supine and the operator sits to the right or left near the head of the table. The caudal hand rests on the table holding the occipital area so that the occipital squama closest to the operator rests on the hyperthenar eminence while the tips of the fingers support the opposite occipital angle (Fig. 10.2).

The cephalad hand rests over the frontal bone so that the thumb lies on one great wing and the tips of the fingers on the other great wing, with as little contact as possible on the frontal bone. If the hand is small, the contacts can be made on the lateral angles of the frontal bone. It is necessary to sit quietly in this position for some minutes until cranial motion is perceived.

As sphenobasilar flexion commences (as a sense of 'fullness' is noted in the palpating hand), apparent occipital movement may be noted in a caudad and anterior direction; simultaneously the great wings seem to rotate anteriorly and caudally around their transverse axis. Encouragement of these motions can be introduced in order to assess any existing restriction. This is achieved by using very light (grams rather than ounces) pressure in the appropriate directions to impede the movement described.

During sphenobasilar extension (as the sense of fullness in the palpating hand recedes), a return to neutral may be noted, as the hands appear to return to the starting position.

Whichever of these motions (flexion, extension) is assessed as being least restricted should then be encouraged. As this is done, a very slight 'yielding' motion may be noted at the end of the range. The tissues should be held in this direction of greatest ease until a sense occurs of the tissues 'pushing back' towards the neutral position. A great deal of sensitivity is needed in order to achieve this assessment and treatment successfully.

Note: It is worth emphasising the author's belief that while the cranial movements described may be palpated and perceived by the sensitive individual, precisely what is moving, and what moves it, remains unproven. The description of cranial motion given above expresses Upledger's (1983) belief as to what is happening (which is widely held to be 'true' in craniosacral circles) and is not established fact (Chaitow 1999).

Jones' cranial methods

The developer of strain/counterstrain, Laurence Jones, has also focused attention on cranial dysfunction (Jones 1981) and suggests specific corrective methods for pain ('tender points') or restrictions (Fig. 10.3).

Locating tender points

Finding the tender points listed below (based on Jones' extensive research and clinical experience) is a matter of gentle fingertip palpation.

Despite there being only a very shallow layer of muscle in most of the locations described, trigger points are commonly located on the cranium, and care is needed as to how much pressure is applied. The suggestion is that the palpating digit should produce just enough discomfort for the patient to register the sensitivity and be able to report on the easing of intensity as positional release is attempted.

How much force?

The author believes that the amount of effort required to produce 'ease' when working on the cranium should be minimal, and should not exceed ounces. The opinions expressed by others are listed below.

- Jones (1981) speaks of 10 lb (5 kg) of pressure and more.
- D'Ambrogio and Roth (1997) suggest no more than 1 lb (0.5 kg) of pressure (this is the degree of force advocated by this text as a maximum, less if possible).

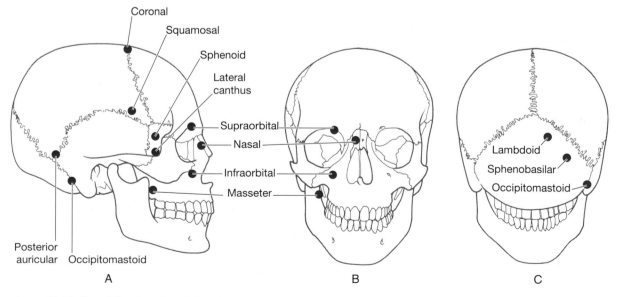

Figure 10.3A, B and C   Jones' cranial tender point locations.

- Upledger (1983), however, believes 5 g of pressure to be adequate.

Varying but light forces are used in order to ease the palpated pain/sensitivity. Once this has been achieved, the instructions in the text to 'hold the position for up to 90 seconds' will be seen. It is worth keeping the words of Upledger in mind, regarding 'sensing' the tissues 'pushing back' at which time it is suggested that the structure be held towards the position of ease. This approach is valid, although there is a difference between the underlying approaches of Jones and Upledger.

While Upledger relates his guidelines to craniosacral therapy, Jones is clear that he does not:

By the time I had begun to adapt my method to treat cranial disorders, I had acquired an abiding faith in the reliability of the tender points to report the efficacy of treatment. I claim no mechanical understanding of the skull, but I am able to relieve most cranial problems simply by relying on feedback from the tender points. The method probably is not comparable to the cranial studies developed by Dr WG Sutherland (cranial osteopath) but it is much easier to learn and it does an excellent job. On these terms I am willing to forego mechanical understanding.

As indicated, the poundage suggested by Jones displays his lack of awareness of (or belief in) the delicacy of the cranial structure, and so the recommended degree of pressure described in the methods outlined below is a scaled down version of Jones' recommendations, and is in line with craniosacral levels of force – ounces or less, rather than pounds.

Treatment of Jones' cranial tender points

Jones reports that suitable treatment of the tender points numbered and described below, by positional release, can positively influence a variety of local problems and sensitivities (pain or sensitivity in the tender points, for example), as well as assisting in the resolution of a number of common complaints (see Box 10.1).

1. Coronal and sagittal tender points The coronal tender point lies on the parietal bone, 1 cm from the anterior medial corner where the coronal and

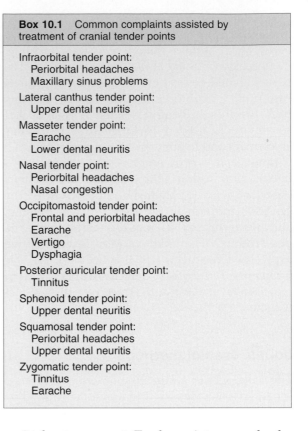

Box 10.1 Common complaints assisted by treatment of cranial tender points

Infraorbital tender point:
    Periorbital headaches
    Maxillary sinus problems
Lateral canthus tender point:
    Upper dental neuritis
Masseter tender point:
    Earache
    Lower dental neuritis
Nasal tender point:
    Periorbital headaches
    Nasal congestion
Occipitomastoid tender point:
    Frontal and periorbital headaches
    Earache
    Vertigo
    Dysphagia
Posterior auricular tender point:
    Tinnitus
Sphenoid tender point:
    Upper dental neuritis
Squamosal tender point:
    Periorbital headaches
    Upper dental neuritis
Zygomatic tender point:
    Tinnitus
    Earache

sagittal sutures meet. Tender points may also be found on either side of the sagittal suture anywhere between the bregma and the lambda. With the patient supine and the operator seated at the head, the tender point is monitored while light pressure is applied caudally to the identical site on the non-affected parietal until sensitivity vanishes from the tender point (Fig. 10.4). This is held for up to 90 seconds.

2. Infraorbital (or maxillary) tender point The infraorbital (or maxillary) tender point is located close to the emergence of the infraorbital nerve (Fig. 10.5). Sensitivity here is commonly associated with sinus headache symptoms. The patient is supine with the operator seated at the head of the table. The interlocked hands of the operator are placed over the face so that the middles of the palms of the hands rest over the cheekbones. Pressure (very light) is applied obliquely, medially and posteriorly, with both hands – as though the heels of the hands are being brought together. Mild discomfort is often noted even with light

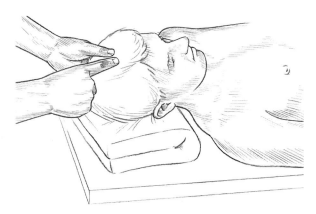

Figure 10.4 Coronal tender point, palpation and treatment contacts and hand positions.

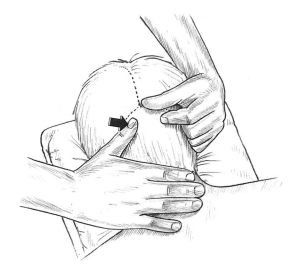

Figure 10.6 Lambdoidal dysfunction palpation and treatment contacts and hand positions.

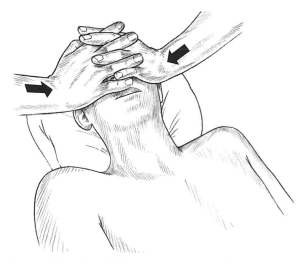

Figure 10.5 Infraorbital tender points, palpation and treatment contacts (only ounces of pressure at most).

pressure (ounces only, not the 8 lb suggested by Jones!). This compressive effort needs to be sustained until a marked feeling of decongestion is reported, along with relief of any sense of pressure previously felt behind the nose.

3. Lambdoidal dysfunction The lambdoidal dysfunction tender point lies on the occipital bone, just medial to the lambdoidal suture approximately 2.5 cm below the level of the lambda, obliquely above and slightly lateral to the inion. Positional release treatment is applied via light compression of precisely the same site on the contralateral side of the occipital bone (Fig. 10.6), until

discomfort vanishes from the palpated tender point. The direction in which pressure is applied can vary from an anterior direction to a medial one, whichever produces ease in the tenderness, involving a light pressure of the treatment area towards the tender point site. The patient should be seated or prone for easy access to the points (tender point and treatment point).

4. Lateral canthus The lateral canthus tender point lies in the temporal fossa, approximately 2 cm lateral to the end of the lateral canthus. The operator is on the ipsilateral side and treatment to the supine patient involves the operator's cephalad hand spanning the frontal bone so that the thumb can rest on the tender point as a monitor (Fig. 10.7). The other hand, using the thenar eminence as a contact, applies superiorly directed pressure towards the palpating thumb, via a contact on the zygomatic bone and the zygomatic process of the maxilla. The palpating cephalad hand exerts light pressure on the frontal bone towards the zygoma, so crowding the tissues and articulations in the area. Varying directions of application of these forces should be attempted until sensitivity in the palpated point eases markedly. The position of ease is maintained for up to 90 seconds.

5. Masseter The masseter tender point lies on the anterior border of the ascending ramus of the

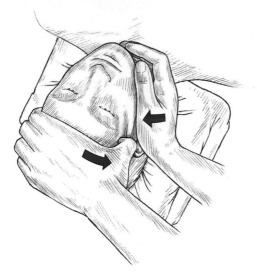

Figure 10.7 Lateral canthus (right side) dysfunction/tender point palpation and treatment contacts and hand positions.

mandible, and may be involved in TMJ dysfunction as well as mandibular neuritis. The patient should be supine, with the jaw slack and the mouth open approximately 1 cm (Fig. 10.8). The operator is seated or stands on the non-affected side, the heel of the caudad hand resting on the point of the chin, applying very light pressure towards the affected side as the index finger of

that hand monitors the tender point. The other hand, which lies on the dysfunctional side of the patient's head (on the parietal/temporal area), offers counterforce to the palpating hand's pressure via the heel of hand which is stabilising the head, while the fingers (which are just above the zygoma) lightly press towards the tender point.

6. Nasal dysfunction The nasal dysfunction tender point is located on the side of the bridge of the nose and, as this is palpated, tenderness is relieved by application of light pressure towards it from the same point on the contralateral side of the nose (Fig. 10.9).

7. Occipito-mastoid The occipito-mastoid tender point lies in a vertical depression just medial to the mastoid process approximately 3 cm superior to its tip. The patient lies supine and the operator holds the head in both hands (Fig. 10.10), with one finger on the tender point. The heels of the hands contact the parietal bones, making absolutely certain that they are superior to the suture line between it and the temporal bones. A very slight (ounces at most) effort is introduced by each hand – one 'screwing' its contact clockwise and the other anticlockwise – until sensitivity vanishes from the tender point. The counter-rotation produced in this way causes

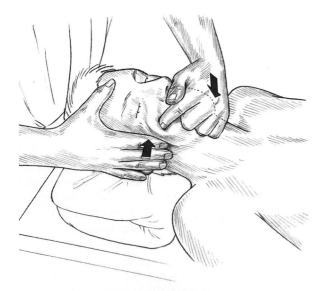

Figure 10.8 Masseter (right side) dysfunction/tender point palpation and treatment contacts and hand positions.

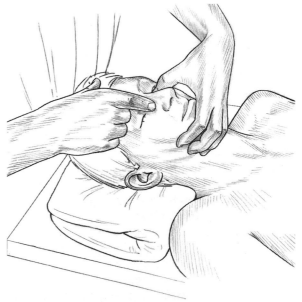

Figure 10.9 Nasal dysfunction/tender (right side) point palpation and treatment contacts and hand positions.

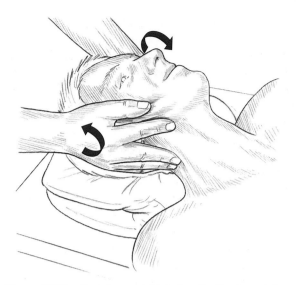

Figure 10.10   Occipito-mastoid dysfunction/tender point palpation and treatment contacts and hand positions.

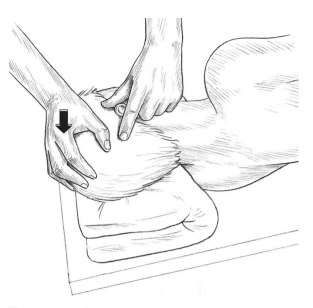

Figure 10.11   Posterior auricular (right side) dysfunction/tender point palpation and treatment contacts and hand positions.

the temporal bones to rotate in opposite directions around a transverse axis. The particular mechanics involved in the dysfunction will determine which side of the head, the ipsilateral or contralateral, requires a clockwise or an anticlockwise rotational effort.

Once the tender point palpates as much less sensitive than previous to the introduction of counter-rotation, this is held for 90 seconds.

8. Posterior auricular The posterior auricular tender point lies in a slight depression approximately 4 cm behind the pinna of the ear, just below its upper border (Fig. 10.11). Treatment requires the patient to be side-lying, with the affected side uppermost, resting on a small cushion which supports both the ear and zygoma of the contralateral side.

Light pressure is applied to the parietal bone to 'bend' the skull 'sideward and over an antero-posterior axis' (Jones' words). Counterpressure can usefully be offered by the other hand. This should remove the pain from the tender point and should be held for up to 90 seconds. Jones reports that tinnitus and dizziness often respond well to easing of tenderness in this point.

9. Sphenobasilar The sphenobasilar tender point lies 2 cm medial to the lambdoidal suture, above the level of the inion. Treatment (Fig. 10.12)

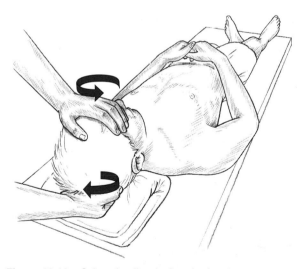

Figure 10.12   Sphenobasilar dysfunction/tender point palpation and treatment contacts and hand positions (use ounces of pressure at most).

involves the operator cupping the occipital bone (patient supine, operator seated at head of table) in one hand and the frontal in the other, tenderness in the point can be monitored by one of the fingers of the inferior hand cupping the occiput. Gentle counter-rotation to the frontal and occipital bones is then introduced, producing torsion through an anteroposterior axis. Counter-rotation in one pair of directions (one hand going clockwise the other counterclockwise) or the other will be found to relieve the tender point sensitivity more effectively than the other, and this should be maintained for 90 seconds. The amount of force introduced in these contacts should be minimal, involving ounces only.

10. Sphenoid The sphenoid (or lateral sphenobasilar) tender point lies on the great wing of the sphenoid, in a depression close to the lateral ridge of the orbit. Jones notes that the temple on the affected side will normally palpate as more prominent than its pair and that the tenderness may relate to tension in the temporalis muscle, as well as to the eccentric stress on the sphenoid.

Positional release treatment is achieved by the application of pressure (light, ounces only) with the heel of one hand from the contralateral great wing towards the monitoring index finger contact on the affected side, which offers counterpressure (Fig. 10.13).

11. Squamosal suture The tender point on the squamosal suture lies on the superior border of the temporal bone and is best palpated from above (Fig. 10.14). The patient should be side-lying with a pillow under the head and the affected side uppermost.

Positional release is achieved by placement of three fingers above and parallel to the temporoparietal articulation, distracting the parietal bone away from the temporal bone. Light pressure only is required (grams or ounces at most). The angle of 'pull' should be varied until the pain noted from pressure on the tender point is reduced markedly or vanishes completely. This is held for 90 seconds or until a 'softening' warmth is noted.

If the tender point is more anterior, closer to the squamosal border, then the contact fingers would be placed on the frontal bone, and it is this which would be distracted obliquely away from the temporal bone in an anterosuperior direction, until pain is reduced or vanishes.

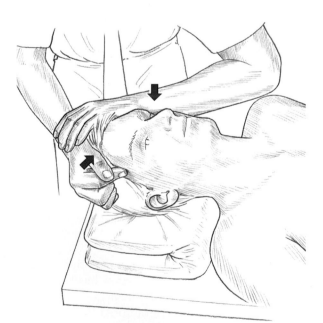

Figure 10.13 Sphenoid (right side) dysfunction/tender point palpation and treatment contacts and hand positions (use very light pressure only).

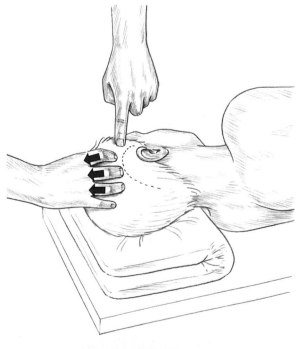

Figure 10.14 Squamosal (right side) dysfunction/tender point palpation and treatment contacts and hand positions.

Jones reports that treating this point often relieves upper dental neuritis.

12. Zygomatic The zygomatic tender point lies just above the zygomatic arch of the temporal bone, about 3 cm anterior to the external auditory meatus. Treatment is identical to that applied to the lateral canthus point except that the 'crowding' forces are applied approximately 4 cm more posteriorly.

POSITIONAL RELEASE METHODS FOR TMJ PROBLEMS

Method 1 DiGiovanna (Scariati 1991) describes a counterstain method for treating tenderness in the masseter muscle (Fig. 10.15). The patient is supine and the operator sits at the head of the table. One finger monitors the tender point in the masseter muscle, below the zygomatic process. The patient is asked to relax the jaw and, with the free hand, the operator eases the jaw towards the affected side until the tender point is no longer painful. This is held for 90 seconds before a return is allowed to neutral and the point repalpated.

Method 2 Upledger uses a positional release via 'decompression' on the TMJ, as a preliminary to application of a gentle traction on the joint in order to disengage over-approximation.

TMJ compression and decompression
(Upledger & Vredevoogd 1983)

The TMJ can be treated by a simple approach involving 'crowding' or compression followed by traction or decompression. The contact (no squeezing just a non-sliding contact) is on the skin. The palms and finger tips are placed on the skin of the cheeks of the supine patient as the operator sits at the head. Light traction on the skin pulls on connective tissue, which is attached to bone. The skin is taken to a point of resistance as the hands are drawn cephalad (taking out the slack). This is held until any sense of the structures moving, or repositioning themselves, ceases – which could take a minute or more (Fig. 10.16A). At this time, skin traction is introduced in a caudad direction, and held at its easy resistance barrier in traction until all restriction has released – which can take some minutes (Fig. 10.16B).

According to Upledger, this approach can produce multiple profound releases throughout the cranial mechanism, including the reciprocal tension membranes and sutures.

Method 3 Goodheart (Walther 1988) describes an in-the-mouth approach using strain/counterstain principles to treat the internal (most likely

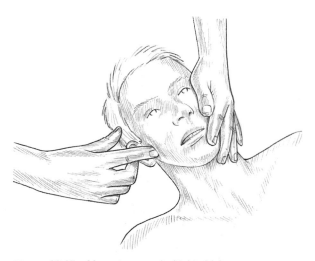

Figure 10.15 Masseter muscle (right side) dysfunction/tender point palpation and treatment contacts and hand positions.

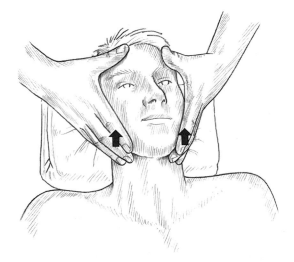

Figure 10.16A TMJ treatment (Upledger & Vredevoogd 1983) crowding/compression stage of treatment.

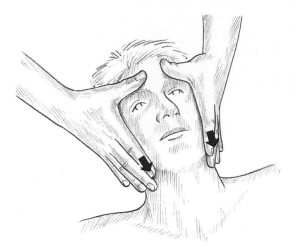

Figure 10.16B Distraction/release phase of treatment.

to be involved in problems associated with jaw closing) or external (most likely to be involved in jaw opening) pterygoid muscles.

The patient is supine and the operator stands to one side. The patient is asked to open the mouth and the operator inserts a gloved index finger (caudad hand) which palpates beyond the last molar on the side on which she is standing:

The operator monitors the pain in the pterygoid muscle area with the index finger. The primary spinal motion for obtaining reduced tenderness in the pterygoid muscle is head and neck hyperflexion, with some lateral flexion and rotation. The position is changed until the maximum amount of pain is reduced in the pterygoid muscle. The patient remains passive while the head and neck are manoeuvered to obtain the relief. When the optimal position is reached the patient takes a deep inspiration and holds it as long as possible. The operator holds the position for 30 or more seconds and then slowly and passively manoeuvres the patient back to neutral.

Re-evaluation is then performed, using digital pressure on the muscle.

These examples indicate the versatility and some of the variations of positional release methods, either being used simplistically as in the first TMJ example, or as part of a treatment sequence which includes stretching/traction subsequent to achievement of 'ease' in the second example, or utilising respiration to reduce the time the position of ease is held, in the third.

REFERENCES

Chaitow L 1999 Cranial Manipulation: Theory and Practice. Churchill Livingstone, Edinburgh

D'Ambrogio K, Roth G 1997 Positional Release Therapy. Mosby, St. Louis

Frymann V 1971 A study of rhythmic motions of the living cranium. *American Osteopathic Association* 70

Greenman P 1989 Principles of Manual Medicine. Williams and Wilkins, Baltimore

Heisey S, Adams T 1993 Role of cranial bone mobility in cranial compliance. Neurosurgery 33(5): 869–877

Jones L 1981 Strain and Counterstrain. American Academy of Applied Osteopathy, Colorado Springs

Lewandoski M, Drasby E et al 1996 Kinematic system demonstrates cranial bone movement about the cranial sutures. J American Orthopic Association 96(9): 551

McPartland J M, Mein J 1997 Entrainment and the cranial rhythmic impulse. Alternative Therapies in Health and Medicine 3: 40–45

Magoun H 1976 Osteopathy in the Cranial Field. Journal Printing Co, Kirksville MO

Marmarou A et al 1975 Compartmental analysis of compliance and outflow resistance of CSF system. J Neurosurgery 43: 523–534

Moskalenko V et al 1961 Cerebral pulsation in the closed cranial cavity. Izvestiia Academii Nauk Biologicheskaia 4: 620–629

Scariati P 1991 In: DiGiovanna E (ed) An Osteopathic Approach to Diagnosis and Treatment. Lippincott, London

Sutherland W 1939 The Cranial Bowl. Free Press Co, Mankato MN

Upledger J, Vredevoogd J 1983 Craniosacral Therapy. Eastland Press, Seattle

Upledger J et al 1979 Strain plethysmography and the cranial rhythm. Proceedings XIIth International Conference in Medicine and Biology, Jerusalem

Walther D 1988 Described in: Applied Kinesiology. SDC Systems, Pueblo

Zanakis N 1996 Studies of CRI in man using a tilt table. J American Osteopathic Association (96)9: 552

11

The Mulligan concept: NAGs, SNAGs, MWMs, etc.

Ed Wilson

It is axiomatic that there is a finite number of manual therapy methods. Mobilisation/manipulation of articular or soft tissue structures forms the bedrock, but the techniques may be performed anywhere along a continuum from light touch to high-velocity thrusts. They may also range from pain-free to pain-provocative in their intended effects.

The actual concepts underpinning the application of techniques are equally varied and depend to a large degree upon the therapist's training and their subsequent clinical experience. However, they all inhabit the same basic paradigm.

Of the multiple varied approaches possible in manual therapy, Mulligan's concepts and methods have many similarities to positional release techniques (PRT), hence the inclusion of this chapter. Both see lightness of touch and an asymptomatic tissue response as fundamental to clinical success. Elimination of symptoms – usually pain or stiffness – before or during functional movement is at their core. Perhaps positional release attaches a greater degree of importance to the physiological consequences of treatment than does Mulligan, who tends towards a more mechanical philosophy. However, others working in the Mulligan tradition have supplemented his work by examining the impact on neural patterning processes of the CNS wrought by his mechanically conceptualised techniques (Wilson 1994, 1997).

The above is discussed more fully later in the chapter, but the similarities between, for example, Mulligan's spinal mobilisation with arm movement and PRT's induration technique

> **Box 11.1** Basic similarities between Mulligan's concept and PRT
>
> ● Repositioning of abnormal tissues (by technique) leads to
> ● Normal output to CNS, which leads to
> ● Defacilitation of CNS, hence
> ● Normal output to tissues and
> ● Normal positioning maintained by neuromuscular control

are immediately apparent (Box 11.1). Both require a sustained, relatively light pressure to perform an intervertebral translation. For Mulligan, however, this is done while the patient carries out active arm movements, i.e. it is not done in preparation for movement, unlike many positional release techniques. These latter techniques typically restore normal function by the elimination of, for example, trigger points, by holding the offending structure in the 'ease' position, achieved by passive repositioning of articular structures. Functional movement is performed afterwards.

Mulligan's (1999) relatively simple but effective treatment techniques involve the repositioning of joint components as (usually) the patient simultaneously carries out their previously symptomatic movement. In some respects they are similar to Kaltenborn's (1980) work and are based on some of his biomechanical principles, but by adding concurrent active movement to passive joint mobilisation, Mulligan has adopted a more functional approach. This chapter serves only as an extended introduction to Mulligan's methods. It is by no means exhaustive: a more comprehensive review can be found in his book (Mulligan 1999).

The basic techniques described below are:

1. NAGs – natural apophyseal glides
2. SNAGs – sustained natural apophyseal glides
3. MWMs – mobilisation with movement
4. SMWLMs – spinal mobilisation with limb movement.

THE CONCEPT

The essential components of Mulligan's concept are as follows.

Pain-free

This is absolutely crucial. The techniques must not reproduce the patient's symptoms. Mild pressure or palpation discomfort may be experienced upon application of the technique, but the symptoms for which the patient has consulted the therapist must not be reproduced by the palpation or the movement.

Positional faults/tracking problems

Mulligan contends that many symptoms (pain, stiffness, weakness) result from joints with subtly malaligned biomechanics, and that these symptoms can be eliminated in many cases by equally subtle repositioning techniques, i.e. they assist in the restoration of biomechanical normality. The key word here is assist: 'force' has no place in Mulligan's vocabulary.

That a normal joint will follow a normal 'track' or 'path' through any particular normal movement is axiomatic (Kapanji 1987). This articular track – incorporating spin, slide, glide, rotation, etc. – is a genetic inheritance and is dependent upon the shape of joint surfaces and articular cartilage, and upon the orientation and attachments of capsule, ligaments, muscles and tendons. To facilitate controlled, free movement while minimising compressive forces is the overall aim of such a design. Any anomalies in the recruitment or coordination of the sequential elements of the movement pattern will be signalled to the central nervous system (CNS), which may well seek to inhibit that inappropriate movement by pain, stiffness or weakness. Thus the therapist is guided as to what is normal movement by its symptom-free status.

Repetition

With the patient and the therapist having been reassured that the biomechanical anomaly has been overcome by the application of a technique and consequent symptom-free movement, it makes sense to bombard the agitated CNS with the normal signals – from the joint and attendant structures – that it has always been patterned to receive. Thus the purpose of symptom-free repetition of movement and mobilisation is ultimately to sedate the CNS, to re-establish dynamic neutral (Hoover 1969). The overlap with positional release concepts can readily be seen here.

Treatment planes

The techniques, of course, must allow for variation in articular structure and types of movement.

Hinge joints

Here the bones lie end-to-end and articulate in the sagittal plane, somewhat like a hinge (Fig. 11.1) Examples would be the elbow and the knee, although the wrist too can be considered to be basically a complex, compound hinge.

With such joint-types the accessory force of the mobilisation is applied at right angles to the movement taking place. In the example of the elbow, a glide laterally of the forearm on a fixed humerus would be applied through the limited range of flexion or extension (see case example in Box 11.7).

Parallel joints

Here the bones lie side-by-side and their articulation is characterised by alterations in that parallel relationship. The radius and ulna or the metacarpals, for example. In treatment situ-

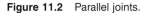

Figure 11.2 Parallel joints.

ations, one of the pair would be stabilised and the other would be repositioned upward or downward as the patient performed active movement (Fig. 11.2).

Spinal facet planes

The angles of spinal facet planes varies from region to region and therefore the angle of the accessory mobilisation must correspond with them. The orientation of C1 and C2 differs from that of C5 and C6, which in turn differs from T6 and T7 (Fig. 11.3).

Indications for use

Because they involve simultaneous joint accessory mobilisation with active movement SNAGs, MWMs and SMWLMs are used exclusively to

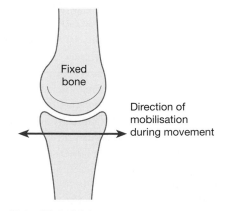

Figure 11.1 Hinge joint.

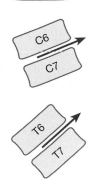

Figure 11.3 Spinal facet planes.

treat movement-generated symptoms. That is, they are not used where the patient complains of resting aches and pains, except perhaps where these are truly of minor significance to the patient, but are exacerbated by active movement. Significant resting symptoms are usually associated with a degree of underlying pathology far beyond that of relatively minor biomechanical abnormalities.

The therapist may be advised to treat the underlying pathology before concerning themselves with limitation of movement, especially as mechanical techniques run the risk of exacerbating the problem, especially if combined with movement. As far as the Mulligan concept is concerned, such a patient would be inappropriate for these techniques because it is highly unlikely that a pain-free status can be achieved, so the approach would be abandoned forthwith.

NAGs and headache techniques, meanwhile, are performed on passive patients and, to a limited extent, stand outside the above strictures, but even they have a mechanical rationale and would be inappropriate for use on a patient whose symptoms were of systemic origin (headache techniques are not used for classical migraine presentations, for example).

However, mild resting aches may simply be indicative of disturbed articular proprioception and inappropriate CNS modulation and are therefore worth considering from a mechanical viewpoint, including adding movement to mobilisation. Overall, the therapist should be guided in the use of Mulligan's techniques by careful consideration of what Maitland (1986) has labelled SIN, i.e. severity, irritability and nature of the presenting symptoms. Inappropriate treatments are performed by even the most expert clinicians sometimes, but at least if the pain-free framework is adhered to then the consequences of such an action should be minimal.

In order to identify which vertebral segment requires treatment by NAGs or SNAGs the rules common to all manual therapy approaches apply, i.e. an interplay between interrogation, observation, palpation and on-going analysis (see Box 11.2).

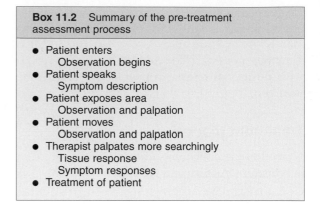

Box 11.2 Summary of the pre-treatment assessment process

- Patient enters
   Observation begins
- Patient speaks
   Symptom description
- Patient exposes area
   Observation and palpation
- Patient moves
   Observation and palpation
- Therapist palpates more searchingly
   Tissue response
   Symptom responses
- Treatment of patient

The patient will describe the location of the primary symptoms and their history, if questioned well. This may support or undermine the therapist's embryonic hypothesis formed as a general observation of gait/posture as the patient entered the room and sat down. Observation of muscle tone, body biomechanics during undressing and the formal, undressed observation phase will further build the hypothesis.

Active and passive spinal movements are then observed and analysed. What is the quality of movement? What is the range? What happens to the symptoms? How do the muscles feel when palpated during the movement?

During this process the therapist is considering the pathologies, physiology and anatomy which makes sense of the data thus far. For example, cervical/shoulder symptoms in the early stages of cervical rotation would implicate an upper cervical spine problem, because not until much later do the lower vertebrae become involved in cervical spine movement.

Thus, the original hypothesis is built upon layer-by-layer, or modified according to findings. Palpation of the vertebrae and surrounding soft tissues for stiffness, deformity and pain response will hopefully confirm the tentative hypothesis and treatment can commence. For NAGs and SNAGs, if the right facet joint between C6/C7 is implicated, the treatment of choice would be a unilateral NAG or SNAG (depending upon the irritability of the problem) at the right articular pillar of C6.

METHODS

NAGs

As previously stated, NAGs are accessory spinal facet mobilisations applied to a passive patient, i.e. the patient does not simultaneously move the affected joint. They can be applied to a spinous process in cases of central or bilateral symptoms, or to articular pillars where unilateral symptoms are dominant. They are posterior to anterior oscillatory glides performed in mid- to end-range, respecting the treatment plane. Failure to respect the facet planes will result in facets merely being compressed and their movement restricted rather than facilitated.

The technique is safe and simple if the pain-free rule is observed, and may be applied to different spinal levels in the same treatment session. Because of the starting position they can only be applied from C2 to approximately T2, depending upon the size of the patient and the span of the therapist's hand, or the length of their arm.

Technique: a central NAG in neutral

With the patient seated, preferably on a chair without arms, they are approached from their right and the (right-handed) therapist's right arm enfolds the patient's head. The patient's forehead should rest comfortably against the therapist's biceps, and their zygomatic arch along the forearm. All serve to stabilise the head. The thumb and fingers of the (right) hand are spread around the patient's occiput and cervical spine, where appropriate, with the exception of the little finger, whose middle phalanx is placed on, and slightly under, the spinous process to be mobilised. For example, if analysis of symptoms allied to palpation has revealed an affected C5/6 articulation, then the little finger would be applied to either the spinous process or articular pillar of C5.

The patient's head is then further stabilised by having it held against the pectoral region of the therapist (female therapists may wish to place a pillow or similar object between themselves and the patient). The patient's body is stabilised by being sandwiched between the chair back and the therapist's hip region (See Fig. 11.4)

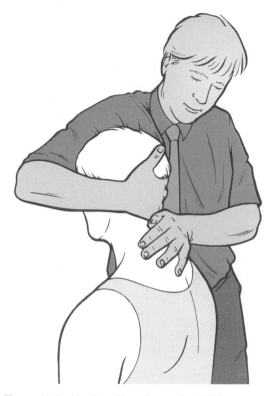

Figure 11.4   Hand positions for cervical NAG.

The thenar eminence of the therapist's left hand is then applied to the middle phalanx of the right, and it is through this phalanx that the mobilisation force is applied (see Fig. 11.5). Note that the right hand does not draw the vertebra forwards; the left hand is the active one. The middle phalanx primarily serves to spread the pressure from the left hand, which is more comfortable than direct thumb pressure on a vertebra, for example.

Rhythmical contraction of the therapist's left biceps brachii and brachialis will now impart an oscillatory force to the vertebra contacted, preferably at a rate of about 2–3 per second. Then after perhaps 20 seconds, re-assess the patient's movements and symptoms.

How long the therapist persists with the NAGs, and in what range, depends upon the patient's original SIN presentation – and to their response to treatment of course. If it seems to be effective very quickly, then leave well alone. In the words of the old adage: don't try to fix what is not broken!

Typical patient

A typical patient is one who presents with pain or stiffness on cervical movement, getting progressively worse as the patient moves further into the affected range (Box 11.3). This accruing of symptoms often indicates multiple levels of involvement, which can be confirmed by palpa-

tion. The patient may have some slight resting ache and a degree of irritability of their symptoms. Often they have been made worse by other, more vigorous, manual therapy techniques, and yet their symptoms would seem to demand a mechanical solution.

Common errors

1. Patient selection. Patients with significant resting aches or pains are unsuitable, as are those whose symptoms, when generated by movement, persist beyond a minute or so.

2. Failure to stabilise the head in the position intended for treatment. Cervical rotation and side-flexion are frequently inadvertently achieved as the therapist's position their right arm around the patient's head.

3. Mobilisation of soft tissue only, i.e. failure to appreciate what is or is not bony contact. The middle phalanx of the finger is, after all, an unusual palpatory tool and must, therefore, be educated by practice and experience.

4. Failure to execute the treatment pressure along the facet or treatment plane.

5. Failure to explain to the patient the overwhelming importance of accurate feedback during the application of the technique to ensure a symptom-free process.

6. Failure to explain the treatment as a whole to the patient. Explaining that their symptoms are essentially benign and are simply due to joint mal-tracking will put them at their ease and encourage normal movement. The assurance from the explanation of their symptoms, and that treatment will cease if symptoms persist, might also recruit the downward inhibitory modulation which can also assist in the alleviation of symptoms (Jones 1992).

NAGs: a summary

1. Oscillatory glides
2. Along treatment planes
3. In mid- to end-range
4. In a weight-bearing, functional position
5. To treat multi-level stiffness
6. Do not reproduce the symptoms complained of by the patient

---

Box 11.3 Case example of NAGs

Patient
A 72-year-old retired woman, an avid gardener and golfer.

Complaint
Inability to extend the cervical spine beyond 30% of its normal range due to central cervical pain at around C5/6 level. Attempting to move beyond that restriction spreads sharp pain into both scapulae. The symptoms were of 3 days' duration following gardening.

Previous treatment
Nil for this episode. Previous episodes had responded to manual therapy after 10–14 days usually.

Presentation
Asymptomatic at rest. Increased thoracic kyphosis and attendant increased cervical lordosis. This was her natural posture and was not antalgic for these symptoms, apparently. Movement restrictions as described above, plus 'tightness' at all other end-ranges. Sore on palpation C4–C6 spinous processes and facet joints. Very stiff C7–T3.

Treatment
Because of the widespread soreness central NAGs were the treatment of choice. However, due to increased cervical lordosis it was very difficult to locate the spinous processes in neutral sitting. To overcome this, the patient's cervical spine was slightly flexed to bring the spinous processes into prominence.

Central NAG C5 mid-range was performed for 20 seconds, after which the patient's symptoms were not manifest until approximately 60% of range. A further 20 seconds of similar NAGs enabled the patient to achieve full range without scapulae pain, but still with some central cervical discomfort.

The application of NAGs was then switched to C7 and T1 for 20 seconds each. This eliminated all symptoms.

Follow-up
The patient remained symptom-free at 2 weeks telephone follow-up.

Note
The final part of the treatment was switched to C7 and T1 because it was felt that their immobility contributed to symptom-generation at the higher levels. This is often the case with kyphotic patients.

7. Are applied from C2–T2, approximately
8. As central or unilateral mobilisations, usually in neutral head position, but they can be progressed into other positions by experienced practitioners.

SNAGs

Method: cervical snags

SNAGs ally active patient movement with the therapist's accessory force and aim at restoring the natural glide of one facet on another during that movement. To this end, the direction of force is always along the treatment (or facet) plane. However, because SNAGs involve active spinal movement too, the therapist must be prepared to 'follow' the chosen plane throughout the movement (see Fig. 11.3, p. 173).

To mimic this facet behaviour it is instructive to place the palm of one hand on the dorsum of the other to represent the planes, then replicate spinal movement with the wrists, observing the alterations in hand orientation as one does so.

Technique: central cervical SNAG in neutral

Like NAGs, the force is applied to the upper of the two vertebrae implicated in the movement dysfunction. With a central SNAG it would be applied to the spinous process, whereas for a unilateral SNAG it would be to the appropriate articular pillar. As a rough rule of thumb for the cervical spine for flexion, extension and side-flexion the direction of force is towards a point between the eyes whereas a unilateral would be directed toward the ipsilateral eye, no matter where in the cervical spine the technique is applied. However, it should be borne in mind that in rotation, the upper cervical facets move much further than the lower cervical facets, and therefore the degree of 'following' the facet is considerably less, and at the end of rotation the lower cervical facets will not lie in line with the eyes. The amount of movement at individual vertebrae can, of course, be palpated beforehand to ascertain the appropriate force direction at any given stage of a movement.

To carry out the technique the patient is again seated and the (right-handed) therapist stands behind. The medial border of the distal phalanx of the right thumb is placed on the spinous process or articular pillar indicated. Like NAGs, the contact digit does not apply the pressure, for in the case of SNAGs the pad of the other thumb is placed over the 'base thumb' and it is the former which applies the pressure (see Fig. 11.5).

How the patient is stabilised depends upon the level of the cervical spine being treated. If it is the upper cervical, then the therapist stabilises the head by laying the lateral border of each index finger along the patient's zygomatic arch. However, if a lower cervical or upper thoracic vertebra is to be mobilised, then most therapists' hands do not have sufficient span to stabilise at the zygomatic level. Instead, the index finger can be laid along the jaw line while the other four fingers drop on to the clavicle to restrain the patient's trunk as the treatment pressure is applied to the spine.

With each SNAG the technique is applied through the previously-painful movement range and back again, often up to and including

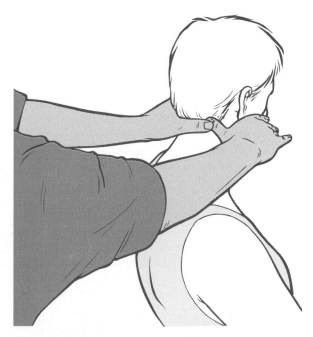

Figure 11.5   Unilateral right C1 SNAG.

end-range and slight overpressure. An accessory mobilisation plus an active movement to end of range obviously entails some risk of exacerbating the symptoms in a notoriously volatile area. In order to minimise this, Mulligan suggests the following protocol.

1. Ensure that the patient understands the importance of the pain-free nature of the treatment, and complies with it.

2. Explain what is being done and why, e.g. joint mal-tracking.

3. Before applying any treatment pressure negotiate with the patient the precise direction and their speed of movement, in order that both can be anticipated accurately as treatment begins.

4. Use the minimum amount of pressure necessary to achieve a pain-free movement. Often the amount needed is barely perceptible to the patient, yet is successful nevertheless.

5. Once the correct amount of pressure and its direction are established and symptom-free movement is achieved, do only three repetitions of that movement with the glide in place. Over-treatment of the cervical spine has more repercussions usually than under-treatment. Subsequent treatment sessions may involve up to 10 repetitions, once the patient has confirmed that no latent symptoms were manifest after session one. Improving but recalcitrant symptoms may benefit from the increased repetitions.

Note

The decision regarding whether to use NAGs or SNAGs on the cervical spine is not entirely clear-cut. The decision made is based upon the patient's symptom presentation (their SIN characteristics) and their findings at assessment. As a guide, use NAGs for irritable conditions and where multiple intervertebral joint dysfunction is apparent, and generalised ache and stiffness present. SNAGs are more appropriate for the 'catch' of pain in a particular part of the movement range (implicating just one joint problem), or for symptoms at the end of range, which NAGs will not really address satisfactorily.

Thoracic SNAGs

Method

Usually applied from T3–T12, the principles which apply to the thoracic spine are the same as those for the cervical. However, the execution is somewhat different. Thumb pressure is uncomfortable here, and is difficult to maintain, so the ulna border of the 5th metacarpal is used in contact with the vertebrae. Patient stabilisation is achieved by either the therapist's other arm or by the use of a seat-belt around the patient's iliac crest. Be sure to avoid the abdomen, as this is uncomfortable for the patient and also distorts movement patterns by acting as a fulcrum around which flexion particularly can take place.

Note that the patient is, where appropriate, seated on the end of a plinth with the legs somewhat abducted. This has the important effect of stabilising the pelvis so that the therapist is certain that the majority of rotation is taking place in the trunk. If the patient cannot straddle the plinth, then an acceptable if less effective alternative is to have the patient seated on the edge of the plinth.

Lumbar SNAGs

Method

Again, the principles common to all SNAGS apply but the application differs a little (see Box 11.4).

Like the thoracic spine, the lumbar spine is mobilised in movement with the ulnar border of the 5th metacarpal, with the exception of L5 (L5/S1 unilaterally), which is inaccessible to such a technique. Instead, at this level the therapist must revert back to thumb pressure.

One further aspect of protocol should be mentioned for the lumbar spine. Mulligan suggests that if the patient's symptoms can be reproduced by carrying out the movement in sitting then they should be treated in sitting to minimise the influence of the hamstrings. Care should be taken to ensure that the patient's feet are supported to avoid loss of balance when treated, which would induce lumbar co-contractions, and that the hips are at more than 90°, otherwise the lumbar spine is encouraged into flexion.

Box 11.4 Case example of lumbar SNAGs

Patient
42-year-old male labourer.

Complaint
Sharp stabbing pain to the right groin with lumbar flexion at mid-range, and with lumbar right lateral flexion just before mid-range. Before and beyond these points the movements were asymptomatic. All other lumbar movements merely felt 'stiff' but were of good range.

The symptoms had persisted for 4 months and there was no known or remembered cause.

Presentation
Movements as above. Some evidence of increased tone in right lumbar musculature. Tender to deep palpation of left L1/L2 facet joint. All other orthopaedic tests relevant to the spine were within normal limits and provoked no symptoms. However, groin symptoms in hip adduction with medial rotation at 90° flexion were made worse by hip joint compression. The symptoms were not reproduced by lumbar flexion in sitting.

Treatment
SNAG L1 unilateral (right) from just before to just beyond mid-range flexion in standing eliminated the symptoms. This was repeated three times and the patient re-tested.

Result
Asymptomatic on lumbar flexion and lateral flexion. Lumbar musculature tone normal. Hip test asymptomatic.

Follow-up
The patient was reassessed two days later. All the symptoms were as the initial presentation except they were much diminished, a mild ache only being produced on testing. The SNAGs were repeated three times, which eradicated the symptoms. Telephone follow-up 1 week later revealed that the patient had remained symptom-free.

Note
It is not unusual for right-sided symptoms to be generated by a left-sided lumbar lesion. The increased muscle tone on the right side of this patient was presumably protective of the left-sided L1/L2 facet. Also, due to shared innervation characteristics it is not unusual for hip tests to be positive even when no hip pathology exists (Bogduk 1987).

Common errors using SNAGs

1. Failure of communication, specifically regarding explanation of treatment, its painfree nature, and the need to establish speed and direction of movement before commencing treatment.

2. Being unaware of differing facet joint angles at different levels of the spine.

3. Over treatment.

4. Lack of familiarity with seat belt use, leading to inability to control the patient comfortably. However, where appropriate the therapists left arm can fulfil this function (see Fig. 11.6). Practising using the seat belt on asymptomatic models is invaluable.

5. Failure to recognise that joint dysfunction is often minimal even where symptoms are significant. The two do not always correlate and minimal treatment pressure is frequently sufficient to eliminate maximal symptoms.

SNAGs: a summary

1. Are weight-bearing and hence functional
2. Incorporate active patient movement, unlike NAGs
3. They are a sustained, not an oscillatory pressure
4. Used to treat one level of spinal dysfunction per treatment session
5. Do not reproduce patient's symptoms
6. Can be central or unilateral. In the case of L5/S1 can be bilateral
7. Can be used diagnostically to confirm level of lesion.

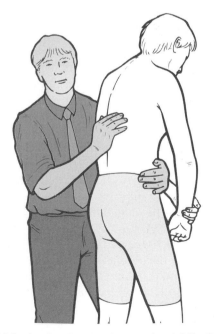

Figure 11.6 Lumbar SNAG using arm for stabilisation.

Headache

Method

The headache technique stands somewhat outside the usual Mulligan protocols for two reasons:

- The patient must be complaining of a current headache in order that the treatment can be proved efficacious. Usually we are not interested in pain or ache at rest.
- The technique employs a sustained glide in neutral on a passive patient and hence falls somewhere between a NAG and a SNAG. Oscillatory glides have no part to play here.

Technique

The patient is counselled as to the technique and its hoped-for effect, and cautioned to report immediately any change of symptoms for good or ill. They are seated, and the therapist approaches the patient exactly as for a NAG (see Fig. 11.4). However, the glide is directed at C2 usually, or C3 occasionally. It begins with the lightest pressure imaginable on the C2 spinous process and the patient reports the effect (see Box 11.5). If none is forthcoming then the pressure is very gradually increased until change is reported. Assuming it is beneficial change, the same precise pressure is maintained until either the headache has gone, or until it ceases improvement. If it ceases improvement then further pressure is added until it changes again, and so on until the headache is successfully eliminated. The pressure is then released and the patient reassessed. If the headache has gone, no further treatment is indicated. If it returns then the procedure is repeated perhaps two or three times until the headache finally goes.

However, if gliding C2 anteriorly below C1 and above C3 (which is what happens with the conventional headache technique) makes the headache worse, then a similar process can be followed on C3 which would have the reverse effect to the C2 glide, i.e. C3 is now moving anteriorly relative to C2, whereas before it was moving backwards relative to C2.

Dizziness

Method

The patient will be complaining of dizziness and/or nausea on movement of the cervical spine, most frequently extension or rotation.

Technique

Having first carefully screened the patient for vertebral artery insufficiency, etc., they are seated and the therapist approaches precisely as for an upper cervical SNAG (see Fig. 11.5). Palpation will have revealed the most likely vertebra for the application of the technique and the SNAG is applied accordingly. Feedback regarding symptom alteration is particularly crucial for this technique at this level and cannot be emphasised enough.

With the SNAG applied, the patient performs the previously symptomatic movement. If successful it is repeated a maximum of three times, and is not repeated in session one even if dramatic improvement is exhibited.

Note

Empirical evidence suggests that with symptoms on extension a C2 central SNAG into extension is the most beneficial.

If rotation is the problem then a unilateral SNAG on the ipsilateral side is recommended. The SNAG pressure is applied to the transverse process of C1, which is located immediately below the mastoid process.

Special notes on headaches and dizziness

These techniques are performed to alter the relationships between C1, C2 and C3 for valid anatomical reasons. Significant areas of the head and face are innervated from these sources, the remainder from various cranial nerves (see Fig. 11.7).

Thus, at surface level there is an intimate relationship between spinal and cranial nerves. Unsurprisingly, their axons terminate intimately too, in the trigemino-cervical nuclei in the upper portion of the cervical spinal cord (see Fig. 11.8).

Box 11.5 Case example of headache

Patient
17-year-old schoolgirl.

Complaint
Constant, severe headache consistent with the cutaneous nerve supply of the greater occipital nerve (C2, 3 dorsal rami). The onset was 2 years before, after being struck on the back of the head by a hockey ball. X-rays were normal.

Previous treatment
Various types of manual therapy practised by different disciplines. All had served to exacerbate her problem, usually a few hours after treatment. They were reported as being quite vigorous in their application.

Presentation
Mechanically normal cervical spine, with only slight 'pulling' at the end of each passive and active test. Thoracic spine, shoulder girdle and glenohumeral tests all normal. Palpation revealed minor stiffness and soreness centrally and bilaterally at C2, and soreness bilaterally along the nuchal line.

Treatment
Mulligan's headache technique, with clear instructions to the patient to relate immediately even the most subtle changes in her symptoms she was seated in her normal, relaxed posture then very gently sustained manual traction was applied to her head to distract the upper cervical facets. This quickly proved to have no therapeutic value and was abandoned.

Next, a very gentle headache SNAG, barely perceptible to the patient, was applied to the spinous process of C2. This has the effect of moving the C2 vertebra anteriorly both below C1 and above C3.

The patient was immediately aware of a 50–60% reduction in her symptoms so the SNAG was maintained at precisely the same pressure. Within approximately 60 seconds her symptoms had disappeared completely and the SNAG was released. Unfortunately, within a few seconds her symptoms returned in their entirety.

The SNAG was therefore reapplied at the previous pressure and sustained until the symptoms again disappeared. However, instead of releasing the SNAG at this moment it was maintained in a pain-free status for a further 60 seconds.

Upon release the patient declared herself symptom-free for the first time in 2 years. It was then agreed that she would be left in the treatment room to sit, read, walk around, drink coffee, etc., and be re-evaluated after half an hour. When this period had elapsed she was still symptom-free. She was then sent home and asked to report back immediately she experienced any headache symptoms.

Results
Eighteen days post-treatment the patient rang the clinic to report the onset of a constant generalised ache in the posterior cervical spine the previous day. There was as yet no recurrence of the headache. She reported that she had fallen off a settee at home and struck the left side of her head on the floor. The next day, the day of the telephone call, she had developed the cervical symptoms.

On re-examination that day her cervical movements were as before but flexion in particular increased her generalised ache a little. Palpation revealed stiffness and soreness at C2 and C3 centrally but not over the facet joints.

In the absence of headache symptoms the choice of treatment for an acute, previously irritable cervical spine was NAGS. These were performed centrally to C2 and C3 for one minute each. The cervical ache was no longer present when the patient was re-evaluated and flexion no longer provoked it.

The patient was again sent away and asked to report any recurrence of relevant symptoms. No contact was made, so prior to writing this case report she was contacted by the author when 4 months had elapsed. She remained symptom-free.

Discussion
A brief perusal of any anatomy textbook, e.g. *Gray's Anatomy*, will demonstrate the relevance of C2 and C3 to headache symptoms. The interesting points raised by this particular case report are:

1. All previous manual therapy intervention had exacerbated her symptoms, yet normal cervical movements failed to do so.
2. The symptoms were eradicated by the most subtle, gentle anterior movement of C2, sustained for only 2 minutes or so. Indeed, it is arguable whether the amount of pressure exerted did in fact elicit any mechanical movement at all. Over the previous 2 years, normal cervical movements must have replicated what the headache SNAG did mechanically. The only difference here was the sustained nature of the therapeutic technique.
3. Other than a possible massive placebo effect, the technique arguably de-facilitated the trigemino-cervico nuclei (Bogduk 1989), and it was the sustained barrage of A beta nerve firing that achieved this. These fibres respond maximally to light touch and pressure, are non-noxious on central states, and are the most rapidly-transmitting nerve fibres present in the human body (Campbell et al 1989). In effect they not only operate the 'pain gate', but also effectively switch off the centrally excited cells after approximately 30 seconds of sustained barrage.

Hence, the normal movement would not replicate this effect, and the more vigorous manual therapy techniques merely provoked central excitability even further.

To conclude, this case report represents the advisability of manual therapists' keeping a pain-free, gentle and brief set of techniques in their repertoire.

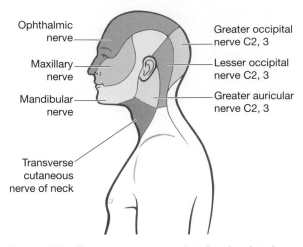

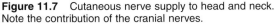

Figure 11.7 Cutaneous nerve supply to head and neck. Note the contribution of the cranial nerves.

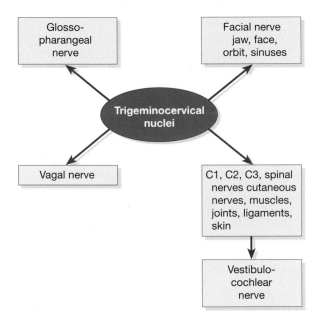

Figure 11.8 Potential links between cervical structures and structures influencing headache and vertigo.

As will be noted, the vertibulo-cochlear nerve is a part of this system. This nerve, an integral part of the system controlling balance, has obvious implications for dizziness. If the trigemino-cervical receptor cells are not in a state of dynamic neutral balance – are facilitated in fact, perhaps by inappropriate afferent discharges from an upper cervical facet joint – then the recep-

tion of efferent inputs from the trigeminal or vertibulo-cochlear nerves may be misinterpreted and the patient could experience headache or dizziness. These symptoms could then be relieved by appropriate techniques directed at the facet joint.

Peripheral mobilisations with movement

Method

As with NAGs and SNAGs, suitable patients for MWMs are those who complain of symptoms (pain, stiffness, weakness) on movement. It is also equally important to explain to the patient what is going to happen and why, and that the pain-free status should be maintained at all times. Spinal conditions are not alone in responding to downward central inhibitory modulation systems. Finally, remember to negotiate both a starting signal for the movement and its velocity.

Four important points regarding methodology should be noted here:

1. With hinge joints, it is the proximal partner which is stabilised and the distal one which is repositioned. This applies to all cases except for when the joint is weight-bearing. In these circumstances the distal partner is obviously fixed by the weight bearing and it is often the proximal partner which is moved.
2. The therapist's hands must be positioned directly above and directly below the hinge joint in order to effect a simple glide. Failure to comply will convert the technique into a collateral ligament stress test (see Fig. 11.9).
3. The oblique nature of the joint lines must be respected, and the accessory treatment force directed along it.
4. Remember, 'less is more' often applies with these techniques. Always try very gentle pressure first. Some joint disturbances are very minor anatomically, even if they display major clinical signs and symptoms.

Methodological protocol for MWMs

1. Establish that the patient's condition is suitable for manual therapy, and in particular for MWM.

2. Explain the technique and the pain-free concept.

3. Establish a starting signal for the movement, and establish the precise direction and velocity of the movement to be performed.

4. Realign the joint, i.e. perform a glide.

5. The patient actively moves the joint into the restricted range with the glide applied.

6. If the symptoms are increased, then the glide is in the wrong direction or the condition is unsuitable. Try the opposite glide direction. If the symptoms are unchanged then abandon MWM and reconsider.

7. If, however, the symptoms are decreased but not eliminated, then the glide is appropriate but needs fine-tuning in terms of angle and pressure, to eliminate the symptoms.

8. Fine-tune the degree of pressure and its angle of application, perhaps adding a degree of rotation if appropriate, until the movement is symptom-free.

9. Maintain glide and repeat symptom-free movement 10 times.

10. Retest movement without glide.
    - Much improved but not symptom-free = 10 more repetitions then retest = MWM into gentle over-pressure at the end of the active range.
    - Unchanged without glide = consider more repetitions or abandonment, depending upon SIN factors.

11. For example, if three sets of 10 × symptom-free repetitions completed with glide, and minor symptoms only remaining = consider strapping and/or home exercises which replicate the glide.

Taping

Controversy surrounds the issue of taping joints, particularly weight-bearing ones (see Box 11.6). The debate centres upon whether taping achieves the desired articular realignment or whether its effects are limited to surrounding soft tissues (the essence of this debate can be found in Herrington & McConnell 1996).

However, perhaps we do not need to refute or confirm either side if we can produce a dialectical argument which unites the opposing factions.

Box 11.6 Joints commonly strapped for MWMs

- Interphalangeal
- Intermetacarpal/intermetatarsal
- Wrist
- Scapula
- Ankle

Taping is mechanical – whether on articular or soft tissue structures – and mechanical techniques inevitably have physiological consequences: they invoke altered neural discharges from the target tissues. These neural discharges have the capacity to act upon the CNS in such a way that its output is affected. Changes in muscle tone may be a consequence, which may in turn subtly alter the biomechanics of the joint or joints upon which the muscle acts. So a soft tissue treatment can have articular consequences, and vice versa. Perhaps taping should be seen simply as a means of achieving asymptomatic status of target tissues, be they articular or soft tissue.

Note

Do not be afraid to admit to a faulty analysis. Many factors may cause or mimic a tracking problem. Abandon MWMs and consider other methods if virtual symptom resolution is not forthcoming relatively quickly.

MWMs: REGIONAL TECHNIQUES

Interphalangeal joint – finger

These are perhaps the best examples of pure hinge joints. The therapist stabilises the proximal phalanx by gripping it lightly from above with the pads of their thumb and index finger of one hand. The pad and index finger of their other hand then execute the glide as the patient flexes or extends the affected joint. Many repetitions can be performed here because it is rare for these joints to be irritable. It is a simple matter to replicate this glide with strapping if required.

Intermetacarpal bones

These form a parallel relationship, so the essence of the technique is to stabilise one bone, then elevate or depress its neighbour in relation to it. A simple index finger/thumb pinch grip is used for both the stabilisation and the glide aspects of the technique.

Remember, if one end of a long bone is elevated then the other end is depressed. When recording the treatment be sure to record where on the glided bone the fingers were placed.

Wrist: symptomatic flexion or extension

The carpus is glided laterally upon the fixed forearm. Therefore, if the carpus and hand are to be 'pushed' laterally then the forearm must be stabilised on its lateral side to counteract that 'push'.

Technique

The therapist enfolds the distal radius and ulna from the lateral side by using their web space primarily. This is a soft, comfortable grip. The web space of their other hand then slides directly on top of the first one but approaching it from the opposite side of the patient's limb. This second hand is the gliding hand and the web space should rest against the pisiform between the distal wrist creases, and should glide the carpus towards the thumb (see Fig. 11.9).

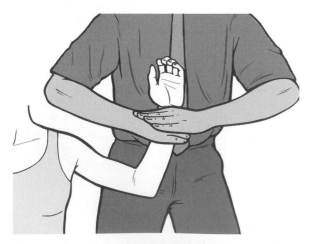

Figure 11.9 Hand positions for wrist joint lateral glide for loss of flexion and extension.

Remember that the wrist-joint line is oblique and direct the glide accordingly.

Remember also that not all wrist flexion/extension takes place between the radius and ulna and the proximal row of the carpus. It may be necessary to experiment with angles and hand positions in order to succeed.

It is possible to strap the wrist to recapture the glide performed by the therapist's hand.

Wrist: resisted pronation and/or supination

The inferior radio-ulnar joint is one where the bones lie parallel to each other, and it is this relationship which is altered. More specifically, it is usually an anterior glide of the ulna on a fixed radius which is required to restore full movement.

Technique

The most comfortable grip is to secure the patient's radial styloid between the therapist's thumb pad and proximal phalanx of the first metatarsal of one hand, and the patient's ulnar styloid similarly with the other hand. As the patient moves into pro/supination, the thumb over the ulnar styloid exerts an appropriate pressure to glide the ulna anteriorly.

If this technique fails or even makes the patient's symptoms worse then, using the same grip, try altering the radio-ulnar relationship in other ways; i.e. bring the ulna posteriorly or fix the ulnar and move the radius instead.

Note The radial artery is vulnerable to pressure during this technique.

Elbow

There are two major conditions to consider at the elbow:

1. Loss of flexion and/or extension
2. Tennis elbow (lateral epicondylagia).

Both utilise a lateral glide technique but the starting positions and mechanisms of treatment differ.

Loss of movement

The humerus is to be fixed and the forearm is to be glided laterally toward the radial head (see Box 11.7). Bear in mind the often quite acutely angled joint line, slanting cephalad from medial to lateral.

The humerus is fixed by the therapist's hand lying along its lateral border, with the thenar eminence on the lateral condyle just above the joint line. The web space of the therapist's other hand is then applied to the upper end of the ulna, just below the joint line, and performs a cephalo-lateral glide as movement through the previously symptomatic range takes place (see Fig. 11.10). Due to the obliquity of the joint line, subtle changes in the direction of the glide may be necessary if a considerable range of movement is traversed.

Note This technique can be performed using a seat-belt to effect the glide. However, this is a difficult technique to master without supervised training.

Tennis elbow

Ideally this technique is performed with the patient in supine lying. Their affected arm is along their trunk, in pronation. The humerus is fixed by the therapist holding it down with their web space positioned just above the elbow joint on the lateral humeral condyle.

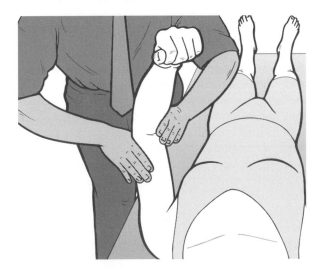

Figure 11.10   Hand positions for elbow MWM.

> **Box 11.7** Case example of peripheral joint (elbow) treatment
>
> **Patient**
> A 26-year-old woman physiotherapist.
>
> **Complaint**
> Inability to extend her right elbow through the last 30° of extension. The patient reported that it felt 'blocked', although not painful unless forced into its end-range zone. This situation had persisted since a fracture of the radial head at the age of 9. There was no resting ache.
>
> **Previous recent treatments**
> 1. Oscillatory mobilisation of the elbow joint as a whole, and of the radial head/capitulum joint and the superior radio-ulnar joint.
> 2. Manipulation.
> Both failed to alter her movement restriction.
>
> **Presentation**
> Active and passive elbow extension seemed to be met by a solid end-feel, although there was some evidence of hyperactivity in the elbow flexors of the upper arm and forearm when end-range was reached.
>
> **Treatment**
> At approximately 10° short of her end-range the humerus was stabilised by the therapist's left hand on the lateral condyle, immediately above the joint line. The therapist's right hand was then placed on the medial condyle of the ulna, immediately below the joint line. Via pressure through the therapist's right hand the forearm was induced to glide laterally in relation to the humerus. The direction of the glide specifically followed the obliquity of the elbow joint as a whole. The patient then attempted to fully extend her elbow.
>
> **Result**
> The patient was immediately able to regain full extension asymptomatically. With the glide maintained in the same precise direction with the same degree of pressure 10 repetitions into full extension were performed. At the end of these repetitions the patient was able to fully extend her elbow without the assistance of the accessory glide. In other words, it was now tracking correctly through the previously restricted range.
>
> **Follow-up**
> The patient remains symptom-free, several months after that treatment.
>
> **Note**
> This case example undermines the widely held belief that adaptive shortening automatically accompanies prolonged movement restriction. It may do, of course, but it is not axiomatic.

The seat-belt is then passed under the forearm of the patient, then over the scapula and acromio-clavicular joint of the therapist's shoulder nearest to the patient's head. The therapist is slightly stooped and the shoulder carrying the seat-belt is over the patient's elbow. With the belt taut it is then a simple matter for the therapist to move into a slightly more upright posture, which has the effect of tightening the belt and gliding the forearm on the fixed humerus (see Fig. 11.11).

With this glide in position the patient is asked to carry out an action previously provocative of their symptoms, e.g. gripping, wrist extension, etc.

To adjust the angle of the glide if the symptoms do not fully disappear initially, the therapist merely leans more forward or backward (minimally) to alter the line of pull of the belt.

Note

1. Tennis elbow is an irritable condition and this should be considered when establishing the number of attempts to be made to achieve the correct glide angle, and how many repetitions of a successful glide might sensibly be attempted.
2. Critics have complained that this technique does not involve movement, merely contraction. However, the common extensor group of muscles crosses the elbow joint and it is seemingly contraction of these muscles which elicits symptoms of terms elbow. Their contraction (acting as stabilisers of the wrist during gripping, of course) will exert a linear movement of the forearm on a fixed humerus and therefore increase intra-articular pressure between the radial head and the capitulum. This is particularly so in full elbow extension (close-pack position) when, coincidentally, tennis elbow symptoms seem to be most pronounced.
3. This technique is of value in tennis elbow conditions of 3 weeks or more standing.
4. If a lateral glide fails to resolve either restricted flexion/extension or a tennis elbow condition, yet clinically a tracking problem or positional fault seems to exist, it is worth applying an anterior or perhaps posterior glide on the radial head as the symptomatic action is performed.

Shoulder

Movements at the glenohumeral joint are enormously complex, involving muscles which attach to the cervical and thoracic spines, the scapula, the pelvic rim, the occiput, the clavicle, the sternum and the upper eight ribs, plus the humerus and forearm of course. A minimum of 40 joints may affect the way the shoulder moves, but although all such joints are amenable to MWMs to enhance shoulder movement, clinically three techniques have proved the most useful.

1. Posterior glide of the head of the humerus

Technique Performed in sitting or standing depending upon the relative heights of patient and therapist, this technique is particularly useful for symptomatic flexion and/or abduction, but it can be used for rotation problems too.

Standing on the opposite side to the patient's affected shoulder, one hand is placed on the patient's upper/mid thoracic region and scapula to counter any trunk rotation or extension. The thenar eminence of the other hand is placed on the greater tubercle of the head of the patient's humerus, with the fingers pointing directly upward. This hand then applies antero-posterior pressure (directed obliquely/lateral to conform with the orientation of the glenoid surface) as the

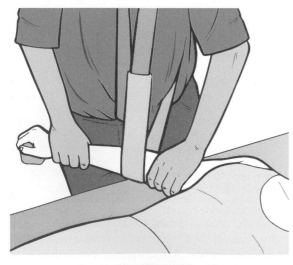
Figure 11.11 Tennis elbow: lateral glide with active gripping.

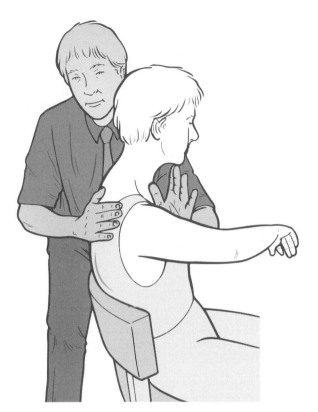

Figure 11.12   Posterior glide of the head of the humerus.

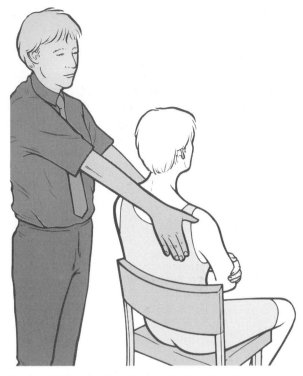

Figure 11.13   Hand position on the scapula prior to patient's arm movement.

patient moves the limb in the required direction (Fig. 11.12).

Note With end-range flexion or abduction it is very easy to roll the gliding hand so that it begins to exert a downward pressure on the humerus instead of a posterior one. Keeping the fingers of the gliding hand pointing upwards will negate this tendency.

2. This shoulder technique is not suitable for taping

Scapula Although not described in Mulligan's book this technique is certainly useful. As with the humeral glide, the therapist stands at the opposite shoulder of the patient, who may be seated or standing. Now, the trunk-restraining hand is placed anteriorly on the sternum or along the clavicle, depending upon the sex of the patient. The other hand, the one which will alter scapular tracking, is placed over the scapula in

such a way that it mimics the shape of the scapula (Fig. 11.13). The thumb lies along the spine of the scapula.

In this way, the scapula can be controlled advantageously during a patient's movement. It can be maintained more caudad where reversed scapulo-humeral rhythm is apparent, or greater approximation of the scapulo-thoracic joint can be maintained where scapula 'winging' is evident. Similarly, scapula rotation can be assisted or resisted as appropriate (see example in Box 11.8).

3. Transverse vertebral glides

This technique falls into the category of Spinal Mobilisation With Arm Movement (SMWAM), but it is appropriate to include it here. It can be performed for shoulder movement restriction in any plane where that movement restrictor has been shown to be of spinal origin (see Box 11.9). The therapist stands behind the seated or standing

---

Box 11.8 Case example of scapula treatment

Patient
52-year-old woman cleaner.

Complaint
Sudden onset of severe left-sided shoulder pain on movement, 4 months before. Symptoms primarily over the acromioclavicular joint area, bicipital groove, and the deltoid insertion on the humerus. Originally diagnosed by her general practitioner as 'frozen shoulder' the diagnosis had been altered to scapulothoracic nerve palsy when pronounced winging of the scapula developed subsequently.

Presentation
Increased thoracic kyphosis and cervical lordosis. Poor left upper trapezius tone. Increased levator scapulae and pectoralis minor tone. Winging of scapula at rest, significantly worsened by the glenohumeral movements of flexion and abduction beyond approximately 40°. Pain accompanied these movements. These movements were described as heavy, painful and weak.

Previous treatment
Anti-inflammatory medication and pendular exercises prescribed by the general practitioner. No benefits had been reported.

Treatment
The scapula technique as described in the text was performed. The purpose was to use mechanical pressure to approximate the scapula to the chest wall and to guide it through a normal pattern during limb movements. It required several attempts to determine the precise amount of pressure required and to coordinate that pressure with guidance of the scapular rotation on movement, but eventually symptom-free flexion was achieved.

Asymptomatic flexion with MWM was repeated eight times and retested. There was an appreciable reduction in the winging both at rest and on movement, but it was still symptomatic beyond 90°. A further three sets of 10 MWMs were performed with a retest between sets, each one exhibiting further improvement.

At the end of treatment with MWMs the mild resting ache had disappeared and there was no winging of the scapula apparent at rest either. However, movement of the limb above 90° flexion was still demonstrating some winging and some symptoms, although markedly reduced in both cases.

The patient was then taught scapula 'setting' exercises to be performed in lying.

Follow-up
Three days later the improvement had been maintained but not improved upon. Three × 10 sets of the treatment described above were performed, which then resulted in asymptomatic unassisted movement into full range with no winging evident.

Result
Two further treatment sessions were required to maintain an asymptomatic status for the patient, the final session taking place 3 weeks after the initial one.

Box 11.9 Case report of SMWAM treatment

Patient
Middle-aged woman physiotherapist.

Complaint
Painful inability to elevate or abduct the left arm above 90°. The situation had persisted for some years since surgery to her left breast and lymphatics.

Previous treatment
Various combinations of massage, mobilisation and stretching.

Presentation
Movement as above. Other arm movements stiff and limited to a minor degree. 'Tight' but not hard end-feel. Trigger points throughout the girdle musculature. Acutely tender T2 spinous process.

Treatment
Spinal mobilisation T2 to right, concurrent with left arm elevation. This permitted almost full pain-free elevation and was repeated three times.

Result
Almost full pain-free range of flexion and abduction.

Follow-up
The patient was seen the next day and had maintained her movement. However, she now had a moderately severe constant resting ache along her inner, upper left arm, which had developed some hours after the treatment. A right transverse glide of T2 sustained for 10 seconds eliminated the ache.

Note
Adaptive shortening had not occurred despite quite extensive scarring. The post-treatment arm pain was presumably somatic referral rather than radicular, since it disappeared so swiftly.

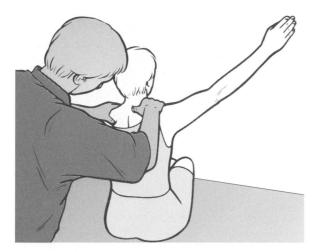

Figure 11.14 Transverse pressure on C7 to the left while the patient swings up the right arm.

patient and with thumb pad or finger against the side of the spinous process (chosen as a result of careful examination and palpation) pushes it transversely away from the side of the affected shoulder (see Fig. 11.14) as the patient moves that shoulder.

Note

- Almost any cervical or thoracic vertebra has the capacity to interfere with shoulder movement.
- Minimal repetitions are indicated (3–4), as this combination of spinal mobilisation plus arm movement can be volatile.

Lower limb

Foot

As the foot is a replica of the hand the same techniques apply here. Therefore, only one technique and application will be described.

Patients who have inversion injuries of the ankle frequently complain of symptoms along the lateral border of the foot. This is not surprising since the fifth metatarsal, too, is vulnerable in such injuries. These symptoms may be apparent during gait or maybe on inversion of the ankle.

Technique The history and presentation of the symptoms suggest malfunction between the fifth and fourth metatarsals. It is then a simple matter to fix the fourth metatarsal between finger and thumb and raise or lower the fifth in relation to it, as the patient performs the appropriate action.

However, if the problem is manifest only in weight-bearing, a better solution may be to strap the fifth metatarsal into the desired position and retest, reversing the strapping if that proves ineffective or exacerbates the situation. Alternatively, consider the relationship between the fifth metatarsal and the cuboid.

Talocrural joint

Plantar flexion In plantar flexion the talus moves anteriorly in relation to the tibial and fibular condyles. If it fails to do so correctly then plantar flexion will be compromised. However, it is not possible to gain purchase on the talus to assist its movement so an alternative must be found.

The patient sits on the bed with the knee on the affected side bent at 90°. The patient's posterior calcaneum is resting on the bed. The therapist stands at the end of the bed and uses one hand to glide the tibia and fibula posteriorly on a talus fixed by its close association with the calcaneous, now jammed against the bed. This effectively brings the talus anteriorly, relative to the tibia and fibula. The therapist's other hand now grips the calcaneous and glides it anteriorly, bringing the talus with it. At this point the patient performs plantar flexion with the above glides in position.

Dorsiflexion This is the reverse of plantar flexion in that the talus moves posteriorly during movement.

The patient is sitting on the bed with the affected foot and ankle just clear of the end of the bed. A rolled towel or similar protects the achilles tendon. The therapist grasps the calcaneous (using a cupped hand as if holding a ball – do not grip with fingers and thumb; it is too painful and will inhibit movement) with one hand and draws it posteriorly, i.e. toward the floor. With the web space of the other hand a posterior glide is exerted on the anterior talus (see Fig. 11.15). However, and this is important, when the patient actively dorsiflexes, the hand on the talus must

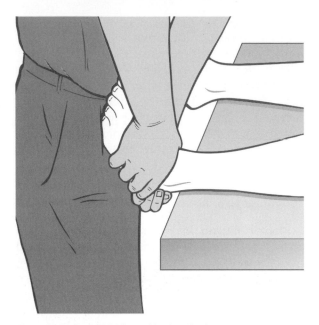

Figure 11.15   MWM for ankle dorsiflexion.

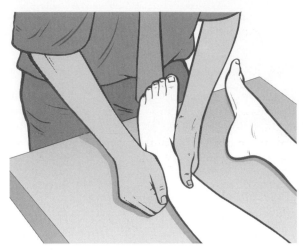

Figure 11.16   MWM for ankle inversion.

be removed or it will compress the network of tendons over the anterior talus as they begin to exert their force on the foot.

Alternative in weight-bearing Having moved from an open-chain to a closed-chain action, this technique differs from that above. Instead the talus is glided posteriorly as before, but now the other hand (or towel, or seat-belt) draws the tibia and fibula forwards over the talus.

Inversion This technique has generated some controversy. The reason will become apparent.

Pain on inversion of the talocrural joint is usually the indicator for the technique, and a 'sprained ankle' the usual cause initially.

Posterior glide of the lateral malleolus is the technique to employ. The patient is sitting on the bed with the affected leg outstretched. The therapist stands at the end of the bed. The calcaneous is supported in one cupped hand, and the thenar eminence of the other is used, first to take up soft tissue slack, then to effect a posterio-cephalad glide of the lateral malleolus, approximately along the line of the anterior portion of the lateral ligament. The patient then carries out the active movement, with the glide in situ of course (see Fig. 11.16).

Note

1. Ankle inversion loss following 'ankle sprain' usually invokes concepts of lateral ligament damage, and yet this technique effectively stresses the anterior portion of the lateral ligament, the portion most often implicated, apparently, in ankle sprains. Herein lies the controversy: stressing the seemingly damaged structure at either acute or chronic phases can dramatically reduce the symptoms during ankle inversion. Mulligan, with some justification, argues it this way: the lateral ligaments are so tough and inelastic that the forces acting upon the ankle during inversion injuries often cause avulsion fractures or malleollar fractures, rather than major ligament damage. If neither fracture occurs and the ligament stays relatively intact, then the forces applied will serve to sublux the malleollus anteriorly. Soreness and swelling would still occur due to disruption of the talocrural joint and the relationship between the tibia and fibula. This might mimic a ligament sprain and potentially confuse the unwary clinician.

2. This technique is readily replicated by strapping. The tape is anchored on the anterior part of the lateral malleolus, which is then glided into its corrected position by the therapist's hand. Their other hand reaches around behind the patient's ankle and pulls the tape into a

spiral, avoiding the achilles tendon as far as possible.

The knee

The knee is a hinge joint with a slight obliquity of joint line, and the techniques are similar to those of the elbow. However, the leg is a much heavier and more unwieldy limb and therefore the seat-belt is used more frequently.

Technique

With the patient sitting or lying on the bed and the knee positioned just short of entering the restricted range, the therapist applies the heel of each hand to opposite sides of the leg, one just above, one just below the joint line. Which is above and which is below depends upon whether a medial or a lateral glide is required, of course. If it is to be a lateral glide then the upper hand will be above the joint line to stabilise the femur, and the lower hand will be below the joint line on the tibia to glide it laterally (Fig. 11.17).

Seat-belt technique

This has the advantage of enabling the therapist to keep one hand free to introduce an element of rotation into the glide if indicated, or to perform over-pressure at the end of range.

The patient is lying prone on the bed. For a lateral glide the therapist stands at the same side

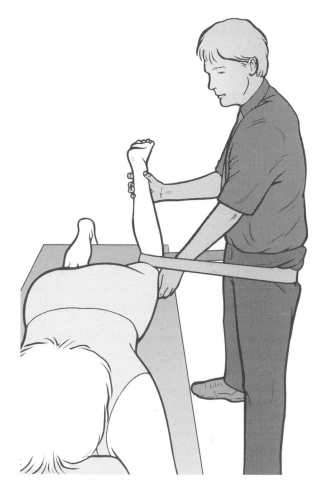

Figure 11.18   Lateral glide of the tibia on the femur.

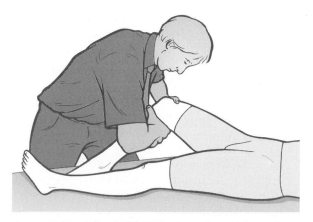

Figure 11.17   Lateral glide of the lower leg with femur fixed.

of the affected knee, level with it, with the seat-belt around the patient's lower leg, just below the knee joint, and around the therapist's hips. The femur is fixed by one hand of the therapist, while the other hand holds the lower leg. By simply pushing against the belt with their hips the therapist will induce a lateral glide at the knee joint through the belt (see Fig. 11.18). For a medial glide the therapist stands on the opposite side of the bed.

Note   The joint cannot be taped, but a home exercise to replicate the glide is applicable either in weight-bearing or non-weight-bearing. It is in fact one of the simplest home exercises to master.

Hip joint

Compared to most other joints the hip is huge, inaccessible and unwieldy. It is a ball and socket joint and really the only MWM available is that of distraction. To an extent this compromises the concept of MWM, because in all other cases joint surfaces have remained in contact, but with altered contact patterns. Nevertheless, the technique of hip distraction is useful and is included here.

Technique

The patient is lying with the affected leg in 90° of flexion at the hip. The seat-belt is passed around their inner, upper thigh as close to the joint as propriety allows. Padding the belt is a necessary kindness here. The seat belt then passes around the therapist's hips, who is standing at the same side as the hip being treated. One of the therapist's hands stabilises the pelvis by pressure on the ileum, just above the acetabulum, while the other hand wraps around the patient's mid thigh to assist with distraction (Fig. 11.19).

Note This starting position and technique is used for flexion, medial rotation and lateral rotation loss.

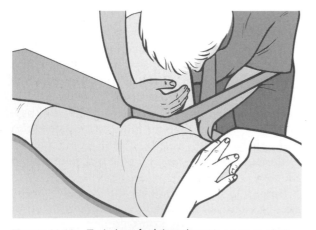

Figure 11.19 Technique for internal rotation with the belt. In this position (without internal rotation) flexion dysfunction can be treated.

Common errors for MWM as a whole

1. Over-treatment. The zeal of the converted is a powerful force!
2. Too aggressive. Always try light pressure/ low amplitude glides first. They can both be steadily increased if light pressure is ineffective.
3. Hands too far from joint line.
4. Inadequate knowledge of functional anatomy. When the initial treatment fails, good anatomical knowledge will enable the therapist to innovate as necessary.
5. Tension. When trying a new, unpractised technique the mental tension of concentration is frequently transmitted to the hands, making them hard and unresponsive.
6. Poor starting position. This prevents the therapist from adequately following joint movements.
7. Poor patient selection. Again either the zeal of the converted wishing to use these techniques on everyone, or just basic lack of experience and knowledge.
8. Poor communication. It is vital that the patient understands and complies with the pain-free concept, and understands the treatment methods.
9. Poor strapping skills. The strapping rapidly becomes ineffective, especially on weight-bearing joints.
10. Lack of follow-up. Always review the patient within 2–3 days, especially if strapping or home exercises are used, to probe for unwanted consequences. Telephone contact will suffice in many cases.

RATIONALE OF THE MULLIGAN CONCEPT

At this point the reader will probably have two questions in mind:

1. How is it possible that the techniques can appear to be instantly successful?
2. Why do the treatment effects persist when the glide is no longer applied, especially in chronic conditions?

In order to explain it is necessary to introduce physiological concepts to complement the mechanical ones on display thus far. The CNS must be invoked since all symptoms emanate from this in effect.

Joint abnormalities, for whatever reason, and no matter how brief or long-standing, create abnormal afferent output which 'agitates', 'facilitates', 'sensitises' the CNS, particularly the wide dynamic range (WDR) cells of the dorsal horn (Woolf 1991). This in turn provokes abnormal efferent discharge to the muscles controlling the joint, creating further muscle imbalance around a joint which is already misbehaving, because of muscle tone problems originally. Thus a vicious circle is formed.

If we break into this circle in such a way that the CNS receives normal afferents and reacts accordingly, then we may generate what appear to be extraordinary mechanical events including immediately enhanced muscle contractile power (Vincenzino et al 1995, Wilson 1997) However, this assumes that there is no major intra-articular or extra-articular pathology affecting the joint. If there is, then leakage of inflammatory exudate will continue to sensitize chemosensitive nerve endings and an abnormal afferent discharge will persist. Similarly if there is, for example, significant joint surface deformity then the abnormal afferent barrage will persist via the mechano-receptors or the pressure sensors in the subchondral bone. Under such circumstances the techniques described will have only a temporary effect at best. However, under appropriate circumstances, realigning joint biomechanics is as good a place as any to break into the circle.

If we then render the movement pain-free, we dam the excitatory barrage. If we add active muscle work, we recruit normal bombardment from their mechano-receptors, etc. If we do it repeatedly we add to the effect.

However, if we have chosen our patient badly we will exacerbate the problem by over-loading highly reactive CNS cells. These simply will not cope and react by creating a shut-down scenario, i.e. increased pain, spasm or inhibition to prevent further noxious afferent discharge – prevent movement that is.

A full explanation to the patient of the problem and the technique, gentle handling and a caring manner recruits the downward inhibitory modulation which further sedates the CNS, and should be utilised in full. So-called placebo has profound physiological effects (Wall 1995).

The resolution of headache and dizziness draws on the same concept of sedating an agitated CNS as was outlined earlier.

Integration with the ideas of other clinicians

It will have become apparent that a combination of Mulligan's technique and/or the concept of the facilitated CNS (Boxes 11.10 and 11.11) can be integrated with the work of other schools.

The summation of effects consequent upon changes in joint motion, afferent discharge alteration, efferent discharge alteration, muscle tone/contractile strength changes and finally pain behaviour, can instigate profound mechanical and physiological benefits for the patient (see Box 11.12).

One, many or all of the above play some part in the concepts of:

- Positional release techniques (this book)
- Muscle energy techniques (Chaitow 1996a)
- The McConnell methods (1986)
- Pathoneurodynamics (Butler 1994) (see Box 11.11)
- Trigger point and myofascial techniques (Chaitow 1988, Chaitow & DeLany 2000)

to name but a few.

No-one owns techniques or concepts and sectarian division helps no-one, least of all the patient. Perhaps the future will bring a holistic unity of concept, even if the techniques diverge somewhat. In the meantime, Mulligan's methods have the concept of 'symptom-free by the application of minimum force' to recommend them.

Box 11.10 Central facilitation for remote effects (Wilson 1997)

Patient
42-year-old businessman.

Complaint
Pronounced limp due to weak calf muscles following immobilisation after a compound lateral dislocation of the right talocrural joint 8 weeks previously.

Presentation
Pronounced limp due to nil push off of the right leg. Calf bulk diminished by approximately 30%. Poor proprioception in right leg standing. Poor-quality heel raise in supported standing with only two repetitions achieved. Tender to deep palpation of right L4/5 and L5/S1.

Treatment
Unilateral SNAG of right L5/S1 in supported standing with attempted heel raise. The patient successfully performed 12 good-quality heel raises before the onset of fatigue. This technique was then repeated for three × 10 repetitions (see Fig. 11.20).

Result
Patient able to perform six good-quality heel raises unaided before fatigue. Markedly better gait over short distances (20 metres approximately). Improved proprioception.

Follow-up
Standard rehabilitation procedures plus the technique as above. The patient also carried out self-SNAG plus heel raise as a home exercise. Return to full activity progressed rapidly and uneventfully.

Note
The shared innervation characteristics of the ankle joint, the calf muscles and the L5/S1 facet joint made this treatment possible. The calf muscle was not particularly weak, merely inhibited, and this inhibition was accessed through the medium of its shared innervation (Bullock-Saxton 1994). Alternatively it could be argued that the bladder meridian was invoked.

(The author has applied this technique many times and found it particularly successful in restoring vastus medialis obliqus performance by stimulation of L1/2 or L2/3 concurrent with attempted knee extension.)

Box 11.11 Peripheral joint mobilisation and its effect on patho-neurodynamics

Patient
38-year-old man professional rally driver.

Complaint
Pain and swelling around the right ankle during weight-bearing after moderate exercise, e.g. golf, hill walking. The situation had persisted for 4 months following a severe ankle sprain. He also complained of right intermittent low back pain and haunch pain.

Previous treatment
Immediate rest, ice, compression, elevation for 2 days followed by ultrasound, joint mobilisation, friction massage and active and passive exercises.

Presentation
Old pitting oedema plus recent swelling around right malleolus. Tender on palpation of lateral malleolus, lateral ligament (anterior portion), achilles tendon, peroneal tendons, and finally right L5/S1, plus the upper quadrant of ankle inversion reproduced his pain at 50% of range. Straight leg raise (SLR) reproduced his ankle and buttock pain at 60°.

Treatment
In sitting, the MWM posterior glide lateral malleolus was performed with concurrent active ankle inversion. This rendered inversion pain-free and was repeated 10 times. On retest without the glide in place both movement and pain had improved markedly. The technique was repeated a further 10 times and retest showed further improvement. A last set of 10 repetitions was deemed enough for that session because of the possible spinal involvement.

After the three sets of 10 repetitions inversion was full and almost pain-free. The SLR was equal to that of the left and provoked no symptoms.

Follow-up
Two days later all the improvements had been maintained and the swelling had diminished considerably too. There was no tenderness on palpation of any of the previously sore structures, including the spine and buttock. SLR was normal. The follow-up treatment required only two sets of 10 repetitions of the previous MWM to render inversion pain-free.

Note
The ankle, the peronei, the achilles tendon, gluteus maximus and the L5/S1 facet joint are united in having L5 and S1 as their primary innervation. The connective tissue supporting the sciatic nerve also receives some innervation from that source (Hromada 1963). Therefore, if the original ankle trauma so sensitised the WDR cells of the L5 and S1 cord segments, then pressure on or movement of any similarly innervated structures would generate neural traffic into those same segments where they might be perceived as pain (Cohen 1995). Normalising ankle joint biomechanics contributed to diminished sensitivity of the spinal receptor cells and raised their pain threshold. Suddenly, the normal afferent discharge from associated structures like the sciatic nerve was perceived as normal and became asymptomatic.

With regard to the swelling, the sympathetic trunk is, of course, linked to the spinal cord segments via the grey rami communicans and they influence each other's level of activity (Lundeberg 1999).

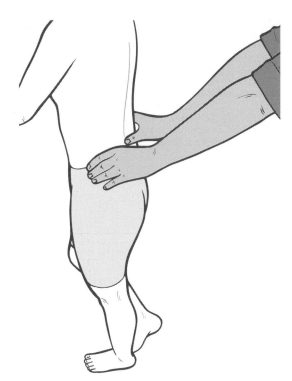

Figure 11.20   Unilateral SNAG with ipsilateral heel raise.

> **Box 11.12**   Benefits to patient post-stroke
> (Contributed by Joan Pollard MCSP SRP)
>
> **Patient**
> A 74-year-old woman.
>
> **Complaint**
> Pain in right hand and shoulder following a left
> cerebrovascular accident (CVA). The patient had high
> tone in the right forearm flexors, biceps, brachioradialis,
> and low tone in the wrist and elbow extensors. The
> hand was held in a position of finger flexion and wrist
> flexion with radial deviation. The shoulder was held in
> internal rotation and adduction due to increased tone in
> pectoralis major and latissimus dorsi. Consequent on
> these facts there was inevitable movement reduction in
> the shoulder, elbow, wrist and fingers.
>
> **Previous treatment**
> Bobath (1979) approach to stroke rehabilitation,
> including active assisted and passive movements of
> the upper limb.
>
> **Treatment**
> The pain in the right hand was principally located
> around the lateral border. Realignment of the fifth
> metacarpal on the fourth by posterior glide, held in
> position by strapping.
>
> **Result**
> Reduction of pain in the hand. Reduction of tone
> through the upper limb. Increased availability of active
> wrist, finger and shoulder movement. Improvement in
> gait, with reciprocal gait pattern and step-through.
>
> **Follow-up**
> Improvement maintained if hand-strapping in place.
> Only pain level and gait improvement remained if the
> strapping was removed.
>
> **Note**
> This case serves to illustrate the far-reaching effects
> of the vicious circle of altered tone to joint
> dysfunction, to pain to altered tone, etc., and the
> significant benefits that can accrue from apparently
> quite insignificant treatment ideas.

REFERENCES

Bobath B 1979 Adult Hemiplegia: Evaluation and Treatment
  2nd Edn. William Heinemann, London
Bogduk N 1986 Cervical causes of headache and dizziness.
  In: Grieve G (ed) Modern Manual Therapy of the
  Vertebral Column. Churchill Livingstone, Edinburgh
Bogduk N 1987 Innervation. Pain patterns and mechanisms
  of pain production. In: Twomey L T, Taylor J R (eds)
  Physical Therapy of the Low Back. Churchill Livingstone,
  Edinburgh
Bogduk N 1989 The anatomy of a headache. Proceedings of
  'Headache and Face Pain Syndrome.' Manipulative
  Physiotherapists Association of Australia
Bullock-Saxton J E 1994 Local sensation changes and altered
  hip muscle function following severe ankle sprain.
  Physical Therapy 74(1): 17–31

Butler D 1994 Mobilisation of the Nervous System. Churchill
  Livingstone, Edinburgh
Campbell J N et al 1989 Peripheral neural mechanisms of
  nociception. In: Wall P D, Melzack R (eds) Textbook of
  Pain 2nd Edn. Churchill Livingstone, Edinburgh
Chaitow L 1988 Soft Tissue Manipulation. Thorsons,
Chaitow L 1996 Muscle Energy Techniques. Churchill
  Livingstone, Edinburgh
Cohen M L 1995 The clinical challenges of secondary
  hyperalgesia. In: Shaclock M O (ed) Moving in on Pain.
  Butterworth Heinemann, London
Herrington L, McConnell J 1996 Exchange of letters. Manual
  Therapy (4): 220–222
Hoover H 1969 Collected Papers. Academy of Applied
  Osteopathy Yearbook, Colorado Springs

Hromada J 1963 The nerve supply of the connective tissue of some peripheral nervous system components. Acta Anatomy 55: 343–351

Jones S L 1992 Descending control of nociception. In: Light A R (ed) The Initial Processing of Pain and its Descending Control: Spinal and Trigeminal Systems. Karger, Basel, p. 203–277

Kapanji I A 1987 The Physiology of the Joints. Volumes 1, 2 and 3. Churchill Livingstone, Edinburgh

Kaltenborn F M 1980 Mobilisation of the Extremity Joints. Dlaff Norus, Oslo

Lundeberg T 1999 Effects of sensory stimulation (acupuncture) on circulatory and immune systems. In: Ernst E, White A (eds) Acupuncture: A Scientific Appraisal. Butterworth Heinemann, London

Maitland G D 1986 Vertebral Manipulation. Butterworth Heinemann, London

McConnell J 1986 The Management of Chondromalacia Patella: a long-term solution. Aust J Physiother 32: 215–223

Mulligan B R 1999 Manual Therapy. Nags, Snags, MWMs, etc. 4th Edn. Plane View Services, Wellington, New Zealand

Vicenzino B et al 1995 Effects of a novel manipulative physiotherapy technique on tennis elbow. Manual Therapy 1(1): 30–35

Wall P D 1995 The placebo response. In: Shacklock M O (ed) Moving in on Pain. Butterworth Heinemann, London

Wilson E 1994 Peripheral joint mobilisation with movement and its effects on adverse neural tension. Manipulative Physiotherapist 26(2): 35–39

Wilson E 1997 Central facilitation for remote effect: treating both ends of the system. Manual Therapy 2(2): 165–168

Woolf C J 1991 Generation of acute pain: central mechanisms. British Medical Bulletin 47(3): 523–533

12

Unloading and proprioceptive taping

Dylan Morrissey

INTRODUCTION

Unloading taping to reduce musculoskeletal pain, and proprioceptive taping to improve movement patterns, are useful empirical adjunctive treatment approaches. It is probable that they operate by similar mechanisms; although the nature of these mechanisms is as yet unproven, hypotheses based on the available literature are presented in this chapter. These concepts are accompanied by clinical guidelines for the application of taping in a variety of situations with accompanying case histories.

Taping can be used in a number of ways to reduce movement-associated pain. Based on a thorough assessment of presenting movement patterns and pain mechanisms, taping can be used as a useful treatment approach in itself, or as a means of maintaining treatment effects. It can be used to provide a physical effect on the tissues that lasts for hours, or even days, supplementing the relatively brief therapist–patient contact.

Taping can be used to affect pain directly by offloading irritable myofascial and/or neural tissues. Taping can also be indirectly used to alter the pain associated with identified faulty movement patterns. These effects are essentially proprioceptively mediated. This is very easily demonstrated in the shoulder girdle; the shoulder area will therefore be used to illustrate this approach. The management of patello-femoral pain by means of taping has also been increasingly investigated in the literature and described elsewhere (McConnell & Fulkerson 1996, Gilleard et al

Table 12.1 Means of pain reduction by taping.

Direct	Indirect (proprioceptively mediated)
Longitudinal offload	Inhibition of overactive movement synergists and antagonists
Transverse offload	Facilitation of underactive movement synergists
	Promotion of optimal interjoint coordination
	Direct optimization of joint alignment during static postures or movement

1998) with evidence for both mechanical and motor control effects of taping on patello-femoral movement and symptoms.

DIRECT METHODS
Longitudinal offload

Painful tissues that are held in tension either because of the unrelieved influence of gravity or because of chronically increased background muscle tone, e.g. due to habitual postures, can often be effectively helped by taping if the tissue can be passively supported in a shortened position. This is particularly useful when addressing symptoms associated with adverse neural dynamics (Fig. 12.1).

It is suggested that free nerve endings and c-fibre endorgans which intertwine with the tissues are irritated by the mechanical and chemical effects of the tissue under tension. This is reduced by holding the tissue in a shortened position therefore reducing pain fibre stimulation (Fig. 12.2).

Transverse offload

A transverse offload approach can be used particularly for myofascial tissues that may be mediated either by similar means to that described above or by a more mechanical effect. Transverse offloading of muscle structures effectively lengthens the muscle being used and may be inhibitory (Fig. 12.3).

A number of suggested techniques mix the two approaches effectively (Fig. 12.4).

INDIRECT METHODS: WITH REFERENCE TO THE SHOULDER GIRDLE

Normal upper limb function is dependent on the ability to statically and dynamically position the shoulder girdle in an optimal coordinated fashion (Glousman et al 1988, Kibler 1998).

Movement faults, for example of the scapulo-thoracic 'joint', have been clinically (Host 1995) and scientifically (Warner et al 1991, Wadsworth & Bullock-Saxton 1997) shown to be strongly associated with common pathologies.

Physiotherapy that aims to improve joint stability, optimal interjoint coordination and muscle function has been shown to be clinically effective in the management of a variety of shoulder presentations (Ginn et al 1997). Proprioception is a critical component of coordinated shoulder girdle movement, with significant deficits having been identified in pathological and fatigued shoulders (e.g. Forwell et al 1996, Voight et al 1996, Warner et al 1996, Carpenter et al 1998). It is

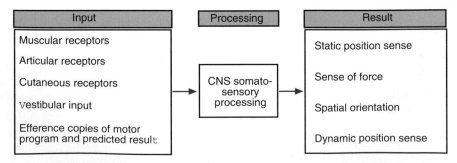

Figure 12.1 Proprioceptive summary. Input from a number of peripheral sources is integrated with expected movement patterns and the commands sent to the periphery with the result being a CNS representation of movement parameters.

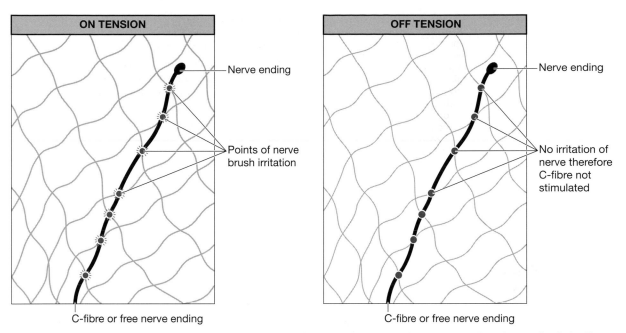

ON TENSION

Nerve ending

Points of nerve brush irritation

C-fibre or free nerve ending

OFF TENSION

Nerve ending

No irritation of nerve therefore C-fibre not stimulated

C-fibre or free nerve ending

Figure 12.2 Free nerve endings piercing the multidirectional fascial planes may be irritated when there is sustained significant tension placed on the tissues. Taping that holds these tissues in a shortened position helps to reduce symptoms associated with movement.

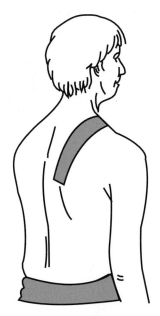

Figure 12.3 Upper trapezius inhibition. From anterior aspect of upper trapezius just above the clavicle over the muscle belly to approximately the level of rib 7 in a vertical line. Once partially attached a firm downward pull is applied and the tail of the tape attached.

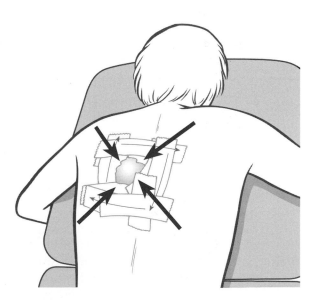

Figure 12.4 The skin over the thoracic spine is gathered centrally in the direction of the large arrows and the skin taped in the direction of the small arrows (see taping guidelines).

an integral goal of rehabilitation programmes to attempt to minimize or reverse these proprioceptive deficits (Magee & Reid 1996, Lephart et al 1997). Taping is a useful adjunct to a patient-specific integrated treatment approach aiming to restore full pain-free movement of the shoulder girdle.

Taping is particularly useful in addressing movement faults at the scapulothoracic, glenohumeral and acromioclavicular joints. The exact mechanisms by which shoulder taping is effective are not yet clear but the suggestion is that the effects are both proprioceptive, mechanical and pain relieving.

Possible physiological mechanisms

Proprioception is a complex process that is difficult to define (Jerosch et al 1996). Essentially, information from mechanoreceptors in the skin, muscles, fascia, tendons and articular structures is integrated with visual and vestibular input at all CNS levels in order to allow perception of

● position sense (static)
● kinesthesia (dynamic)
● force detection.

Proprioception is particularly important for upper limb interjoint coordination (Sainburg et al 1993) due to the complexity of the kinetic chain, the relative lack of osseous stability and the precision of the tasks performed. The literature focuses on the role of articular and myofascial structures in contributing to shoulder girdle proprioception while cutaneous input is regarded as having a lesser role (e.g. Jerosch et al 1996, Warner et al 1996, Lephart et al 1997, Carpenter et al 1998).

Recent research, however, suggests that, in the normal ankle joint, facilitation of proprioceptive cutaneous input by means of taping is effective in improving reaction speed and position awareness (Robbins et al 1995, Lohrer et al 1999). There is also some evidence that taping the patella can influence the relative onset of activity of the vastus lateralis and vastus medialis obliquus during quadriceps activation (Gilleard et al 1998). This may be cutaneously mediated.

Taping as a form of proprioceptive biofeedback?

A potential mechanism by means of which proprioceptive shoulder taping may be effective is via augmented cutaneous input (Figs 12.5–12.7)

Tape is applied in such a way that there is little or no tension while the body part is held or moved in the desired direction or plane. The tissues will therefore develop more tension when movement occurs outside these parameters. This tension will be sensed consciously, thus giving a stimulus to the patient to correct the movement pattern. Over time and with sufficient repetition and feedback, these patterns can become learned components

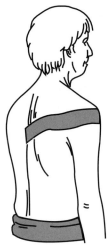

Figure 12.5 Retraction of the shoulder. From the anterior aspect of the shoulder, 2 cm medial to the joint line, around deltoid muscle just below acromial level to T6 area without crossing midline. Tape pull is into retraction.

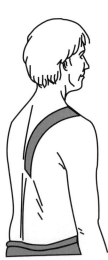

Figure 12.6 Retraction/upward rotation. From anterior shoulder just below the coracoid to low thoracic (T10) area. The initial pull on the tape is up and then back as the tape comes over the midline.

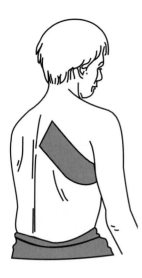

Figure 12.7 Serratus anterior facilitation and inferior angle abduction. From 2 cm medial to the scapula border, following the line of the ribs down to the mid-axillary line. Four one-third overlapping strips are applied with the origin and insertion pulled together and bunching the skin.

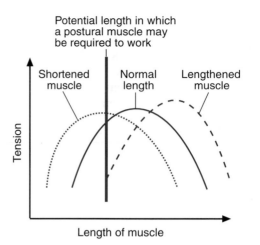

Figure 12.8 Length–tension curves. Although lengthened muscle has the capability to generate more force, postural muscles frequently need to be able to generate most force in inner range positions in which case it is often desirable that they are relatively short.

of the motor engrams for given movements. This process therefore represents cutaneously mediated proprioceptive biofeedback.

Taping as a means of altering muscle function

Mechanically, if taping can be applied in such a fashion that a chronically inhibited (underactive) muscle is held in a shortened position (Fig. 12.8), there will be a shift of the length–tension curve to the left, and greater force development in the inner range through optimised actin–myosin overlap during the cross-bridge cycle (Fig 12.7).

Similarly, if taping can be applied in such a fashion that a relatively short, overactive, muscle is held in a lengthened position, there will be a shift of the length–tension curve to the right, and lesser force development through decreased actin–myosin overlap during the cross-bridge cycle at the point in joint range at which the muscle is required to work (Fig. 12.3)

The taping method used to inhibit upper trapezius activity (as in Fig. 12.3) has been investigated in a pilot study (O'Donovan 1997) and shown to have a significant inhibitory effect on the degree of upper trapezius activity in relation to lower trapezius during elevation.

This is demonstrated as soon as the tape is applied. Clinical effects of taping the shoulder girdle can be significant and immediate, espe-cially in promoting altered movement patterns and allowing earlier progression of rehabilitation. Recent study has shown that the pull involved in applying the second of the two tapes is critical to the electromyographic and mechanical positional changes observed during successful taping application (Brown 1999). The mechanisms by which the above study results, and the clinical effects seen during application, merit further investigation.

Taping guidelines: shoulder as an example

It is essential to be clear about the aims of taping in order to ensure optimal results:

- In the case of the shoulder this would be assessed for its habitual resting position and for movement faults contributing to the symptom presentation.
- The skin would then be prepared by removal of surface oils and body hair.
- The shoulder would be actively positioned in the desired position by the patient with the guidance of the therapist, or passively if the patient is unable to maintain the desired position.

- A hypoallergenic mesh tape would be applied without tension (e.g. Mefx, Molnlycke, Sweden).
- A robust zinc oxide tape (Strappal, Smith and Nephew, UK) would then be applied from the anterior aspect of upper trapezius, just above the clavicle, to approximately the level of rib seven, in a vertical line, with a little tension and the comparable movement sign reassessed for the effect of the intervention.
- Further tapes may then be applied as necessary.
- The taping is continued until the patient has learnt to actively control movement in the desired fashion, or the effects on symptoms are maintained when it is not worn.

Skin reactions

If the client develops a skin reaction this can either be due to an allergic reaction, a 'heat rash', or because the tape is concentrating too much tension in one area. Tension concentrations usually occur around the front of the shoulder.

Heat rashes tend to be localized to the area under the tape and settle quickly. Allergic reactions are more irritating and widespread, and must be treated with great caution as reapplication is likely to lead to a more severe reaction due to immune sensitisation.

Scapulohumeral function

The scapulothoracic joint gains some stability in relation to medially directed forces from the clavicular strut via the acromioclavicular joint. This still allows a large range and amplitude of translatory and rotary movement that is primarily produced, controlled and limited by the axioscapular myofascial structures (Kibler 1998).

Compromised thoracoscapulohumeral rhythm results in the potential for impingement due to downward rotation of the glenoid associated with tipping or winging.

An anterior tilt of the glenoid is regarded as being a significant occult instability risk (Kibler 1998) (Box 12.1). The scapulohumeral joint relies heavily on the passive stability provided by the

---

Box 12.1

Downward rotation occurs about an axis located one-third of the length of the spine of the scapula lateral to the proximal end of the spine of the scapula. Tipping is when the inferior angle protrudes from the chest wall and the coracoid is pulled down and medially as compared to winging where the entire medial border of the scapula lifts off the chest wall.

---

capsuloligamentous structures and the dynamic stability provided by the rotator cuff (Glousman et al 1988, Harryman et al 1990, 1992; Terry et al 1991; Payne et al 1997).

This stability is crucially dependent on intact proprioception (Nyland 1998). Disruption by trauma or repetitive disadvantageous movement patterns can result in impingement or instability either in isolation or more commonly in combination (Warner et al 1995).

An example of how taping can be used in the management of a patient with excessive tipping of the scapula is presented in case history

---

Box 12.2 Case history: direct longitudinal offload

A 34-year-old woman presented with acute discogenic low back and long leg sciatic pain, due to an exacerbation of existing low back pain caused by sleeping awkwardly on a long-haul airplane journey.

The presentation was both severe and irritable, to the extent that she had to be examined in sidelying, in order to avoid exacerbation.

A key comparable sign was a 20° straight leg raise reproducing all her leg and back pain symptoms.

Application of longitudinal offload taping along the course of the sciatic nerve, and its common peroneal branches, reduced her symptoms on SLR and increased the pain-free range to 45° in conjunction with manual therapy techniques.

This allowed her to walk far more normally with markedly reduced pain.

The V-shaped tapes were placed at the base of the fibula, at the head of the fibula, two-thirds of the way down the posterior aspect of the thigh and at the top of the posterior aspect of the thigh. These were applied in the order stated. Interestingly, an initial attempt to apply the tape in a reverse order was not successful (Fig. 12.9)

This taping was used throughout the first 2 weeks of her management by which time she was significantly better and able to discontinue that aspect of her treatment.

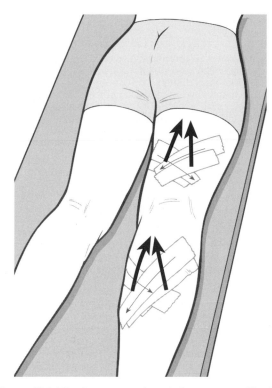

Figure 12.9 The tissues over the sciatic nerve are offloaded superiorly in the direction of the large arrows and the skin taped in the direction of the small arrows (see taping guidelines).

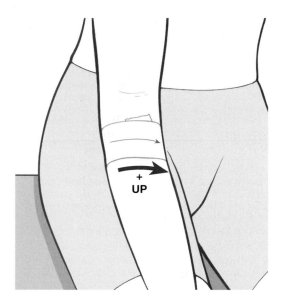

Figure 12.10 The skin and muscle tissue overlying the common extensor origin is lifted and pulled medially in the direction of the large arrows and the skin taped in the direction of the small arrows (see taping guidelines).

Box 12.3 Case history: direct transverse offload

A recreational racquet sports player presented with lateral elbow pain with clear local soft tissue components as well as a positive radial nerve tension test and low cervical facet joint stiffness.

Static resisted contraction (SRC) of the common extensor origin muscles and extensor carpi radialis brevis in particular was comparable (Fig. 12.10).

As part of the management a transverse offload tape was applied to the common extensor origin with immediate reduction of symptoms from SRC and improved grip strength, through reduction of pain inhibition.

This remained part of her management until return to sport when it was replaced with an 'aircast' lateral epicondyle brace, which can be used to similar effect.

Box 12.4. An example of how taping can be used to elevate a depressed scapula and stabilize a traumatically unstable acromioclavicular joint is presented in case history 4 (Box 12.6). The case histories have been deliberately chosen to show a range of taping techniques that can be used either in conjunction with other modalities and methods, or in isolation.

CONCLUSION

Management of complex neuromusculoskeletal dysfunction and pathology and pain syndromes requires a multifactorial approach based on individual assessment. Strategies used to reduce pain, increase mobility, improve movement co-ordination and improve strength may be augmented by the use of taping used to offload tissues or to improve movement patterns by proprioceptive means.

Taping is a particularly useful treatment adjunct as it has the particular advantage of lasting well beyond the patient–therapist contact, thus extending the duration of therapeutic stimulus. Repetition and long duration experience of altered movement is essential in altering established motor engrams and overcoming the effects of established inhibition or pain presentations.

Box 12.4 Case history

This case represents a particular example of inhibition of overactive movement synergists and antagonists and facilitation of underactive movement synergists.

A 33-year-old cricketer presented complaining of persistent and progressive shoulder pain of non-specific onset but particularly related to bowling and throwing. He had experienced episodes of pain towards the end of the previous season, which had not interfered with participation nor persisted after the end of the season. He had experienced problems from the start of the current season which had progressed to the extent that he was no longer able to bowl or throw overarm, had pain persisting between games, while overhead activities of daily living were compromised.

Assessment showed clear impingement features including:

● localized pain to the front of the shoulder
● a painful arc on mid-range elevation that was associated with marked protraction and tipping (Norkin & Levangie 1992) of the scapula and accentuated on slow eccentric elevation
● generalized loss of thoracic extension and rotation focused at T5 ± 7
● a positive empty-can test (Magee & Reid 1996) (a static resisted contraction of abduction with the arm medially rotated and held at 90° of abduction in the scapular plane)
● general restriction of glenohumeral accessory joint glides

● restricted medial rotation with scapulothoracic relative flexibility on the kinetic medial rotation test (Comerford 1992, Morrissey 1998)
● painful, weak static resisted abduction and lateral rotation
● tight overactive pectoralis minor as demonstrated by the shoulder girdle not being able to lower to the supporting surface when the
● patient was supine and gentle pressure was applied anteroposteriorly through the coracoid process.

An initial treatment plan was formulated including: thoracic manipulation (HVLA thrust) to increase the available thoracic extension during elevation; pectoralis lengthening using trigger point treatment and specific soft-tissue mobilization to decrease the active scapula tipping; local soft-tissue deinflammation with ice; and scapula setting – initially in neutral but then incorporated into dynamic movement. It was decided to emphasize upward rotation and retraction as he demonstrated an excessively protracted, tipped scapula during elevation.

The scapula setting (Box 12.5) proved difficult for the patient to master so the shoulder was taped (Figs 12.5 and 12.6). This resulted in an immediate improvement in the patient's ability to set the scapula and an improved scapulohumeral rhythm associated with a marked decrease in the painful arc symptoms. The taping was reapplied for 3 weeks while his treatment and rehabilitation were progressed to the extent that he had achieved satisfactory control of scapula movement during functional activities and had begun to resume some of his sporting activities.

Box 12.5

Scapula setting has been defined as 'Dynamic orientation of the scapula in a position so as to optimise the position of the glenoid and so allow mobility and stability of the gleno-humeral joint' (Mottram 1998).

Box 12.6 Case history

This case represents a particular example of promotion of optimal interjoint coordination as well as direct optimisation of joint alignment during static postures or movement.

A 23-year-old rugby player presented 2 weeks after a shoulder pointer (fall onto the point of the shoulder causing an inferior blow to the acromium) and resultant acromioclavicular joint sprain. Assessment showed a visible joint step with upper trapezius spasm accentuating this via its attachment to the lateral third of the clavicle (Johnson et al 1994). Range of movement was markedly reduced and the patient complained of constant pain aggravated by any movement. He was still using a sling. The scapula was noted to be in a downward rotated, depressed position thus accentuating the step and resultant acromioclavicular joint pain.

The initial treatment therefore aimed to decrease the resting joint pain using large amplitude joint mobilizations and interferential therapy, which was partially successful.

In order to further reduce the resting pain and affect the pain on movement it was necessary to improve the symmetry of the joint by decreasing upper trapezius activity and facilitating upward rotation and elevation of the scapula. This was done using tape (Figs 12.11 and 12.12) and reinforced with soft-tissue techniques (trigger point massage and specific soft-tissue mobilization) to the upper trapezius (see Figs 12.3, 12.5, 12.11, 12.12).

An immediate improvement in symmetry was noted and a marked increase in pain-free ROM. He was able to discard the sling. Taping remained an integral part of the treatment until he was able to actively set the scapula independently.

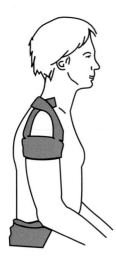

Figure 12.11 Elevation of the shoulder girdle. (1) Anchor strip applied at level of deltoid tuberosity, encircling two-thirds of the circumference of the arm; (2) elevatory strips applied from posterior arm/deltoid to the anterolateral aspect of the base of the neck; (3) elevatory strips applied from anterior arm/deltoid to the posterolateral aspect of the base of the neck; (4) locking strip over tape 1.

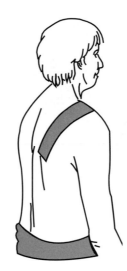

Figure 12.12 AC joint relocation; from coracoid process over the distal end of the clavicle with a downward pull applied just before the tail of the tape is attached to level of rib 6 in vertical line. Only ever applied after successful application of elevatory taping (Fig. 12.11).

REFERENCES

Brown L 1999 The effect of taping the glenohumeral joint on scapulohumeral resting position and trapezius activity during abduction. Unpublished MSc Thesis, University College London

Carpenter JE et al 1998 The effects of muscle fatigue on shoulder joint position sense. American Journal of Sports Medicine 26: 262–265

Comerford M 1992 Postgraduate course notes

Forwell LA et al 1996 Proprioception during manual aiming in individuals with shoulder instability and controls. Journal of Orthopaedic and Sports Physical Therapy 23: 111–119

Gilleard W et al 1998 The effects of patellar taping on the onset of VMO and VL muscle activity in persons with patello-femoral pain. Physical Therapy 78: 25–32

Ginn L et al 1977 A randomized, controlled clinical trial of a treatment for shoulder pain. Physical Therapy 77: 802–811

Glousman R et al 1988 Dynamic electromyographic analysis of the throwing shoulder with gleno-humeral instability. Journal of Bone and Joint Surgery 70A: 220–226

Harryman DT II et al 1990 Translation of the humeral head on the glenoid with passive gleno-humeral motion. Journal of Bone and Joint Surgery 72A: 1334–1343

Harryman DT II et al 1992 The role of the rotator interval capsule in passive motion and stability of the shoulder. Journal of Bone and Joint Surgery 74A: 53–66

Host H 1995 Scapular taping in the treatment of anterior shoulder impingement: case report. Physical Therapy 75: 803–811

Howell S et al 1988 Normal and abnormal mechanics of the gleno-humeral joint in the horizontal plane. Journal of Bone and Joint Surgery 70A: 227–232

Jerosch J et al 1996 Proprioception and joint stability. Knee Surgery, Sports Traumatology Orthroscopy 4: 171–179

Johnson G et al 1994 Anatomy and actions of trapezius muscle. Clinical Biomechanics 9: 44–50

Kibler WB 1998 The role of the scapula in athletic shoulder function. American Journal of Sports Medicine 26: 325–337

Lephart SM et al 1997 The role of proprioception in the management and rehabilitation of athletic injuries. American Journal of Sports Medicine 25: 130–137

Lohrer H et al 1999 Neuromuscular properties and functional aspects of taped ankles. American Journal of Sports Medicine 27: 69–75

McConnell J, Fulkerson 1996 The knee: patello-femoral and soft tissue injuries. In: Zachazewski et al JE (eds) Athletic injuries and rehabilitation. Saunders, Philadelphia

Magee DJ, Reid DC 1996 Shoulder injuries. In: Zachazewski JE et al (eds) Athletic injuries and rehabilitation. Saunders, Philadelphia

Morrissey D 1998 The kinetic medial rotation test of the shoulder: a normative study. Unpublished MSc thesis, University College London

Mottram S 1997 Dynamic stability of the scapula. Manual Therapy 2: 123–131

Norkin CC, Levangie PK 1992 Joint Structure and Function: A Comprehensive Analysis. FA Dacis, Philadelphia

Nyland JA 1998 The human glenohumeral joint: a proprioceptive and stability alliance. Knee Surgery Sports Traumatology, Arthroscopy 6: 50–61

O'Donovan N 1997 Evaluation of the effect of inhibitory taping on EMG activity in upper and lower trapezius during concentric isokinetic elevation of the upper limb. Unpublished MSc Physiotherapy thesis, University College London

Payne L et al 1997 The combined static and dynamic contributions to subacromial impingement: a biomechanical analysis. American Journal of Sports Medicine 25: 801–808

Robbins S et al 1995 Ankle taping improves proprioception before and after exercise in young men. British Journal of Sports Medicine 29: 242–247

Sainburg RL et al 1993 Loss of proprioception produces deficits in interjoint co-ordination. Journal of Neurophysiology 70: 2136–2147

Stokes M, Young A 1984 Investigations of quads inhibition: implications for clinical practice. Physiotherapy 70: 425–428

Terry G et al 1991 The stabilizing function of passive shoulder restraints. American Journal of Sports Medicine 19: 26–34

Voight ML et al 1996 The effects of muscle fatigue on and the relationship of arm dominance to shoulder proprioception. JOSPT 23. 348–352

Wadsworth DJS, Bullock-Saxton JE 1997 Recruitment patterns of the scapular rotator muscles in freestyle swimmers with sub-acromial impingement. International Journal of Sports Medicine 18: 618–624

Warner J et al 1995 Patterns of flexibility, laxity and strength in normal shoulders and shoulders with instability and impingement. American Journal of Sports Medicine 18: 366–374

Warner J et al 1991 Scapulo-thoracic motion in normal shoulders and shoulders with gleno-humeral instability and impingement syndrome. Clinical Orthopaedics and Related Research 285: 191–199

Warner J et al 1996 Role of proprioception in patho-etiology of shoulder instability. Clinical Orthopaedics and Related Research 330: 35–39

INDEX

Related Journals from Harcourt Publishers

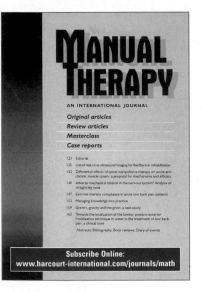
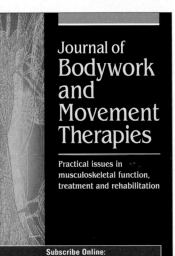
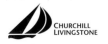
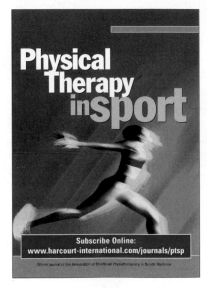
CHURCHILL
LIVINGSTONE

Journals Marketing Department, Harcourt Publishers Ltd, 32 Jamestown Road, London NW1 7BY, UK
tel: +44 (0)20 8308 5790   fax: +44 (0)20 7424 4433   Call toll free in the US: 1-877-839-7126
e-mail: journals@harcourt.com   www.harcourt-international.com